Clinical Neurology

Clinical Neurology

Peter Gates MBBS, FRACP

Associate Professor of Neurology, University of Melbourne
Director of Stroke, Director of Neuroscience and a
Director of Physician Training at Barwon Health, Geelong, Victoria

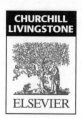

CHURCHILL
LIVINGSTONE

ELSEVIER

Sydney Edinburgh London New York Philadelphia St Louis Toronto

Churchill Livingstone
is an imprint of Elsevier

Elsevier Australia. ACN 001 002 357
(a division of Reed International Books Australia Pty Ltd)
Tower 1, 475 Victoria Avenue, Chatswood, NSW 2067

ELSEVIER

National Library of Australia Cataloguing-in-Publication Data

---

Author: Gates, Peter.

Title: Clinical Neurology: a primer / Peter Gates.

ISBN: 9780729539357

Notes: Includes Index

Subjects: Neurology. Nervous system—diseases.

Dewey Number: 616.8

Publisher: Sophie Kaliniecki
Developmental Editor: Sabrina Chew and Neli Bryant
Publishing Services Manager: Helena Klijn
Project Coordinator: Eleanor Cant and Geraldine Minto
Edited by Linda Littlemore
Proofread by Kerry Brown
Cover and internal design by Stan Lamond from Lamond Art & Design
Index by Michael Ferreira
Typeset by TNQ Books and Journals
Printed by China Translation & Printing Services Ltd.

Contents

Foreword

There have been many attempts over the years to distil the knowledge needed for medical students and young doctors to begin to engage in neurological diagnosis and treatment. This book by Professor Peter Gates is one of the best books developed to date. Peter Gates is an outstanding clinical neurologist and teacher who has been acknowledged in his own university as one of the leading teachers of undergraduates and registrars in recent times. He takes a classical approach to neurological diagnosis stressing the need for anatomical diagnosis and to learn as much as possible from the history in developing an understanding of likely pathophysiologies and aetiologies. In this book he sets out the lessons of a lifetime spent in clinical neurology and distils some of the principles that have led him to become a master diagnostician.

The first chapter is devoted to neuroanatomy from a clinical viewpoint. The concept of developing diagnosis through an understanding of the vertical and horizontal meridians of the nervous system is developed and intriguingly labelled under latitude and longitude. All the key issues around major anatomical diagnosis are distilled in a very understandable way for the novice. This chapter (and subsequent chapters) is widely illustrated with case studies and the illustrations are excellent. Key points are emphasised and important clinical questions stressed. A great deal of thought has gone into the clinical anecdotes chosen to illustrate major diagnostic issues. These reflect the learnings of a lifetime spent in neurological practice.

Subsequent chapters take the reader through the neurological examination and major neurological presentations and neurological disorders. Key aspects are illustrated with great clarity. This is a book that can be consulted from the index to get points about various disorders and their treatments but, more importantly, should be read from cover to cover by young doctors interested in coming to terms in a more major way with the diagnosis and treatment of neurological disorders. It also contains a lot of material that will be of interest to more experienced practitioners. The book has a clinical orientation and the references are comprehensive in listing most of the relevant key papers that the reader who wishes to pursue the basis of clinical neurology further may wish to consult. The final chapter is an excellent overview of how one can approach information gathering and keeping up-to-date using the complex information streams available to the medical student and young doctor today.

This book is clearly aimed at medical students and young doctors who have a special interest in developing further understanding of the workings of the nervous system, its disorders and their treatments. I would recommend it to senior medical students, to young doctors at all stages and also to those beginning their neurological training. It also has some information that may be of interest to the more senior neurologist in terms of developing their own approach to teaching young colleagues. It is the best introduction to the diagnosis and treatment of nervous system disorders that I have seen for many years and contains a font of wisdom about a speciality often perceived as difficult by the non-expert.

Professor Edward Byrne AO
Vice-Chancellor and President
Monash University
Melbourne
Australia

Foreword

Preface

This book was written with two purposes in mind: firstly, it is an introductory textbook of clinical neurology for medical students and hospital medical officers as well as neurologists in their first year(s) of training and, secondly, it is designed to sit on the desk of hospital medical officers, general practitioners and general physicians to refer to when they see patients with the common neurological problems.

This book is the culmination of 25 years of clinical practice and teaching in neurology and is an attempt to make neurology more understandable, enjoyable and logical.

The aim is to provide an approach to the more common neurological problems starting from the symptoms that are encountered in everyday clinical practice. It describes how best to retrieve the most relevant information from the history, the neurological examination, investigations, colleagues, textbooks and the Internet.

This book in no way attempts to be a comprehensive textbook of neurology and as such is not intended for the practising neurologist. There are and will always be many excellent and comprehensive books on neurology.

There are chapters on the examination technique as well as a DVD that demonstrates and explains the normal neurological examination together with some abnormal neurological signs.

Investigations and treatments in the text will very quickly be out of date but the basic principles of clinical neurology developed more than 100 years ago are still relevant now and will be for many years to come. The clinical neurologist is like an amateur detective and uses clues from the history and examination to answer the questions: 'Where is the lesion?' and 'What is the pathology?'

Although it is not intended for the experienced neurologist, the author is aware of some neurologists who have found some of the techniques in this textbook (e.g. the Rule of 4 of the brainstem) useful in their teaching.

The original title of this book was *Neurology Demystified*, after a general physician commented to the author that the 'Rule of 4' of the brainstem had demystified the brainstem for the general physician. It encapsulates what this author has been attempting to achieve over the past 30 years of teaching neurology: to make it simpler and easier to understand for students, hospital medical officers, general practitioners and general physicians.

One of the most rewarding things in life is teaching those who are interested in learning and to see the sudden look of understanding in the eyes of the 'student'.

Acknowledgements

I would like to thank my colleagues John Balla, Ross Carne, Richard Gerraty and Richard McDonnell for reviewing sections of the manuscript. At Elsevier, I also wish to thank Sophie Kaliniecki for accepting my book proposal, Sabrina Chew, Eleanor Cant and Linda Littlemore for all the support and encouragement they provided during the writing of the manuscript, and also to Greg Gaul for the illustrations. I would particularly like to thank Stephen Due and Joan Deane at the Geelong Hospital library who have been a tremendous support over many years, especially but not only during the writing of this book. Also, I thank the radiologists and radiographers at Barwon Medical Imaging for providing most of the medical images. My thanks also to the many patients and friends who generously consented to have pictures or video taken to incorporate in this book. Kevin Sturges from GGI Media Geelong, a friend and technological whiz, helped me with all the images and video production.

Thank you also to the students and colleagues who anonymously reviewed the manuscript for their many wonderful suggestions and words of encouragement.

I have indeed been fortunate to have been taught by many outstanding teachers during my training and, although to name them individually runs the risk of omission and causing offence, there are a few that I would like to acknowledge: Robert Newnham, rheumatologist at the Repatriation General Hospital in Heidelberg who, in 1975, first taught the symptom-oriented approach while I was a final-year medical student; at St Vincent's Hospital in Melbourne the late John Billings, neurologist, who introduced me to the excitement of neurology and John Niall, nephrologist, for challenging me to justify a particular treatment with evidence from the literature; Arthur Schweiger, John Balla, Les Sedal, Rob Helme, Russell Rollinson and Henryk Kranz (neurologists) for the opportunity to enter neurology training at Prince Henry's Hospital Melbourne where John Balla encouraged me to write my first paper; Lord John Walton, neurologist, for the opportunity to work and study in Newcastle upon Tyne; Peter Fawcett, neurophysiologist, for the opportunity to study neurophysiology; Dr Mike Barnes, neurologist in rehabilitation, who helped in 1983 at the Newcastle General Hospital to make the video of John Walton taking a history.

I also wish to thank Henry Barnett, neurologist, in London, Ontario, for the opportunity to work on the EC-IC bypass study; and Dave Sackett, Wayne Taylor and Brian Haynes in the department of epidemiology at McMaster University for opening my eyes to clinical epidemiology and evidence-based medicine. And last but not least my long standing friend Ed Byrne, currently Vice-Chancellor of Monash University, for the appointment at St Vincent's Hospital in Melbourne on my return from overseas and for his friendship and wise council over many years.

This book is dedicated to my children, Bernard, Amelia and Jeremy, and my wife Rosie, for without their support over the many years this project would not have been possible.

Reviewers

Charles Austin-Woods BSc(Hons), MBBS
Registrar, Wollongong Hospital, Wollongong, NSW

Cheyne Bester BSc(Hons)

Benjamin C Cheah BSc(Hons), BA
Prince of Wales Medical Research Institute
Prince of Wales Clinical School, University of New South Wales, Sydney, NSW

Hsu En Chung BMedSc, MBBS
Junior Medical Officer, Austin Health, Melbourne, Vic

Richard P Gerraty MD, FRACP
Neurologist, The Alfred Hospital, Melbourne, Vic
Associate Professor, Department of Medicine, Monash University

Matthew Kiernan DSc, FRACP
Professor of Medicine – Neurology, University of New South Wales
Consultant Neurologist, Prince of Wales Hospital, Sydney, NSW

Shane Wei Lee MBBS(Hons), PostGradDip (surgical anatomy)
Resident, Royal Melbourne Hospital, Melbourne, Vic

Michelle Leech MBBS(Hons), FRACP, PhD
Consultant Rheumatologist, Monash Medical Centre
Associate Professor and Director of Clinical Teaching Programs, Southern Clinical School, Monash University, Melbourne, Vic

Sarah Jensen BMSc, MBBS
Junior Medical Officer, The Canberra Hospital, ACT

James Padley PhD, BMedSc(Hons)
4th year medical student, University of Sydney, Sydney, NSW

Claire Seiffert BPhysio(Hons), MBBS
Junior Medical Officer, Wagga Wagga Base Hospital, Wagga Wagga, NSW

Selina Watchorn BA, BNurs, MBBS
Junior Medical Officer, The Canberra Hospital, ACT

John Waterston MD, FRACP
Consultant Neurologist, The Alfred Hospital, Melbourne, Vic
Honorary Senior Lecturer, Department of Medicine, Monash University

chapter 1

Clinically Oriented Neuroanatomy:

'MERIDIANS OF LONGITUDE AND PARALLELS OF LATITUDE'

Although most textbooks on clinical neurology begin with a chapter on history taking, there is a very good reason for placing neuroanatomy as the initial chapter. It is because *clinical neurologists use their detailed knowledge of neuroanatomy not only when examining a patient but also when obtaining a neurological history* in order to determine the site of the problem within the nervous system. This chapter not only describes the neuroanatomy but attempts to place it in a clinical context.

The 'student of neurology' cannot be expected to remember all of the detail but needs to understand the basic concepts. This understanding, combined with the correct technique when taking the neurological history (see Chapter 2, 'The neurological history') and performing the neurological examination (see Chapter 3, 'Neurological examination of the limbs', Chapter 4, 'The cranial nerves and understanding the brainstem', and Chapter 5, 'The cerebral hemispheres and cerebellum'), together with the illustrations in this chapter will enable the 'non-neurologist' to localise the site of the problem in most patients almost as well as the neurologist. It is intended that this chapter serve as a resource to be kept on the desk or next to the examination couch.

To help simplify neuroanatomy the concept of the **meridians of longitude and parallels of latitude** is introduced to liken the nervous system to a map grid. The site of the problem is where the meridian of longitude meets the parallel of latitude. Examples will be given to explain this concept.

It is also crucial to understand the difference between upper and lower motor neurons. The terms are more often (and not unreasonably) used to refer to the central and peripheral nervous systems, CNS and PNS, respectively. More specifically, upper motor neuron refers to motor signs that result from disorders affecting the motor pathway above the level of the anterior horn cell, i.e. within the CNS, while lower motor neuron refers to motor symptoms and signs that relate

- The hallmark of clinical neurology is to evaluate each and every symptom in terms of its nature (i.e. weakness, sensory, visual etc) and its distribution in order to decide where the lesion is.
- The nature and distribution of the symptoms and signs (if present), i.e. the neuroanatomy, point to the site of the pathology in the nervous system. They rarely if ever indicate the nature of the underlying pathology.

TABLE 1.1   Upper and lower motor neuron signs

	Upper motor neuron signs	**Lower motor neuron signs**
Weakness	The UMN pattern*	Specific to a nerve or nerve root
Tone	Increased	Decreased
Reflexes	Increased	Decreased or absent
Plantar response	Up-going	Down-going

*The muscles that abduct the shoulder joint and extend the elbow and wrist joints are weak in the arms while the muscles that flex the hip and knee joints and the muscles that dorsiflex the ankle joint (bend the foot upwards) are weak in the legs.

to disorders of the PNS, the anterior horn cell, motor nerve root, brachial or lumbrosacral plexus or peripheral nerve (see Table 1.1). The alterations in strength, tone, reflexes and plantar responses (scratching the lateral aspect of the sole of the foot to see which way the big toe points) are different in upper and lower motor neuron problems.

The reason why this is so important is highlighted in Case 1.1.

> The pathology is always at the level of the lower motor neuron signs.

CASE 1.1   A patient presents with difficulty walking

Often the non-neurologist directs imaging at the region of the lumbosacral spine, but this will only detect problems affecting the peripheral nervous system (including the cauda equina) between the 3rd lumbar nerve root (L3) and the first sacral (S1) nerve root. The patient is then referred for a specialist opinion and, when the patient is examined, there are signs of an upper motor neuron lesion that indicate involvement of the motor pathway (meridian of longitude) in the central and *not* the peripheral nervous system.

The lesion *has to be above the level of the 1st lumbar vertebrae*, the level at which the spinal cord ends. Imaging has been performed below this level and thus missed the problem. The appropriate investigation is to look at the spinal cord above this level.

CONCEPT OF THE MERIDIANS OF LONGITUDE AND PARALLELS OF LATITUDE

The meridians of longitude
- The descending motor pathway from the cortex to the muscle
- The ascending sensory pathway for pain and temperature
- The ascending sensory pathway for vibration and proprioception

> The nervous system can be likened to a map grid (see Figure 1.1). Establishing from the history and examination the 'meridians of longitude' and 'parallels of latitude' will localise the pathological process.

The ascending sensory pathways extend from the peripheral nerves to the cortex.[1]

---

1 The spinothalamic pathway may only extend to the deep white matter.

The parallels of latitude
CENTRAL NERVOUS SYSTEM
- Cerebral cortex
- Cranial nerves of the brainstem

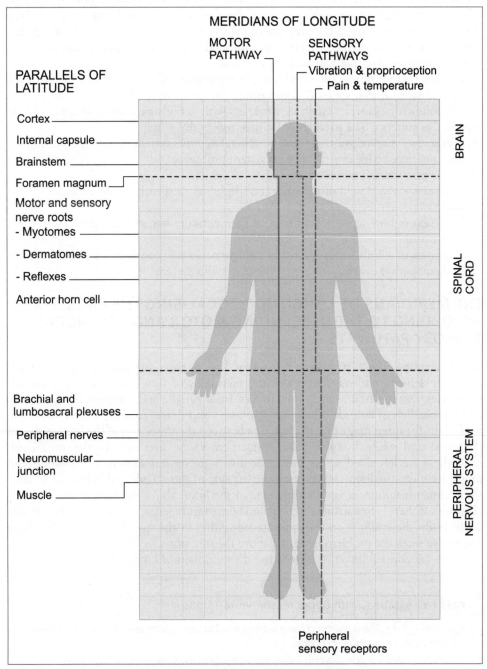

FIGURE 1.1 Meridians of longitude and parallels of latitude

Note: The motor pathway and the pathway for vibration and proprioception cross the midline at the level of the foramen magnum while the spinothalamic tract crosses immediately it enters the spinal cord.

PERIPHERAL NERVOUS SYSTEM
- Nerve roots
- Peripheral nerves

If the patient has weakness the pathological process must be affecting the motor pathway somewhere between the cortex and the muscle while, if there are sensory symptoms, the pathology must be somewhere between the sensory nerves in the periphery and the cortical sensory structures. The presence of motor and sensory symptoms/signs together immediately rules out conditions that are confined to muscle, the neuromuscular junction, the motor nerve root and anterior horn cell.

It is the pattern of weakness and sensory symptoms and/or signs together with the parallels of latitude that are used to determine the site of the pathology.

The following examples combine weakness with various parallels of latitude to help explain this concept. The parallels of latitude follow the + sign.

- Weakness + marked wasting – the peripheral nervous system, as marked wasting does not occur with central nervous system problems
- Weakness + cranial nerve involvement – brainstem
- Weakness + visual field disturbance (not diplopia) or speech disturbance (i.e. dysphasia) – cortex
- Weakness in both legs + loss of pain and temperature sensation on the torso – spinal cord
- Weakness in a limb + sensory loss in a single nerve (mononeuritis) or nerve root (radiculopathy) distribution – peripheral nervous system

THE MERIDIANS OF LONGITUDE: LOCALISING THE PROBLEM ACCORDING TO THE DESCENDING MOTOR AND ASCENDING SENSORY PATHWAYS

The descending motor pathway (also referred to as the corticospinal tract) and the ascending sensory pathways represent the meridians of longitude. The dermatomes, myotomes, reflexes, brainstem cranial nerves, basal ganglia and the cortical signs represent the parallels of latitude. The motor pathways and dorsal columns both cross at the level of the **foramen magnum**, the junction between the lower end of the brainstem and the spinal cord, while the spinothalamic tracts cross soon after entering the spinal cord.

If there are left-sided upper motor neuron signs or impairment of vibration and proprioception, the lesion is either on the left side of the spinal cord below the level of the foramen magnum or on the right side of the brain above the level of the foramen magnum. If there is impairment of pain and temperature sensation affecting the left side of the body, the lesion is on the opposite side either in the spinal cord or brain. If the face is also weak the problem has to be above the mid pons.

Cases 1.2 and 1.3 illustrate how to use the meridians of longitude.

CASE 1.2 A patient with upper motor neuron signs

A patient has weakness affecting the right arm and leg, associated with increased tone and reflexes (upper motor neuron signs).

- This indicates a problem along the motor pathway in the CNS, either in the upper cervical spinal cord on the same side above the level of C5 or on the left side of the brain above the level of the foramen magnum (where the motor pathway crosses).

CASE 1.2 A patient with upper motor neuron signs—cont'd

- If the right side of the face is also affected, the lesion cannot be in the spinal cord and must be in the upper pons or higher on the left side because the facial nerve nucleus is at the level of the mid pons. In the absence of any other symptoms or signs this is as close as we can localise the problem. It could be in the midbrain, internal capsule, corona radiata or cortex.
- The presence of a left 3rd nerve palsy is the parallel of latitude and would indicate a left midbrain lesion (this is known as Weber's syndrome). Dysphasia (speech disturbance) or cortical sensory signs (see Chapter 5) are other parallels of latitude and would indicate a cortical lesion.

CASE 1.3 A patient with weakness in the right hand without sensory symptoms or signs

A patient has weakness in the right hand in the absence of any sensory symptoms or signs. In addition to the weakness the patient has noticed marked wasting of the muscle between the thumb and index finger.

- Weakness indicates involvement of the motor system and the lesion has to be somewhere along the 'pathway' between the muscles of the hand and the contralateral motor cortex. The absence of sensory symptoms suggests the problem may be in a muscle, neuromuscular junction, motor nerve root or anterior horn cell, the more common sites that cause weakness in the absence of sensory symptoms or signs. Motor weakness without sensory symptoms can also occur with peripheral lesions.
- Wasting is a lower motor neuron sign, a parallel of latitude, and clearly indicates that the problem is in the PNS (marked wasting does not occur with problems in the neuromuscular junction or with disorders of muscle; it usually points to a problem in the anterior horn cell, motor nerve root, brachial plexus or peripheral nerve). Plexus or peripheral nerve lesions are usually, but not always, associated with sensory symptoms or signs.
- The examination demonstrates weakness of all the interosseous muscles, the abductor digiti minimi muscle and flexor digitorum profundus muscle with weakness flexing the distal phalanx of the 2nd, 3rd, 4th and 5th digits, which are referred to as the long flexors. All these muscles are innervated by the C8–T1 nerve roots, but the long flexors of the 2nd and 3rd digits are innervated by the median nerve while the long flexors of the 4th and 5th digits are innervated by the ulnar nerve. The parallel of latitude is the wasting and weakness in the distribution of the C8–T1 nerve roots.

The motor pathway

The motor pathway (see Figure 1.2) refers to the corticospinal tract within the central nervous system that descends from the motor cortex to lower motor neurons in the ventral horn of the spinal cord and the corticobulbar tract that descends from the motor cortex to several cranial nerve nuclei in the pons and medulla that innervate muscles plus the motor nerve roots, plexuses, peripheral nerves, neuromuscular junction and muscle in the peripheral nervous system.

The motor pathway:
- arises in the motor cortex in the precentral gyrus (see Figure 1.5) of the frontal lobe

> The motor pathway crosses the midline at the level of the foramen magnum (the junction of the spinal cord and the lower end of the medulla).

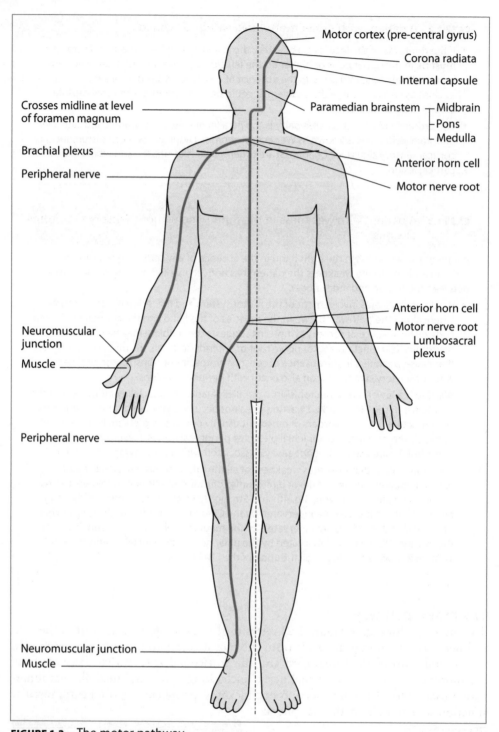

FIGURE 1.2 The motor pathway
Note: The pathway crosses at the level of the foramen magnum where the spinal cord meets the lower end of the medulla.

- descends in the cerebral hemispheres through the corona radiata and internal capsule
- passes into the brainstem via the crus cerebri (level of midbrain) and descends in the ventral and medial aspect of the pons and medulla
- descends in the lateral column of the spinal cord to the anterior horn cell where it synapses with the lower motor neuron
- leaves the spinal cord through the anterior (motor) nerve root
- passes through the brachial plexus to the arm or through the lumbosacral plexus to the leg and via the peripheral nerves to the neuromuscular junction and muscle.

> If a patient has symptoms or signs of weakness, the problem must be somewhere between the muscle and the motor cortex in the contralateral frontal lobe (see Figure 1.2).

The sensory pathways

There are two sensory pathways: one conveys vibration and proprioception and the other pain and temperature sensation and both convey light touch sensation.

PROPRIOCEPTION AND VIBRATION

The pathway (see Figure 1.3):
- arises in the peripheral sensory receptors in the joint capsules and surrounding ligaments and tendons (proprioception) or in the pacinian corpuscles in the subcutaneous tissue (vibration) [1]
- ascends up the limb in the peripheral nerves
- traverses the brachial or lumbosacral plexus
- enters the spinal cord through the dorsal (sensory) nerve root
- ascends in the *ipsilateral* dorsal column of the spinal cord with the sacral fibres most medially and the cervical fibres lateral
- ascends in the medial lemniscus in the medial aspect of the brainstem via the thalamus to the sensory cortex in the parietal lobe.

Abnormalities of vibration and proprioception may occur with peripheral neuropathies but rarely are they affected with isolated nerve or nerve root lesions.

> - The dorsal columns cross the midline at the level of the foramen magnum.
> - If the patient has impairment of vibration and/or proprioception, the problem is either on the ipsilateral side of the nervous system below or on the contralateral side above the foramen magnum (see Figure 1.2).

PAIN AND TEMPERATURE SENSATION

The spinothalamic pathway (see Figure 1.4):
- includes the nerves conveying pain and temperature that arise in the peripheral sensory receptors in the skin and deeper structures [1]
- coalesces to form the peripheral nerves in the limbs or the nerve root nerves of the trunk
- from the limbs, traverses the brachial or lumbosacral plexus
- enters the spinal cord through the dorsal (sensory) nerve root
- ascends in the spinothalamic tract located in the anterolateral aspect of the spinal cord, with nerves from higher in the body pushing those from lower laterally in the spinal cord

- ascends in the lateral aspect of the brainstem to the thalamus.

Although there is some debate about whether they then project to the cortex, abnormal pain and temperature sensation can occur with deep white matter hemisphere lesions.

If the history and/or examination detects unilateral impairment of the sensory modalities affecting the face, arm and leg, this can only localise the problem to above the 5th cranial nerve nucleus in the mid pons of the brainstem on the contralateral side to the symptoms and signs, i.e. there is no 'parallel of latitude' to help localise the problem more accurately than that. The presence of a hemianopia and/or cortical sensory signs would be the parallels of latitude that would indicate that the pathology is in the cerebral hemispheres affecting the parietal lobe and cortex.

Case 1.4 illustrates a patient with both motor and sensory pathways affected.

> The spinothalamic tracts cross the midline almost immediately after entering the spinal cord.
>
> If a patient has impairment of pain and temperature sensation, the lesion must either be in the ipsilateral peripheral nerve or the sensory nerve root or is contralateral in the CNS between the level of entry into the spinal cord and the cerebral hemisphere (see Figure 1.4).

CASE 1.4 A woman with difficulty walking

A 70-year-old woman presents with difficulty walking due to weakness and stiffness in both legs. There is no weakness in her upper limbs. She has also noticed some instability in the dark and a sensation of tight stockings around her legs. The examination reveals weakness of hip flexion associated with increased tone and reflexes and upgoing plantar responses. There is impairment of vibration and proprioception in the legs and there is decreased pain sensation in both legs and on both sides of the abdomen up to the level of the umbilicus on the front of the abdomen and several centimetres higher than this on the back.

- The weakness in both legs indicates that the motor pathway (meridian of longitude) is affected.
- The alteration of vibration and proprioception also indicates that the relevant pathway (another meridian of longitude) is involved.
- The increased tone and reflexes are upper motor neuron signs and, therefore, the problem must be in the CNS not the PNS, either the spinal cord or brain.
- The fact that the signs are bilateral indicates that the motor pathways on both sides of the nervous system are affected and the most likely place for this to occur is in the spinal cord, although it can also occur in the brainstem and in the medial aspect of the cerebral hemispheres. (For more information on the cortical representation of the legs, not illustrated in this book, look up the term 'cortical homunculus' which is a physical representation of the primary motor cortex.)
- The impairment of pain sensation is the 3rd meridian of longitude and indicates that the spinothalamic tract is involved.
- The upper motor neuron pattern of weakness and involvement of the pathway conveying vibration and proprioception simply indicate that the problem is above the level of L1, but the sensory level on the trunk at the level of the umbilicus is the parallel of latitude and localises the lesion to the 10th thoracic spinal cord level (see Figures 1.12 and 1.13).

This is not an uncommon presentation, and it is often taught that a thoracic cord lesion in a middle-aged or elderly female is due to a meningioma until proven otherwise.

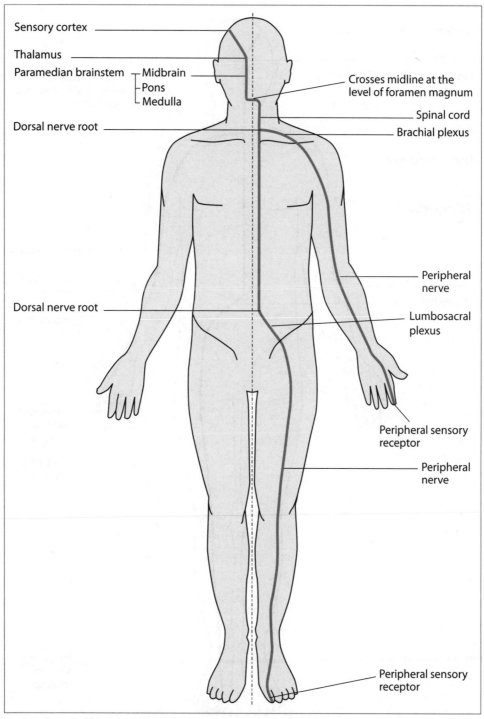

FIGURE 1.3 Pathway conveying proprioception and vibration

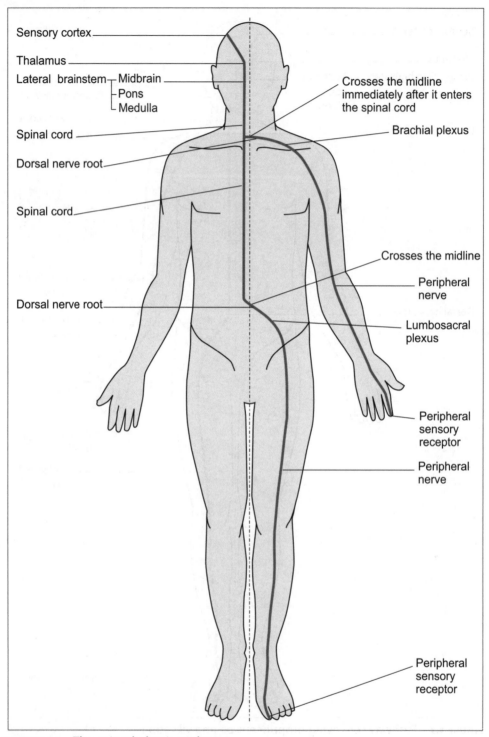

FIGURE 1.4 The spinothalamic pathway

THE PARALLELS OF LATITUDE: FINDING THE SITE OF PATHOLOGY WITHIN THE STRUCTURES OF THE CENTRAL AND PERIPHERAL NERVOUS SYSTEMS

The parallels of latitude refer to the structures within the CNS and PNS that indicate the site of the pathology. For example, if the patient has a hemiparesis and a non-fluent dysphasia, it is the dysphasia that indicates that the weakness must be related to a problem in the dominant frontal cortex.

In the CNS the parallels of latitude consist of:

- the cortex – vision, memory, personality, speech and specific cortical sensory and visual phenomena such as visual and sensory inattention, graphaesthesia (see Chapter 5, 'The cerebral hemispheres and cerebellum')
- the cranial nerves of the brainstem (see Chapter 4, 'The cranial nerves and understanding the brainstem') – each cranial nerve is at a different level in the brainstem and thus represents a parallel of latitude. For example, if the patient has a 7th nerve palsy the problem either has to be in the 7th nerve or in the brainstem at the level of the pons. The nerve roots and peripheral nerves are the parallels of latitude in the PNS:
- The motor and sensory nerves when affected will result in a very focal pattern of weakness and/or sensory loss that clearly indicates that the problem is in the peripheral nerve (see Chapter 11, 'Common neck, arm and upper back problems' and Chapter 12, 'Back pain and common leg problems with or without difficulty walking').
- The nerve roots include
  - **myotomes** – motor nerve roots supplying muscles produce a classic pattern of weakness of several muscles supplied by that nerve root; specific nerve roots are part of the reflex arc and if, for example, the patient has an absent biceps reflex the lesion is at the level of C5–6
  - **dermatomes** – areas of abnormal sensation from involvement of sensory nerve roots (see Figures 1.12, 1.13 and 1.22).

Parallels of latitude in the central nervous system

If a patient has a problem within the CNS, involvement of either the cortex or the brainstem will produce symptoms and signs that will enable accurate localisation. For example, the patient who presents with weakness involving the right face, arm and leg clearly has a problem affecting the motor pathway (the meridian of longitude) on the left side of the brain above the mid pons. The presence of a left 3rd nerve palsy (the parallel of latitude) would indicate the lesion is on the left side of the mid-brain while the presence of a non-fluent dysphasia (another parallel of latitude) would localise the problem to the left frontal cortex. Case 1.5 illustrates how to use the parallels of latitude in the CNS.

CASE 1.5 A man with right facial and arm weakness, vision and speech impairment

A 65-year-old man presents with weakness of his face and arm on the right side together with an inability to see to the right and, although he knows what he wants to say, he is having difficulty expressing the words. He also has, when examined, impairment of vibration and proprioception sensation in the right hand.

- The weakness of his face and arm indicate a lesion affecting the motor pathway or meridian of longitude on the left side of the brain above the mid pons.

> **CASE 1.5** A man with right facial and arm weakness, vision and speech impairment—cont'd
>
> - The difficulty expressing his words indicates the presence of a non-fluent dysphasia (the parallel of latitude), accurately localising the problem to the left frontal cortex.
> - The inability to see to the right is another parallel of latitude and it reflects involvement of the visual pathways from behind the optic chiasm to the left occipital lobe in the left hemisphere, resulting in a right homonymous hemianopia (this is discussed in Chapter 5, 'The cerebral hemispheres and cerebellum').
> - The impairment of vibration and proprioception in the right hand indicates that the parallel of latitude conveying this sensation is affected. Since the other symptoms and signs point to a left hemisphere lesion, the abnormality of vibration and proprioception indicates involvement of the parietal lobe, and this also would indicate that the visual disturbance is almost certainly in the left parietal lobe and not the occipital lobe. This sort of presentation is very typical of a cerebral infarct affecting the middle cerebral artery territory (see Chapter 10, 'Cerebrovascular disease').

THE HEMISPHERES

Figure 1.5 is a simplified diagram showing the main lobes of the brain and the cortical function associated with those areas. If the patient has cortical hemisphere symptoms and signs this clearly establishes the site of the pathology in the cortex of a particular region of the brain.

THE BRAINSTEM

Figure 1.6 shows the site of the cranial nerves in the brainstem with the numbers added: the 9th, 10th, 11th and 12th cranial nerves at the level of the medulla; the 5th, 6th, 7th and 8th at the level of the pons; and the 3rd and 4th at the level of the midbrain (see Chapter 4 for a detailed discussion of the brainstem and cranial nerves). Also note that the 3rd, 6th and 12th cranial nerves exit the brainstem close to the midline while the other cranial nerves exit the lateral aspect of the brainstem.

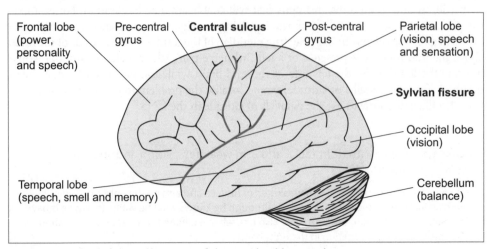

FIGURE 1.5 The left lateral aspect of the cerebral hemisphere

Note: The central sulcus separates the frontal lobe from the parietal lobe (see Chapter 5, 'The cerebral hemispheres and cerebellum').

The presence of cranial nerve signs, except for a 6th or a 3rd nerve palsy in the setting of downward transtentorial herniation of the brain due to a mass above the tentorium, which can sometimes be a false localising sign (where the pathology is not in the nerve or brainstem), means the pathology MUST be at the level of that cranial nerve either in the nerve itself or in the brainstem.

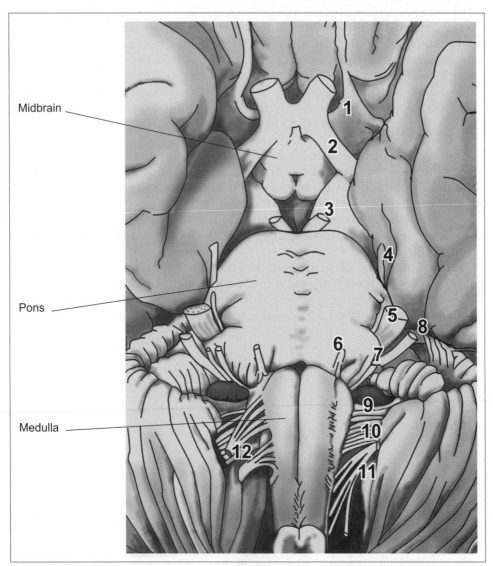

FIGURE 1.6 The ventral aspect of the brainstem showing the cranial nerves

Reproduced and modified from *Gray's Anatomy*, 37th edn, edited by PL Williams et al, 1989, Churchill Livingstone, Figure 7.81 [2]

This view is looking up from underneath the hemispheres. The cerebellum can be seen either side of the medulla and pons, the olfactory nerves (labelled 1) lie beneath the frontal lobes, and the under surface of the temporal lobes can be seen lateral to the 3rd and 4th cranial nerves.

1 = Olfactory, 2 = ophthalmic, 3 = oculomotor, 4 = trochlear, 5 = trigeminal, 6 = abducent, 7 = facial, 8 = auditory, 9 = glossopharyngeal, 10 = vagus, 11 = spinal accessory and 12 = hypoglossal

Parallels of latitude in the peripheral nervous system
CRANIAL NERVES

In Figure 1.7 the important points to note are:

- The 1st division of the trigeminal nerve extends over the scalp to somewhere between the vertex and two-thirds of the way back towards the occipital region where it meets the greater occipital nerve supplied by the 2nd cervical nerve root. In a trigeminal nerve lesion the sensory loss will not extend to the occipital region, whereas with a spinothalamic tract problem it will.
- The 2nd and 3rd (predominantly the 3rd) cervical sensory nerve root supplies the angle of the jaw helping to differentiate trigeminal nerve sensory loss from involvement of the spinothalamic/quintothalamic tract. The angle of the jaw and neck are affected with lesions of the quinto/spinothalamic tract. Sensory loss on the face without affecting the angle of the jaw indicates the lesion is involving the 5th cranial nerve.
- The upper lip is supplied by the 2nd division and the lower lip by the 3rd division of the trigeminal nerve.
- The trigeminal nerve ends in front of the ear lobe.

The corneal reflex afferent arc is the 1st division of the trigeminal nerve; the nasal tickle reflex is the 2nd division (see Chapter 4, 'The cranial nerves and understanding the brainstem').

The anatomies of the muscles to the eye, the visual pathway and the vestibular pathway are discussed in Chapter 4, 'The cranial nerves and understanding the brainstem'.

The purpose of the illustrations in the remainder of this chapter is to serve as a reference point for future use, and it is not anticipated that the reader will remember them all. With this textbook at the bedside the clinician can quickly refer to the illustrations to work out the anatomical basis of the pattern of weakness or of sensory loss.

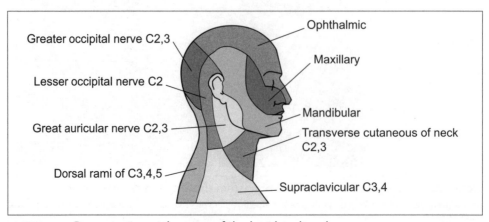

FIGURE 1.7   Dermatomes and nerves of the head and neck

Reproduced from *Gray's Anatomy*, 37th edn, edited by PL Williams et al, 1989, Churchill Livingstone, Figure 7.242 [2]

Note: The ophthalmic, maxillary and mandibular nerves are the three components of the 5th cranial nerve, the trigeminal nerve.

THE UPPER LIMBS
Brachial plexus
The most important aspects to note in Figure 1.8 are:
- The suprascapular nerve and the long thoracic nerve arise from the nerve roots (C5, C6 and C7) proximal to the junction of C5 and C6, helping to differentiate between a brachial plexus lesion at the level of C5–C6 and a nerve root lesion.
- The radial nerve arises from C5, C6 and C7.
- The median nerve arises from C5, C6, C7, C8 and T1.
- The ulnar nerve arises from the 8th cervical and 1st thoracic nerve roots. The clinical features of ulnar nerve lesions and pathology affecting the C8–T1 nerve roots are very similar, and a detailed examination is usually required to differentiate between these two entities.

Motor nerves and muscles of the upper limb
AXILLARY AND RADIAL NERVES
Figure 1.9 shows the muscles innervated by the axillary and radial nerves. The important points to note are:
- The axillary only supplies the deltoid muscle, not the other muscles (supraspinatus, infraspinatus and subscapularis) around the shoulder that collectively form the rotator cuff. Weakness isolated to the deltoid will indicate an axillary nerve lesion (occasionally seen with a dislocated shoulder).

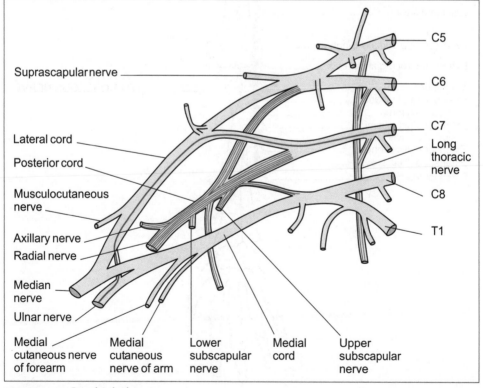

FIGURE 1.8 Brachial plexus

Reproduced and modified from *Gray's Anatomy,* 37th edn, edited by PL Williams et al, 1989, Churchill Livingstone, Figure 7.243 [2]

Note: For simplification, the names of a number of nerves have been removed as they are rarely examined in clinical practice.

- The branches of the radial nerve to the triceps muscle arise from above the spiral groove of the humerus. The spiral groove is a common site for compression and thus the triceps is not affected.
- The branches to the brachioradialis, extensor carpi radialis longus and extensor carpi radialis brevis arise proximal to the posterior interosseous nerve, these will

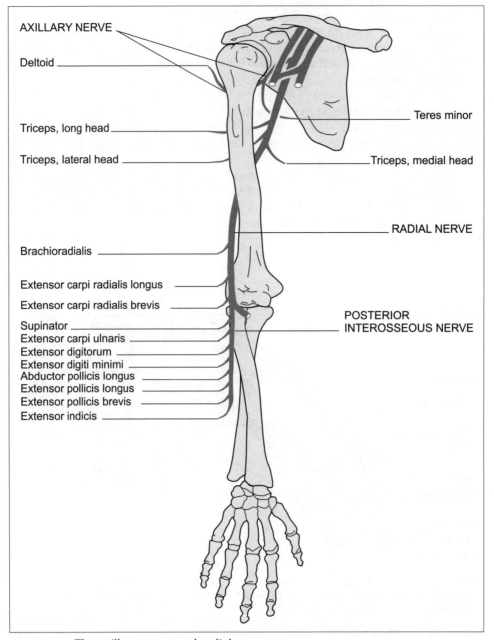

FIGURE 1.9   The axillary nerve and radial nerves

Reproduced from *Aids to the Examination of the Peripheral Nervous System*, 4th edn, Brain, 2000, Saunders, Figure 15, p 12 [3]

be affected by a radial nerve palsy but spared if the problem is confined to the posterior interosseous nerve.

MEDIAN NERVE

Figure 1.10 shows the muscles supplied by the median nerve. The points to note are:
- The branches to the flexor carpi radialis (flexes the wrist) and flexor digitorum superficialis (flexes the medial four fingers at the proximal interphalangeal joint) arise near the elbow, proximal to the anterior interosseous nerve.

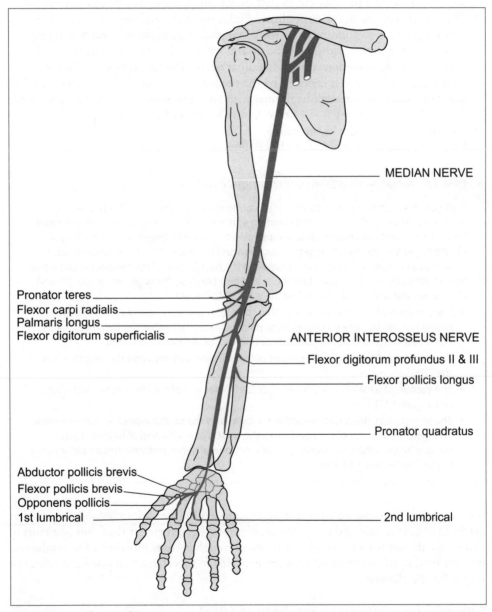

Pronator teres
Flexor carpi radialis
Palmaris longus
Flexor digitorum superficialis

MEDIAN NERVE

ANTERIOR INTEROSSEUS NERVE
Flexor digitorum profundus II & III
Flexor pollicis longus

Pronator quadratus

Abductor pollicis brevis
Flexor pollicis brevis
Opponens pollicis
1st lumbrical

2nd lumbrical

FIGURE 1.10   The median nerve

Reproduced from *Aids to the Examination of the Peripheral Nervous System,* 4th edn, Brain, 2000, Saunders, Figure 27, p 20 [3]

- The anterior interosseous nerve supplies the flexor pollicis longus (flexes the distal phalanx of the thumb), the pronator quadratus (turns the wrist over so that the palm is facing downwards) and the lateral aspect of the flexor digitorum profundus (flexes the distal phalanges of the 2nd and 3rd digits).
- The nerve to abductor pollicis brevis, the muscle that elevates the thumb when the hand is fully supinated (palm facing the ceiling), arises at or just distal to the wrist in the region of the carpal tunnel.

ULNAR NERVE

Figure 1.11 shows the muscles innervated by the ulnar nerve. The points to note are:
- The branches to the flexor carpi ulnaris (flexes the wrist) and medial aspect of the flexor digitorum profundus (flexes the distal phalanges of the 4th and 5th digits) arise just distal to the medial epicondyle and will be affected by lesions at the elbow, a common sight of compression of the ulnar nerve. The lateral aspect of flexor digitorum profundus is innervated by the median nerve and, thus, flexion of the 2nd and 3rd distal phalanges will be normal with an ulnar nerve lesion at the elbow while they will be affected by C8–T1 nerve root or lower cord brachial plexus lesions.
- All other branches arise in the hand.
  Case 1.6 illustrates a problem with the ulnar nerve.

CASE 1.6 A man with weakness in his right hand

A 35-year-old man presents with weakness confined to his right hand. This has been present for some time and he has noted thinning of the muscle between his thumb and index finger. He has also noticed pins and needles affecting his little finger, the medial half of his 4th finger and the medial aspect of his palm and the back of the hand to the wrist. The examination reveals reduced pain sensation in the distribution of the symptoms and weakness of abduction of the medial four digits and also bending the fingertips of the 4th and 5th but not the 2nd or 3rd fingers. The thumb is not affected.

- The presence of weakness indicates that the motor pathway (meridian of longitude) is affected and the altered sensation to pain indicates that either the peripheral nerve, nerve root or spinothalamic pathway to that part of the hand is affected.
- The presence of wasting is the parallel of latitude and indicates that the problem is in the PNS.
- The pattern of weakness clearly represents involvement of the ulnar nerve at the elbow (see Figure 1.11).
- The sensory loss affecting the medial 1½ digits and the medial aspect of both the palm and the dorsal aspect of the hand up to the wrist is also a parallel of latitude as the sensory loss is within the distribution of a peripheral nerve and indicates an ulnar nerve lesion (see Figures 1.14 and 1.15).

The remaining illustrations show the areas supplied by the various sensory nerves that detect light touch, pain and temperature. Neurologists remember these but 'students of neurology' do not need to remember them, although by remembering a few landmarks it is not hard to fill in the gaps. They are included in this chapter to provide a reference source for the clinician.

Cutaneous sensation of the upper limbs and trunk

Below each illustration are the one or two important features that are most useful at the bedside.

The dermatomes are higher on the back than they are on the front of the trunk. Sensory loss that is at the same horizontal level on both the anterior and posterior aspects of the trunk is not related to organic pathology and is more likely to be of functional origin.

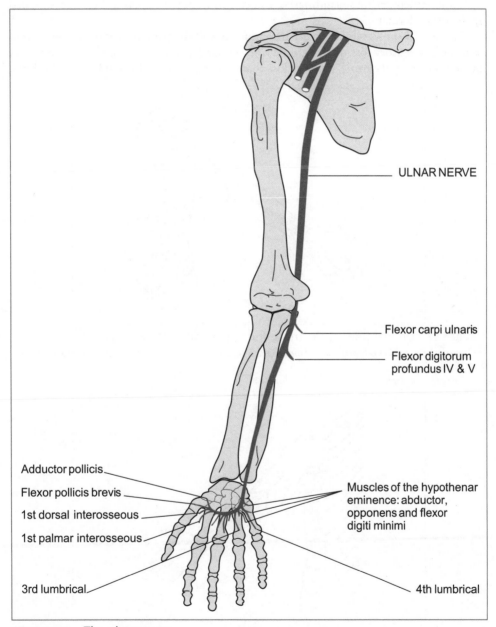

ULNAR NERVE

Flexor carpi ulnaris

Flexor digitorum profundus IV & V

Adductor pollicis

Flexor pollicis brevis

1st dorsal interosseous

1st palmar interosseous

3rd lumbrical

Muscles of the hypothenar eminence: abductor, opponens and flexor digiti minimi

4th lumbrical

FIGURE 1.11 The ulnar nerve

Reproduced from *Aids to the Examination of the Peripheral Nervous System,* 4th edn, Brain, 2000, Saunders, Figure 36, p 26 [3]

The areas of sensation in the upper limb and trunk supplied by the sensory nerve roots, the dermatomes, are shown in Figures 1.12 and 1.13. A simple method of remembering the dermatomes is:

- The arm–C7 affects the 3rd finger, C6 is lateral to this and C8 is medial to this.
- The trunk–T2 is at the level of the clavicle and meets C4; T8 is at the level of the xiphisternum (the lower end of the sternum), T10 is at the level of the umbilicus and T12 is at the level of the groin.

If you remember these landmarks, you can work out the areas in between supplied by the other dermatomes.

Figure 1.13 shows why it is very important to roll the patient over or sit them up to examine any sensory loss on the trunk. *The dermatomes are higher on the back than they are on the front of the trunk.* Sensory loss that is at the same horizontal level on both the

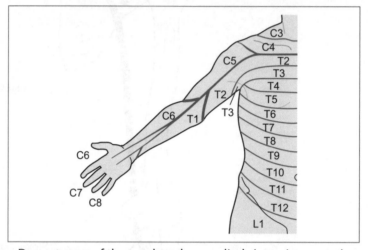

FIGURE 1.12   Dermatomes of the trunk and upper limb (anterior aspect)

Reproduced from *Aids to the Examination of the Peripheral Nervous System,* 4th edn, Brain, 2000, Saunders, Figure 87, p 56 [3]

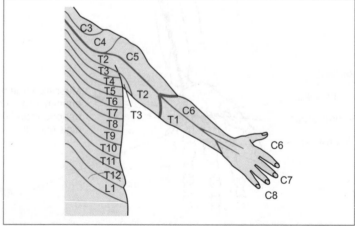

FIGURE 1.13   Dermatomes of the trunk and upper limb (posterior aspect)

Reproduced from *Aids to the Examination of the Peripheral Nervous System,* 4th edn, Brain, 2000, Saunders, Figure 88, p 57) [3]

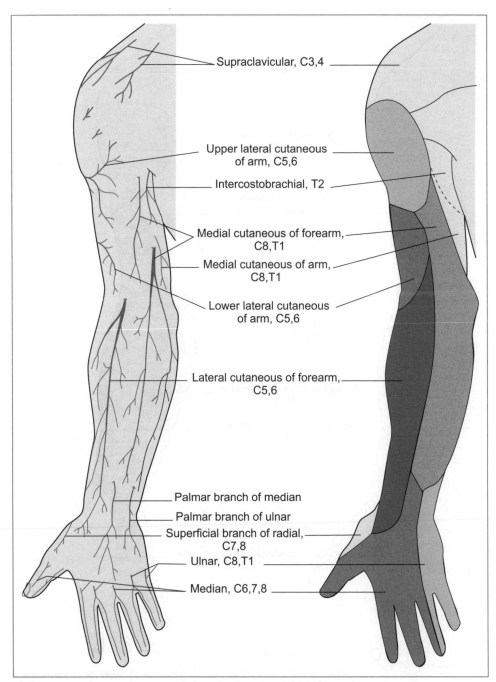

FIGURE 1.14 Sensory nerves of the upper limbs (anterior aspect)

Reproduced from *Gray's Anatomy*, 37th edn, edited by PL Williams et al, 1989, Churchill Livingstone, Figure 7.244 [2]

Note: The nerve root origin of the nerves is also shown. Note that the median nerve supplies the lateral 3 ½ digits while the ulnar nerve supplies the medial 1½ digits.

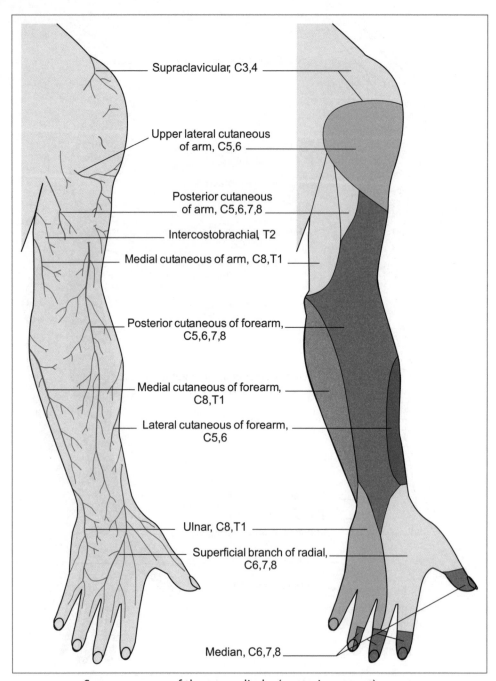

FIGURE 1.15   Sensory nerves of the upper limbs (posterior aspect)

Reproduced from *Gray's Anatomy,* 37th edn, edited by PL Williams et al, 1989, Churchill Livingstone, Figure 7.245) [2]

Note: The nerve root origin of the nerves is also shown.

anterior and posterior aspects of the trunk is not related to organic pathology and is more likely to be of functional origin.

THE LOWER LIMBS
Lumbar and sacral plexuses
Unlike the brachial plexus, there is little in the lumbosacral plexus (Figure 1.16) that helps localise whether the problem is in the lumbosacral plexus or the nerve roots. It is important to note that the sciatic nerve arises from predominantly the 5th lumbrical at the 1st and 2nd sacral nerve roots.

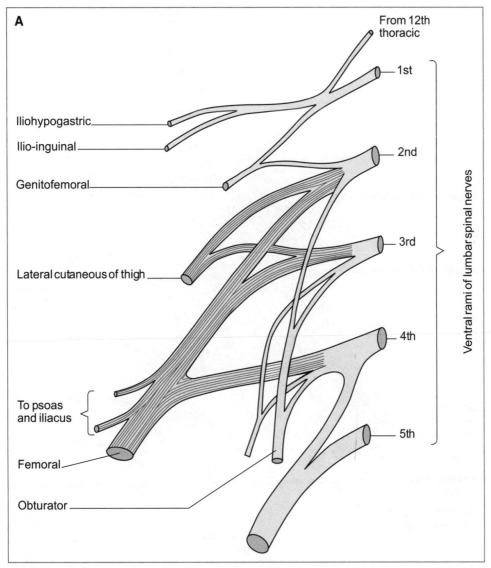

FIGURE 1.16   A Lumbar plexus

Note: The main nerve to arise from the lumbar plexus is the femoral nerve. It is formed from the 2nd, 3rd and 4th lumbrical nerve roots.

The motor nerves and muscles of the lower limb

FEMORAL NERVE

The point to note (see Figure 1.17) is that the common peroneal nerve arises from the sciatic nerve above the popliteal fossa and above the level of the neck of the fibula, a common site for compression, and that there are no branches between where it arises and the neck of the fibula.

SCIATIC NERVE

The point to note is that the tibialis posterior muscle is supplied by the posterior tibial nerve while the tibialis anterior muscle is supplied by the common peroneal nerve (see

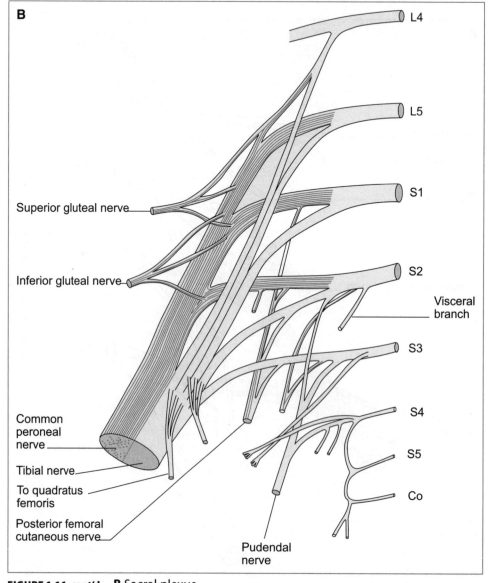

FIGURE 1.16, cont'd   B Sacral plexus

Reproduced from *Gray's Anatomy*, 37th edn, edited by PL Williams et al, 1989, Churchill Livingstone, Figures 7.252 and 7.256 [2]

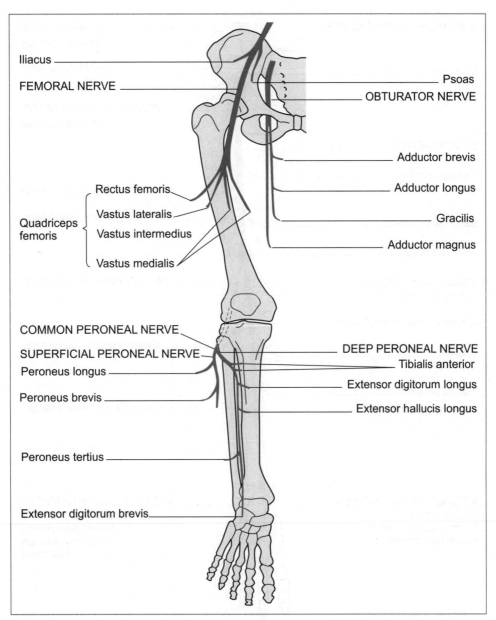

FIGURE 1.17 The femoral nerve, obturator nerve and common peroneal nerve of the right lower limb

Reproduced from *Aids to the Examination of the Peripheral Nervous System*, 4th edn, Brain, 2000, Saunders, Figure 46, p 32 [3]

Figure 1.18). Examining these muscles individually in patients with a foot drop helps to differentiate between a common peroneal nerve palsy and an L5 nerve root lesion. Inversion is stronger in a common peroneal nerve lesion while eversion is stronger with an L5 nerve root lesion. (See Chapter 12, 'Back pain and common leg problems with or without difficulty walking'.)

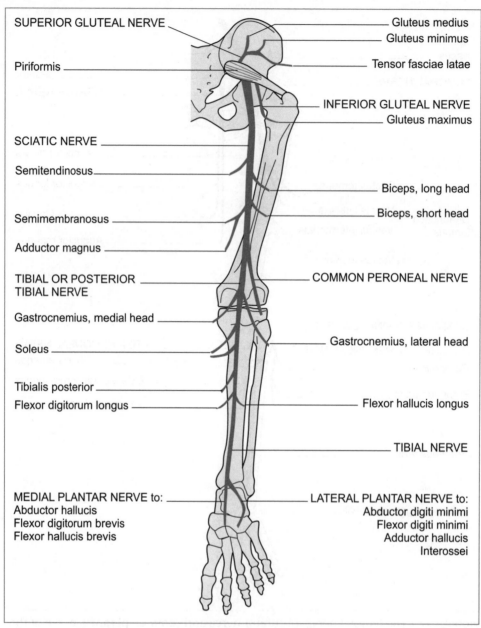

FIGURE 1.18 The sciatic nerve and posterior tibial nerve

Reproduced from *Aids to the Examination of the Peripheral Nervous System,* 4th edn, Brain, 2000, Saunders, Figure 47, p 33 [3]

Cutaneous sensation of the lower limbs

As discussed with reference to the upper limbs and trunk, Figures 1.19–1.22 are supplied as a reference source along with some important clinical clues.

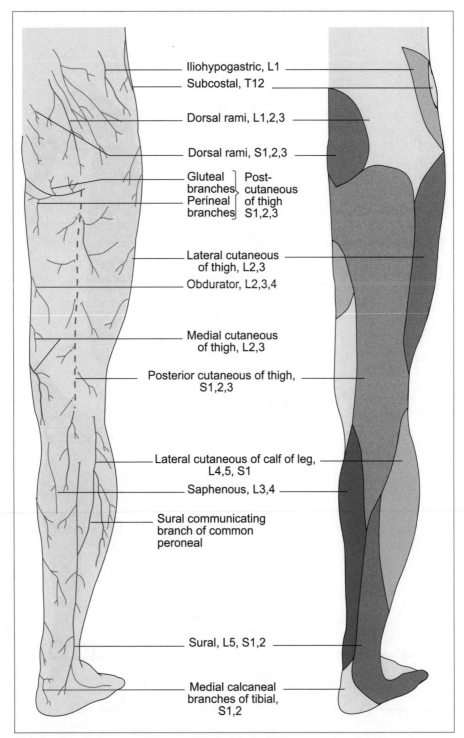

FIGURE 1.19 The sensory nerves of the lower limbs (posterior aspect)

Reproduced from *Gray's Anatomy,* 37th edn, edited by PL Williams et al, 1989, Churchill Livingstone, Figure 7.258) [2]

Note: The nerve root origin of the nerves is also shown.

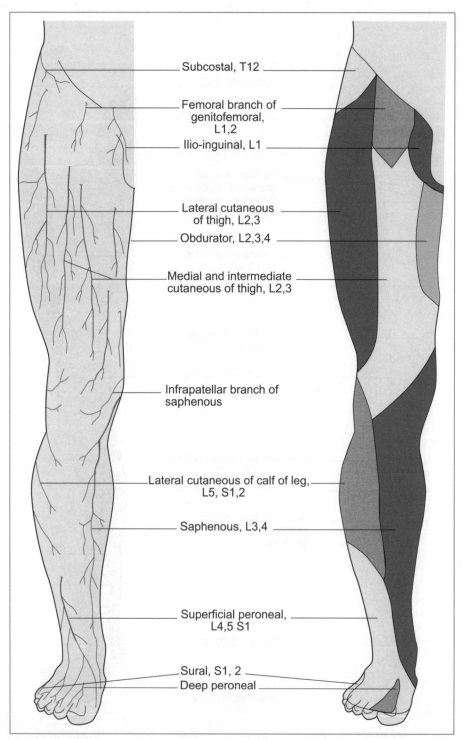

FIGURE 1.20   The sensory nerves of lower limbs (anterior aspect)

Reproduced from *Gray's Anatomy*, 37th edn, edited by PL Williams et al, 1989, Churchill Livingstone, Figure 7.254 [2]

Note: The nerve root origin of the nerves is also shown.

USEFUL LANDMARKS FOR REMEMBERING CUTANEOUS SENSATION

Rather than trying to remember all the dermatomes, the following landmarks can be used.

- T12 is at the level of the groin (see Figure 1.12).
- L3 crosses the knee (see Figure 1.22).
- S1 supplies the outside of the foot (see Figure 1.22).

REFERENCES

1 Brodal A. Neurological anatomy, 2nd edn. London: Oxford University Press; 1969:807.
2 Williams PL et al (eds). Gray's anatomy 37th edn. London: Churchill Livingstone; 1989.
3 Brain. Aids to the examination of the peripheral nervous system, 4th edn. Edinburgh: Saunders; 2000.

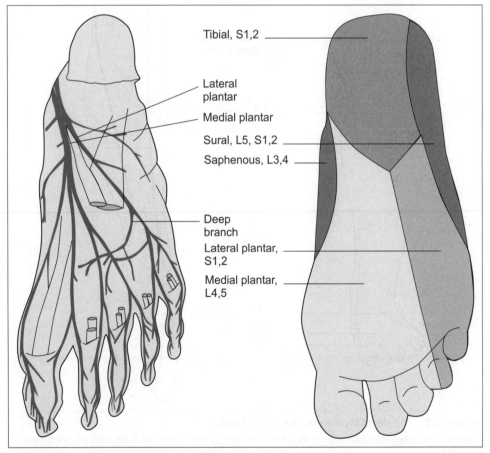

FIGURE 1.21   The sensory nerves affecting the soles of the feet

Reproduced from *Gray's Anatomy*, 37th edn, edited by PL Williams et al, 1989, Churchill Livingstone, Figure X, p Y [2]

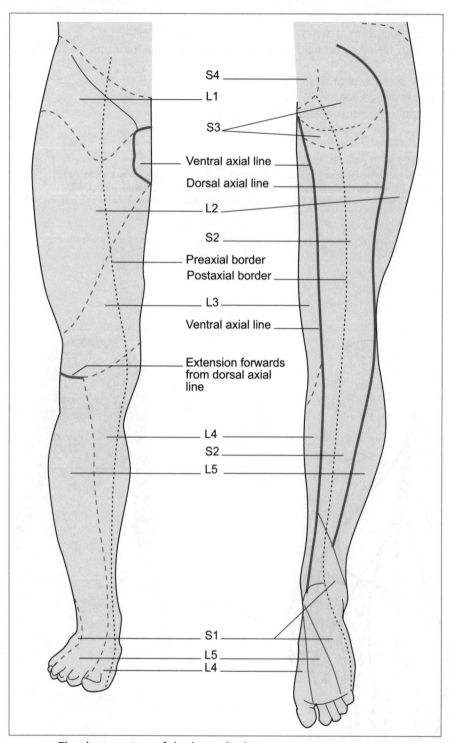

S4

L1

S3

Ventral axial line

Dorsal axial line

L2

S2

Preaxial border

Postaxial border

L3

Ventral axial line

Extension forwards
from dorsal axial
line

L4

S2

L5

S1

L5

L4

FIGURE 1.22 The dermatomes of the lower limbs

Reproduced from *Aids to the Examination of the Peripheral Nervous System,* 4th edn, Brain, 2000, Saunders, Figure 89, p 58 [3]

Note: T12 meets L1 at the groin, L3 crosses the knee and L5 affects the outside of the shin and the dorsal aspect of the foot. If you remember these landmarks you can work out the area in between supplied by the other dermatomes.

chapter 2

The Neurological History

This chapter will endeavour to provide a basic understanding of the principles of history taking so that the time spent on the ward learning how to take a history can be more effective, more interesting and more enjoyable. In particular, the pivotal aspects of clinical neurology will be discussed.

- **Where is the lesion?** Is the problem in the cerebral hemispheres, brainstem, cerebellum, spinal cord, nerve roots, brachial or lumbosacral plexus, peripheral nerve, neuromuscular junction or muscle? When considering the nature (i.e. whether it is weakness, sensory symptoms or visual or speech disturbances) and the distribution of the weakness and sensory symptoms in terms of which parts of the body are affected, thinking about the underlying neuroanatomy will help to localise the problem within the nervous system.

- **What is the pathology?** Establish the mode of onset and progression of the illness.

Almost invariably *the difference between making the correct diagnosis and not* is a direct consequence of the time spent taking a very detailed history. The most common mistake that inexperienced clinicians make when taking a history is that they elicit the nature of the symptoms but do not clarify the exact distribution or how the symptoms evolved. Migraine, subarachnoid haemorrhage, meningitis and a hangover will all present with headache, nausea, vomiting and photophobia. It is not the symptoms that indicate the likely diagnosis but rather the way in which those symptoms have evolved.

Using the techniques described in this chapter, there is no reason why an inexperienced student or hospital medical officer cannot obtain the same history as an experienced clinician. There is always an experienced clinician on the other end of a telephone who can be more helpful if given a good history.

Consider Cases 2.1 and 2.2.

In both of these cases the referring physician has used the nature of the symptoms, the age of the patient and the past and family history to make a diagnosis. In the first case the clinician has assumed that patients of this age are likely to suffer from a stroke and that the presence of multiple risk factors for cerebral vascular disease means that the patient's symptoms are due to cerebral ischaemia. In fact this patient's symptoms evolved over several weeks and were related to a malignant tumour. In the second case the past

---

CASE 2.1

Dear Dr,
Thank you for admitting this 65-year-old man with a stroke. He presents with left-sided weakness. He has a past history of hypertension, diabetes and hypercholesterolaemia. He is a smoker and his father and older brother both died of a stroke.
Yours sincerely,

CASE 2.2

Dear Dr,
Thank you for seeing this 25-year-old man with migraine. He has headache, nausea, vomiting and photophobia. He had migraine in childhood and his mother and sister both suffer from migraine.
Yours sincerely,

---

and family history of migraine was used to make a diagnosis of migraine. This patient's symptoms were of instantaneous onset and were related to a ruptured berry aneurysm causing subarachnoid haemorrhage (bleeding into the subarachnoid space – the space beneath the outer lining of the brain, referred to as the dura mater, and the surface of the brain).

A past history of a medical problem does not preclude the patient suffering from a totally unrelated illness. The approach of using the past history to influence the diagnosis of the current problem often leads to a delay in diagnosing new problems in patients with chronic diseases. In most instances 'prior probability' is correct, and this can lull clinicians into thinking that they are clever when in fact it was difficult for them to be wrong even if they did not obtain a detailed history. Typical examples of this are an older person with a hemiparesis with the most likely cause being a stroke and the general practitioner (GP) who diagnoses most patients as having a tension-type headache and is correct the vast majority of the time simply because most patients attending a GP with headache do in fact suffer from tension-type headache.

> • A past history of an illness or risk factors for an illness only increase the likelihood that the patient has a particular problem; they should not be used to make a diagnosis.
>
> • The nature and distribution of the symptoms can only localise the problem within the nervous system and cannot infer a particular pathological diagnosis.

The age of the patient and the past, family and social history simply increase the likelihood of a particular illness being present. This information should be regarded as '**circumstantial evidence**'. As in law, where many innocent people have been found guilty on the basis of circumstantial evidence, in medicine many incorrect diagnoses have been made using the age of the patient and the past, family, social and medication history to make a diagnosis.

Spencer [1] stated that it is not possible to learn how to take an effective history from a textbook. The clinical environment is the only setting in which the skills of history taking, physical examination, clinical reasoning, decision making, empathy and professionalism can be taught and learnt as an integrated whole. Although this is correct, one could use the analogy of learning to play golf: you can either hack away for years to teach yourself or you can have lessons that will make the practice more effective.

Traditionally, students have been taught to ask a long list of neurological questions about headache, dizziness, weakness, numbness etc in the forlorn hope that, after this 'fishing expedition' (also referred to as 'looking for the pony'[1]) [2], a

---

[1] 'Looking for the pony' comes from a Christmas tale of two brothers, one of whom was an incurable pessimist and the other an incurable optimist. On Christmas day, the pessimist was given a room full of new toys and the optimist a roomful of horse manure. The optimist threw himself into the muck and began burrowing about in it. When his horrified parents extricated him from the excrement and asked why on earth he was thrashing about in it, he joyfully cried, 'With all this horse manure, there's got to be a pony in here somewhere!'

diagnosis will be apparent. In other words, in the hope of finding the diagnosis ('the pony'), one collects a large list of answers to numerous specific questions that largely relate to the nature of the symptoms with little understanding about what the answers represent. It has been suggested that students should be taught to take a history this way and then taught not to take it that way. I disagree. I would like to recommentd that students should be taught how to take a history in a way that is meaningful to them rather than just collecting useless information they do not know how to use.

PRINCIPLES OF NEUROLOGICAL HISTORY TAKING

When obtaining the history from a patient with a neurological problem it is important to establish whether the problem is:
* a monophasic illness
* intermittent symptoms or recurrent episodes.

An alternative method of obtaining the history in patients presenting with intermittent disturbances of neurological function or recurrent episodes, e.g. epilepsy or headache, is recommended. In essence, with intermittent disturbances it is better to obtain a blow-by-blow description of several individual episodes. This alternative approach is described in Chapter 7, 'Episodic disturbances of neurological function' and Chapter 8, 'Seizures and epilepsy'.

Having established that the problem is a monophasic illness, the three basic principles of history taking are simple:

1 *Define the likely underlying pathological basis by eliciting the mode of onset, progression and duration of each and every symptom* (i.e. the time course of the illness).
2 *Establish the site of the disorder within the nervous system by determining the nature and distribution of symptoms.*
3 *Elicit other facts that may either establish a cause for the problem or, more importantly, influence subsequent management of the patient.* This includes the family history, past history, coexistent medical problems, prescribed drugs and natural remedies the patient is taking, social factors and the patient's concerns.

Difficulties making a diagnosis are almost always the result of failure to establish the mode of onset, progression and duration of symptoms.

Some patients are not capable of giving an accurate history. This is often (but not always) due to the presence of an inability to speak the language, dementia, confusion or amnesia. In these circumstances it is necessary to question a relative or an eyewitness. If that is not possible, one has no choice but to use circumstantial evidence (the past and family history) and prior probability (certain conditions affect particular people of a certain sex and age) to come to a likely diagnosis.

THE UNDERLYING PATHOLOGICAL PROCESS: MODE OF ONSET, DURATION AND PROGRESSION OF SYMPTOMS

Different pathological processes evolve over variable periods of time and it is this variability that can be used to determine the most **likely pathology**. Three modes of onset can be loosely defined: sudden onset within seconds to minutes, gradual onset over hours to days and a very gradual onset over months to years (see Figure 2.1). The expression 'mode of onset' refers to the time for all symptoms to FULLY develop in terms of either their intensity and/or their distribution.

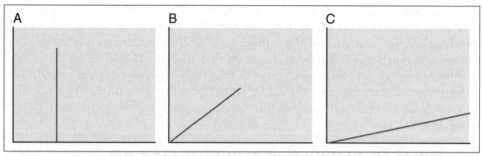

FIGURE 2.1 The three 'modes of onset' of an illness: **A** acute, seconds to minutes; **B** subacute, hours to days; **C** chronic, months to years

The pathological processes that reflect these modes of onset are:

A Instantaneous – seconds, rarely minutes
- Electrical: an epileptic seizure or an arrhythmia such as a tachyarrhythmia (fast heart beat), bradyarrhythmia (slow heart beat) or complete heart block (no impulse between the right atrium and ventricles, the Stokes–Adams attack)
- Vascular: subarachnoid haemorrhage, cerebral embolus
- Mechanical: trauma, a slipped intervertebral disc or positional vertigo

B Subacute – hours to days
- Infective: meningitis, encephalitis
- Inflammatory: multiple sclerosis, acute inflammatory neuropathies
- Metabolic disorders: hyponatraemia, diabetic coma

C Chronic – months to years
- Neoplastic: benign and occasionally malignant tumours
- Degenerative: cervical spondylitic myelopathy and the various genetic disorders
- Chronic endocrine problems: hypothyroidism, Cushing's disease, pituitary disorders
- Chronic inflammatory/infective processes: polymyositis, chronic inflammatory demyelinating peripheral neuropathies, cryptococcal or tuberculous meningitis

The majority of diseases that clinicians encounter fit into one of these three basic patterns, but it is important to remember that *they are only a guide* and there are always exceptions to the rule.

Exceptions to the rule include:
- Symptoms such as diplopia (double vision) and vertigo will, as a result of their very nature, always begin abruptly and need not necessarily indicate a pathological process with a vascular or mechanical basis (see the section 'The nature and distribution of symptoms').
- At time, neoplastic disorders can present with a very rapid evolution of symptoms as a result of a seizure and the rapid onset of a focal neurological deficit after the seizure; tumours can also appear to evolve more rapidly when there is a superimposed mechanical shift due to the mass effect.
- Vascular disorders can have a slower onset: for example, the stroke-in-evolution that may or may not be stepwise; the intracerebral haemorrhage that evolves over many minutes; the subdural that develops over hours to days (although here the bleeding results in a mass lesion); or the giant aneurysm that behaves as a tumour with symptoms due to the mass.
- In older patients with a chronic disease the deterioration is so slow that it is assumed that their increasing disability is simply related to old age until there is a sudden crisis, such as a fall where they are unable to get up. Patients present under these circumstances with an apparent illness of sudden onset, where

in reality it is simply the 'straw that broke the camel's back' phenomenon. The true nature is only clarified when a careful and detailed history of slowly evolving disability is obtained.

THE NATURE AND DISTRIBUTION OF SYMPTOMS

Neurologists use the nature of the symptoms and their distribution over the body to determine which part of the nervous system is involved in the disease process. In doing this it is important to remember that many patients use terms differently from the medical profession and, therefore, it is important to clarify what the patient means.

There are two circumstances where it is not possible to establish the exact time of onset of the initial symptom(s):

- Firstly, if the symptoms are present on awakening, even if the patient awoke at an unusual hour, unless you can determine that the symptoms awoke the patient (and this is very unlikely). The best estimate for the onset is the time between falling asleep and awakening.

- Secondly, if the symptoms are only noticeable when there is an external stimulus (e.g., the patient becomes aware of numbness only when they touch their face).

In this situation it *is imperative to elicit whether the symptoms have progressed since first noticed.* Progression can either be more intense symptoms or spread of the symptoms to other parts of the body.

Symptom clarification

Symptom clarification involves having the patient qualify exactly what they mean when they describe their symptoms. The term *collapse* in the toilet can be anything from a severe bout of diarrhoea to sudden death. The complaint of weakness or numbness does not necessarily imply a loss of strength or sensation, respectively. It is not unusual for patients with a facial nerve palsy (Bell's palsy) to describe their face as numb when in fact it is actually weak. The term *weakness* is used by some patients to describe a loss of function regardless of the cause, and actual weakness can be described as a feeling of heaviness, numbness or even a loss of feeling. When some patients say they have double vision what they mean is that their vision is blurred, not that they see two objects! Dizziness is another very vague term that means different things to different patients.

When clarifying the nature of symptoms, the following sample questions may be helpful:
- By weakness, do you mean an actual loss of strength?
- You said you had double vision – do you mean you actually saw two objects and, if you did, were they side-by-side or one above the other?
- When you say you are dizzy, what do you mean? Do you have a feeling of light-headedness or is it a sensation that the room or your head is spinning?
- When you say your speech is slurred, do you mean it sounds as if you are intoxicated (this would be the description of dysarthria) or do you mean that either you have difficulty finding the words that you want to say or, even though you can think of what you want to say, you are unable to actually say those words (this is the description of dysphasia)?

The nature of symptoms

Some symptoms can point to involvement of a specific part of the nervous system, others only indicate a particular pathway or system within the nervous system, while others are so non-specific that they have no value in localising the problem.

SYMPTOMS THAT LOCALISE TO A PARTICULAR PART OF THE NERVOUS SYSTEM

- Unilateral visual loss indicates that either the ipsilateral eye or optic nerve is affected.[2]
- Visual loss affecting both temporal fields (lateral vision): optic chiasm.[3]
- Hemianopia (loss of vision to one side): the optic radiation or occipital cortex.
- Vertical diplopia: brainstem, specifically the midbrain, 3rd or 4th cranial nerve (very rarely due to local muscle; superior and inferior recti or superior and inferior oblique muscle problems in the orbit).
- Horizontal diplopia: brainstem, specifically the pons, 6th cranial nerve or median longitudinal fasciculus (very rarely due to local muscle; medial or lateral rectus problems within the orbit).
- The 'pill-rolling' tremor at rest of Parkinson's: basal ganglia – specifically the subthalamic nucleus.
- Variability of weakness with exercise suggests the neuromuscular junction and myasthenia gravis or Lambert–Eaton syndrome.[4] Increased weakness with exercise indicates possible myasthenia gravis, while increased strength (and increased reflexes if examined before and after exercise) with exercise the Lambert–Eaton syndrome.
- A loss of speech is referred to as aphasia, while impairment of speech is referred to as dysphasia affecting the production and/or comprehension of written or spoken language. This almost invariably indicates a dominant hemisphere problem, usually cortical. Very rarely, a subcortical or even a thalamic problem can cause dysphasia.

SYMPTOMS THAT ONLY POINT TO INVOLVEMENT OF A PARTICULAR PATHWAY

- Vertigo (room or head spinning): vestibular system, anywhere from the inner ear through the vestibular nerve to the brainstem and the central vestibular cortex in the temporal lobe
- Weakness: motor pathway between the cerebral cortex and the muscle
- Altered sensation: sensory pathways between the peripheral nerves and the cerebral cortex
  Note: Spontaneous symptoms such as tingling or paraesthesia imply a sensory problem but do not differentiate between the pathways of pain and temperature and those of vibration and proprioception. Symptoms, such as a limb that feels but does not look swollen, skin that is stretched tight or that feels as if there is a tight stocking or glove around the limb, and instability in the dark or when the eyes are closed, are characteristic of the problems affecting the proprioceptive pathways. An inability to feel the temperature or to experience pain clearly points to involvement of the spinothalamic pathways.
- Marked wasting or fasciculations (visible twitching) of muscles: the lower motor neuron from the anterior horn cells in the spinal cord through the anterior nerve roots, brachial or lumbrosacral plexus and peripheral nerves

---

[2] A note of caution: patients can confuse a visual loss to one side of their vision (a hemianopia) with a monocular or unilateral visual loss. For example, when the patient has visual symptoms on the right, they sometimes assume it is in the right eye. It may, however, be in the right visual field. It is important to clarify whether the patient could see all or only one half of an object; it would be helpful if they had covered each eye in assessing their vision, but most patients do not do this.

[3] Optic chiasm lesions are extremely rare and most patients are not aware of the bilateral visual disturbance.

[4] Fatigue- and exercise-induced worsening of symptoms is very common in many chronic neurological disorders and does not imply problems at the neuromuscular junction.

NON-SPECIFIC SYMPTOMS

- Dysarthria: has no localising value (other than it clearly indicates the problem is above the level of the foramen magnum). It can result from non-dominant hemisphere lesions, deep dominant hemisphere lesions, brainstem pathology and problems affecting the 9th, 10th and 12th nerves, the neuromuscular junction and even disorders of muscle. Neurologists can often differentiate between the different causes of dysarthria but this is difficult for non-neurologists.
- Anosmia: is the loss of the sense of smell; if it is of neurological origin it points to involvement of the olfactory pathway, but in most patients it does not relate to any disorder of the nervous system but is rather due to local nasal pathology.
- Exacerbation of symptoms from heat and exercise: transient worsening of symptoms with heat or exercise that is not relieved by immediate rest is very common with many neurological disorders. One of the most common conditions in which this is a feature is multiple sclerosis.
- Ataxia (or unsteadiness on the legs): is a very non-specific symptom. Although it suggests a cerebellar problem, it can also be present in patients with arthritis in the joints of the legs, weakness or a proprioceptive disturbance in the legs and in patients with vertigo that is vestibular and not cerebellar in origin. A useful question to ask is whether the instability relates to a feeling of instability in the head, indicating probable involvement of the vestibular system, hypotension or a cerebellar problem, or to a sense of unsteadiness in the legs in the absence of any altered sensation in the head, suggesting a problem of weakness or sensory disturbance in the legs.
- Pain: is most often related to non-neurological disorders. If it is of neurological origin, it is almost invariably an indication of involvement of the peripheral nervous system as central pain syndromes are exceedingly rare. Central pain syndromes develop after thalamic infarction in which there is pain in the distribution of the contralateral hemi-sensory loss.
- Urinary or bowel sphincter disturbance: sphincter disturbance is a prominent symptom of intrinsic spinal cord problems (as opposed to extrinsic cord compression in which sphincter disturbance develops late), sacral nerve root lesions or autonomic nervous system involvement. However, in females urinary incontinence is more often of gynaecological origin and not related to a neurological problem.
- Dysphagia: (or difficulty swallowing) can occur with brainstem (medulla) or hemisphere problems and is therefore in itself a poor localising symptom.

Weakness with sensory symptoms immediately indicates that the problem CANNOT be related to diseases of muscle, the neuromuscular junction or anterior horn cell within the spinal cord, as these sites result in pure motor syndromes.

The distribution of symptoms

As already discussed in Chapter 1, 'Clinically oriented neuroanatomy', ALWAYS think about the underlying neuroanatomy that the nature and distribution of symptoms represents. In most instances the history can assist in establishing whether the pathology is affecting the brain or spinal cord (in the central nervous system) or peripheral nervous system.

As you take the history, think of the nervous system as a map grid with the **meridians of longitude** and **parallels of latitude** that were discussed in Chapter 1, 'Clinically oriented neuroanatomy'. Although the neurological examination is far more important when it comes to accurate localisation, many patients present with transient neurological symptoms and there may not be any neurological signs. For example, establishing from the history that a patient has weakness affecting the entire left side of the body including the face clearly indicates that the problem must be in the central nervous system and on the contralateral side above the mid pons.

> By defining the meridians of longitude and the parallels of latitude that the symptoms (and subsequently the signs, if present) represent, it is possible to localise the site of the problem in the nervous system in most patients.

PATTERNS OF WEAKNESS

If the symptom is weakness, ask questions to define the exact pattern of weakness. If it is confined to one limb, ascertain if it is the whole limb or only part of the limb that is affected. If the whole limb is weak, this is more suggestive of a central nervous system problem. If only part of the limb is weak, then it is more likely (but not always) related to involvement of the peripheral nervous system (nerve root, an individual nerve, the brachial plexus in the arm or lumbosacral plexus in the leg). Establish what part of the limb is weak. Muscle wasting and/or fasciculations (involuntary twitching of parts of muscles) are both occasionally observed by patients and localise the problem to the lower motor or peripheral nervous system.

An example of how the pattern of weakness can help to localise the problem while taking a history is shown in Case 2.3.

The patterns of weakness that indicate involvement of a particular part of the nervous system include:

- Weakness confined to one limb: weakness affecting the entire arm or the entire leg, particularly when it begins suddenly, is most likely to be due to a central rather than a peripheral nervous system problem. The history is not particularly useful when there is a focal weakness in a limb. Focal weakness in a limb can be either of central or peripheral nervous system origin and a neurological examination is needed to sort out the various causes. On the other hand, establishing exactly what part of the limb is weak can narrow down the possibilities if the problem is in the PNS.
  - Weakness of the hand or forearm: C7, C8, T1 nerve root, median, ulnar or radial nerve (Case 2.4 illustrates weakness in the right arm accompanied by some sensory loss.)
  - Weakness of the upper arm or shoulder: C5–C6 nerve root, axillary, musculocutaneous or suprascapular nerve problems
  - Weakness of the upper leg: L2, L3, L4 nerve root or femoral nerve
  - Weakness the lower part of the leg: L5–S1 nerve root, sciatic, common peroneal or posterior tibial nerve problem.

CASE 2.3 A 55-year-old man presents with 'right-sided weakness'

If the weakness involves the whole leg, then it most likely reflects an upper motor neuron or central nervous system problem, above the level of L2 in the lumbar spinal cord. If the ipsilateral arm is affected, this places the pathology above the level of C5 in the cervical spinal cord and, if the ipsilateral face is also affected, the lesion is above the facial nerve nucleus in the contralateral mid pons of the brainstem. In the absence of any additional symptoms, this is as far up as we can localise the problem. On the other hand, if the patient has impaired speech in the form of dysphasia, this indicates involvement of the speech cortex. The right-sided weakness is the meridian of longitude indicating involvement of the motor pathway. The dysphasia is the parallel of latitude indicating involvement of the cortical structures that form the basis of speech.

- Hemiparesis: the abrupt onset of weakness of the arm and leg with or without facial involvement is almost certainly a central nervous (upper motor neuron) system problem. Most often it is related to a problem in the contralateral hemisphere, less likely the contralateral brainstem and very rarely in the ipsilateral spinal cord above the level of C5. Slowly evolving hemiparesis could be of central or peripheral nervous system origin.
- Paraparesis: weakness confined to both legs is most often related to a spinal cord problem or a lower motor neuron problem such as a peripheral neuropathy.
- Quadriparesis: four-limb weakness indicates a cervical spinal cord problem above the C5 level, less often a peripheral neuropathy or muscle disease.

Obviously, once a patient has symptoms affecting the cranial nerves, vision, speech, hearing, vertigo, memory or cognition, the problem CANNOT be confined to the spinal cord.

PATTERNS OF SENSORY SYMPTOMS

When a patient complains of numbness in a hand, all we can ascertain from this is that the problem must be somewhere between the peripheral nerve and the contralateral cerebral cortex. On the other hand, if we then ask the patient to clarify the exact area of numbness we can ascertain whether the numbness is in the distribution of a single nerve or nerve root or whether in fact it involves one of the sensory pathways, differentiating between sensory symptoms arising in the peripheral versus the central nervous system, respectively.

For example, a patient complains of numbness in the hand. If the numbness affects the medial 1½ fingers on both the palmar and dorsal aspects of the fingers and the medial aspect of the hand up to the wrist, this pattern of sensory loss is typical of an ulnar lesion (see Figures 1.14 and 1.15). A second example is the patient who

---

CASE 2.4 A young man with weakness in the right arm and focal sensory loss

A 20-year-old man has fallen asleep in a chair after a heavy night of drinking. He awakens the next morning and notices severe weakness in his right arm. He is unable to extend his wrist and fingers and his hand grip is very weak. He is not aware of any pain but there is a small area of sensory loss between his thumb and index finger. He is right-handed and his speech is normal.

- The patient has noticed his symptoms on waking and therefore the exact mode of onset cannot be determined except to say that they arose sometime between when he fell asleep and when he woke. The onset therefore could have been very sudden or it could have come on gradually over minutes or hours.
- The patient has a focal weakness in the right arm with an inability to extend the wrist and fingers. This occurs with a stroke, a radial nerve palsy or with a C7 radiculopathy. The weakness is usually mild with a C7 radiculopathy and usually there is associated pain. Severe weakness in the right hand in a right-handed person due to a central nervous system problem will almost invariably be associated with a severe speech disturbance and a wrist drop is unusual for a stroke. However it is the very focal sensory loss between the first and second fingers that enables the correct diagnosis of a radial nerve palsy. As shown in Figure 1.15, the area of skin between the first and second digits is supplied by the superficial radial nerve. C7 radiculopathy would produce sensory loss affecting the middle three digits of the hand.

CASE 2.5   A woman with numbness and tingling

A 25-year-old woman presents with a gradual onset of numbness and tingling commencing in the toes and spreading over 3 days to affect her body from the breasts down. She has also noticed difficulty urinating and has been constipated.

- The distribution of the sensory symptoms clearly indicates involvement of the sensory pathways because they affect both the legs and the trunk and cannot represent problems associated with individual nerves or nerve roots.

- Sensory symptoms do not occur on the entire trunk in problems affecting the peripheral nervous system, but sensory disturbance on either side of the midline can be seen in, for example, diabetic truncal neuropathy. This gives a band of sensory loss extending a few centimetres on either side of the midline rather than sensory loss affecting the whole of the trunk.

- The sensory symptoms extend up to the level of the breasts, which is consistent with a lesion at the level of T4 in the thoracic spinal cord. The disturbance of sphincter function also indicates that the problem is in the spinal cord. The mode of onset is gradual over several days and this suggests an inflammatory or infective process.

---

complains of numbness in the leg, which in itself cannot help localise the problem, whereas numbness confined to the lateral aspect of the thigh below the groin and above the knee is the area supplied by the lateral cutaneous nerve of the thigh (see Figure 1.20). Case 2.5 illustrates numbness originating from a central nervous system problem.

Sensory symptoms affecting the ipsilateral leg, arm and the face indicate a lesion above the contralateral 5th nerve nucleus in the brainstem.

Patients are often referred with suspected tarsal tunnel syndrome due to compression of the medial or lateral plantar nerves at the level of the medial malleolus when they have symptoms affecting the top as well as the sole of the foot, clearly indicating that the problem is beyond the distribution of the medial or lateral plantar nerves, which only supply the sole of the foot, and therefore the problem cannot be tarsal tunnel syndrome.

PAIN

In most instances pain is unrelated to a neurological problem. Pain in the region of a joint made worse by moving that joint reflects local joint pathology. Pain with localised tenderness is related to a process at the site of tenderness, e.g. acute gout in a joint.

When pain does reflect a neurological problem, defining the exact distribution of the pain can be very helpful in localising the problem. Pain radiating from the neck down the arm to the thumb indicates probable involvement of the C6 nerve root. This is often termed referred pain as the site of the pain is not at the site of the pathological process but is referred to another part of the body. Pain confined to one or more branches of the trigeminal nerve on the face indicates involvement of that nerve (although dental pain is also confined to the distribution of the trigeminal nerve as all the dentures are supplied by the nerve), whereas pain beyond the distribution of the trigeminal nerve clearly excludes trigeminal neuralgia (see Chapter 9, 'Headache and facial pain'). Case 2.6 illustrates how the distribution of pain and reduced sensation can aid in diagnosis.

CASE 2.6   An older man with severe pain radiating from his right buttock to the ankle

A 70-year-old man experiences the sudden onset, while bending over in the garden, of severe pain radiating from his right buttock down his right leg to the ankle. He retires to bed and, when he stands the following morning, he has difficulty walking because he cannot lift his right foot. When he touches his right leg he notices that there is reduced sensation affecting the top of his foot and the lateral aspect of his shin.

- The mode of onset of his pain is sudden and occurs while the patient is bending over, suggesting a mechanical problem. The weakness of dorsiflexion of the right foot is in keeping with either an L5 radiculopathy or a common peroneal nerve lesion. The presence of the pain is more in keeping with a radiculopathy and, of course, the pattern of sensory symptoms is clearly in the distribution of the L5 nerve root (see Figure 1.22).
- This is a classical presentation of sciatica. Exactly why the weakness and sensory disturbance develops some hours later when clearly the nerve root is compressed by the disc at the time of the original injury is unclear.

PAST HISTORY, FAMILY HISTORY AND SOCIAL HISTORY

At the beginning of this chapter it was stated that the family history, past history or social history should not be used to make a diagnosis unless there is absolutely no alternative. These aspects of the history support the diagnosis that is made from an analysis of the presenting symptoms as outlined above.

Another important point is that, although patients may state that there is a past or family history of a particular illness, the diagnosis may have been incorrect. This is another reason why the past and family history should not be used to make a diagnosis. It is very important to be certain that there is either proof of the diagnosis or symptoms that are consistent with that diagnosis. This is particularly so with a past or family history of an illness such as migraine, for which there is no test to confirm the diagnosis. In many instances on detailed questioning the prior headaches do not fulfil the criteria for migraine as defined by the International Headache Society [3]. Many relatives are told that the cause of death was a heart attack when patients suffer sudden death or succumb during sleep without any pathological confirmation of the diagnosis.

- Unfortunately, many erroneous diagnoses are sustained by simply accepting the patient's statement that they or a relative had a particular illness in the past.

- Beware of new symptoms or an alteration in the rate at which the illness is worsening in patients with chronic neurological disorders, as this often indicates the presence of a second disorder.

In many patients with chronic neurological diseases, there is a tendency for both the patient and the inexperienced practitioner to assume that all new symptoms relate to that chronic neurological illness. However, a diagnosis of Parkinson's disease does not exclude the patient from suffering a stroke, spinal cord compression or some other neurological problem. In a patient with a chronic slowly progressive neurological problem, *the vital clue that there may be an additional illness is a sudden change in the rate of progression of the disability*. An example of this seen by the author is a patient with slowly progressive difficulty walking over years related to Parkinson's disease who developed a rapid decline in function from walking to being bedridden within 6 months due to dermatomyositis. Another example is a patient with slowly progressive Parkinson's disease who develops rapidly worsening walking related to increasing leg weakness due to spinal cord compression.

THE PROCESS OF TAKING THE HISTORY

Most often patients come to the consultation with a preconceived idea about what they intend to say, some with many, many pages of notes. After the initial introductions, *it is very important to allow the patient time to describe the symptoms without interruption*, recording brief comments that you can explore later. If you interrupt the patient at this early stage a vital piece of information may be forgotten while another patient may feel 'cheated' and complain that the doctor did not listen to what they

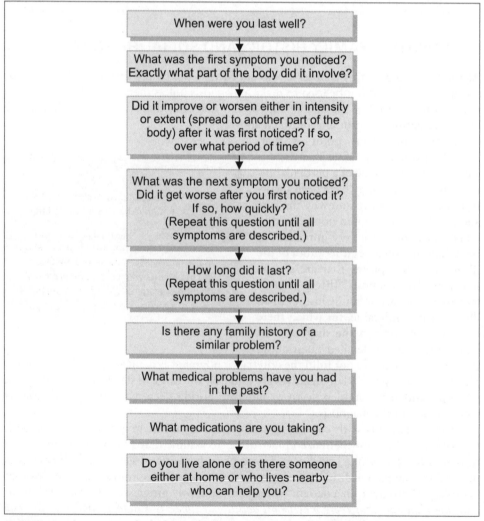

FIGURE 2.2   A suggested method of asking questions of patients who have a monophasic illness

had to say! This usually takes a few minutes. In many cases, one has a few clues after the patient's initial comments but often there is a lot of information that does not help in determining the nature of the problem. At some stage it is necessary to clarify (where possible):
- the mode of onset and progression of the symptoms
- the exact nature and distribution of the symptoms
- the past, family, social and medication history that may influence subsequent management.

This is best achieved by using the approach illustrated in Figure 2.2.

The DVD contains a lecture explaining the principles in this chapter and Lord John Walton, who at the time was Professor of Neurology at Newcastle upon Tyne (UK), taking a history from a patient. It should be noted that he asks repeated questions to establish exactly when the patient first noticed the symptoms. In this instance the patient only became aware of a problem when she sat on a cold surface, thus the time of onset of the initial symptoms cannot be established exactly. Further questioning elicits that the problem progressed after it was first noticed. In this manner he is identifying the possible pathological process(es) he needs to consider by establishing the fact that the problem is progressive over several days. He also clarifies with the patient the exact nature and distribution of symptoms, thus defining the site of the problem within the nervous system. He next asks about symptoms in the past history that would indicate any previous neurological illness or symptoms that may relate to the current illness. Unfortunately, this latter aspect does require prior knowledge and experience. Although he comments at the end that this is a pattern he recognises, it can be seen that his method of taking the history reflects the principles espoused in this chapter.

As stated earlier, it is not possible to learn how to take an effective history by reading a textbook. It is anticipated that students armed with the information in this chapter will find their time on the wards taking histories from patients with neurological disorders more rewarding and interesting.

REFERENCES

1 Spencer J. Learning and teaching in the clinical environment. BMJ 2003; 326(7389):591–594.
2 Sackett DL, Haynes RB, Tugwell P. Clinical diagnostic strategies. In: Sackett DL, Haynes RB, Tugwell P (eds). Clinical epidemiology: A basic science for clinical medicine. 1st edn. Boston: Little, Brown and Company; 1985:11.
3 International Headache Society. The international classification of headache disorders, 2nd edn. Cephalgia 2004; 24:24–37.

chapter 3

Neurological Examination of the Limbs

Learning how to perform a neurological examination requires repeated practice. Practice without an understanding of how to examine the various aspects of the nervous system and how to interpret the findings is akin to practising golf without having had lessons – useless. This chapter describes how to examine the limbs and interpret the findings. As it is very difficult to learn examination technique from a textbook, a video of the technique is included on the accompanying DVD.

Apart from a few pathognomonic signs that distinguish one disease from another, for example the tremor, rigidity and bradykinesia implicating Parkinson's disease with involvement of the substantia nigra or basal ganglia, in most instances the neurological examination *does not* establish the aetiology or cause of the problem. It simply localises the part of the nervous system affected by the pathological process.

The principal purpose of the examination is to determine whether the patient has **lower motor neuron (LMN)** signs or, more specifically, signs that indicate involvement of the peripheral nervous system (anterior horn cells, nerve roots, brachial or lumbosacral plexus, peripheral nerve, neuromuscular junction or muscle) or **upper motor neuron (UMN)** signs that indicate involvement of the central nervous system (brain, cerebellum and spinal cord). These were briefly discussed in Chapter 2, 'The neurological history', and, because they are absolutely crucial, they will be discussed in more detail in this chapter (see Table 3.1).

Although there are many ways to examine a patient, the following method is used by many neurologists and is the one recommended by this author.

THE MOTOR EXAMINATION

The examination of the motor system involves:
- inspecting for wasting and fasciculations in the muscles
- looking for changes in tone and reflexes
- testing strength
- checking the plantar responses.

The examination should start with inspection for wasting and fasciculations. This author then examines the tone, followed by strength, then the reflexes and the plantar responses. The exact order is not important.

Many examiners will perform a screening test of the upper limbs by observing patients elevating their arms and holding them horizontally straight out in front, initially with their eyes open and then subsequently closed (see Figure 3.1). The palms can be turned either down or up – it does not matter – although occasionally having

TABLE 3.1	The neurological findings in upper versus lower motor neuron lesions	
	Upper motor neuron lesion	**Lower motor neuron lesion**
Wasting	Usually no wasting but there may be mild wasting with long standing problems	No wasting in the very early stages but usually associated with significant wasting
Power	Weakness of extensor muscles in the arms* and flexor muscles in the legs**	The pattern of weakness reflects that part of the LMN that is affected
Tone	Increased +/– clonus	Decreased
Reflexes	Increased	Decreased or absent
Plantars	Up-going (extensor)	Down-going
Sensory findings	Sensory level	Focal sensory loss reflecting involvement of a nerve root, plexus or peripheral nerve

*Shoulder abduction, elbow extension, wrist and finger extension in the arms.
**Hip flexion, knee flexion and foot dorsiflexion in the legs. The tone may not be increased and the reflexes can be absent in acute spinal cord lesions referred to as spinal shock. Clonus is a series of involuntary repetitive movements of the ankle, up and down, induced by suddenly pushing the foot upwards while the leg is extended [1]. The test is less painful if it is performed with the knee slightly flexed.

- The pathology is always at the level of the LMN signs and at or above the uppermost limit of the UMN signs.

- In most instances the neurological examination *does not* establish the aetiology or cause of the problem. It simply localises the part of the nervous system that is affected by the pathological process.

- If the history has been obtained using the method described in Chapter 2, 'The neuro-logical history', the nature and distribution of the symptoms should provide an idea as to whether there will be upper or lower motor neuron signs.

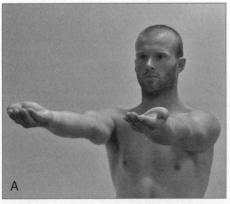
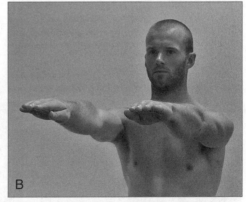

FIGURE 3.1 Screening test of the upper limbs with hands outstretched: **A** with palms up; **B** with palms down

the palms turned upwards seems a more sensitive technique.[1]

The arm(s) will:
- drift downwards if there is weakness
- drift upwards and often outwards if there is a proprioceptive or parietal lobe problem

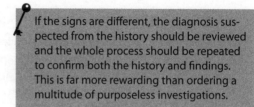

If the signs are different, the diagnosis suspected from the history should be reviewed and the whole process should be repeated to confirm both the history and findings. This is far more rewarding than ordering a multitude of purposeless investigations.

- oscillate up and down with a cerebellar disturbance if the patient is asked to elevate the limbs briskly, which can be missed if the movement is too slow.

Inspection for wasting and fasciculations

The muscles of the upper arm, forearm, hand, thigh, anterior tibial compartment and calves are examined for wasting and/or fasciculations. Fasciculations are visible spontaneous contractions or twitching of muscle fibres that are innervated by a single motor unit [1]. It may be necessary to spend several minutes carefully examining the muscles in order to detect fasciculations. It is easy to be certain that wasting is present when it is very severe, but with milder degrees of wasting one is less certain that there is a lesion involving the peripheral (LMN) nervous system. Some patients are very thin, and inexperienced clinicians may incorrectly suspect wasting when examining the small muscles of the hands, particularly in older patients. If the wasting affects one arm or one leg a comparison can be made with the contralateral limb. The muscles, if wasted, will initially lose their rounded appearance and appear flattened.

The reliable signs of muscle wasting are (Figure 3.2):
- loss of the visible bulge that occurs when the thumb is adducted towards the index finger – the first dorsal interosseous muscle
- prominence of the anterior border of the tibia – tibialis anterior muscle
- prominence of the spine of the scapula – supraspinatus and infraspinatus muscles
- scalloped appearance just above the patella as if a bite has been taken out of the muscle – quadriceps.

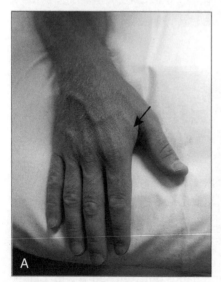
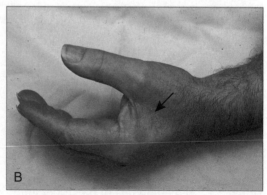

FIGURE 3.2 The first dorsal interosseous muscle: **A** no wasting; **B** wasting

1 Unproven personal observation.

Looking for changes in tone

There are two different ways to test for tone, depending on whether the problem is affecting the motor system or the extrapyramidal system (the latter is discussed in Chapter 13, 'Abnormal movements and difficulty walking due to central nervous system problems').

> Tone is tested using quick movements when the motor system is being assessed.

TESTING FOR INCREASED TONE RELATED TO AN UPPER MOTOR NEURON PROBLEM

It is important to first check with the patient whether a quick movement of the arm or leg would cause pain.

- Arms. Tone is tested with the forearm semi-pronated and the elbow flexed at 90° (refer to Figure 3.3A). The examiner holds the elbow with one hand and then places the other hand in the hand of the patient as if they were shaking hands. The test is performed with a quick supination of the forearm. If there is increased tone there will be a discernible catch. Very occasionally, when the tone is markedly increased, repetitive contractions may occur, and this is referred to as **clonus**.
- Legs. Tone is tested with the leg lying flat on the bed and slightly externally rotated and with the knee flexed very slightly. The examiner places their hands behind the leg just above the knee and attempts to quickly elevate the leg. If there is increased tone, the heel will lift up off the bed. The leg may lift off the bed in patients who are very anxious and who find it difficult to relax – slight external rotation of the leg prior to the quick movement helps in this situation and eliminates the false impression of increased tone in anxious patients. The other test for increased tone in the legs is ankle clonus, where the leg is slightly

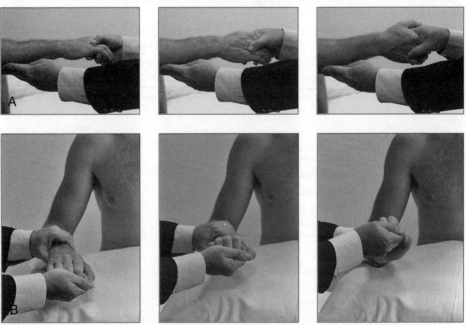

FIGURE 3.3 How to test tone in the upper limbs: **A** motor system; **B** extrapyramidal system

flexed at the knee with the ankle plantar-flexed. The examiner places their left hand behind the knee and grasps the foot with their right hand and forcibly dorsiflexes the foot. Repetitive contractions while the examiner holds the foot in dorsiflexion is a sign of increased tone, referred to as ankle clonus.

TESTING FOR INCREASED TONE RELATED TO AN EXTRAPYRAMIDAL PROBLEM

To test the upper limbs (Figure 3.3B), the forearm and hand are pronated and the examiner holds the middle of the forearm with one hand and holds the hand of the patient in a monkey grip. The patient's hand is compressed into the wrist as the wrist is slowly flexed and extended. This technique will elicit the classical cog-wheel rigidity seen with *extrapyramidal problems*.

To test the lower limbs, the leg is flexed at the knee and the examiner holds the leg behind the knee. Using the other hand the examiner grasps the foot and slowly dorsiflexes and plantar-flexes the ankle, looking for the cog-wheel rigidity. The two techniques for testing tone are demonstrated on the DVD.

Testing muscle strength

Use simple language that the patient can understand. The extent of muscle testing can be varied, depending on whether the history suggests an UMN problem or a LMN problem. In patients with involvement of the central nervous system or corticospinal tract, specific patterns of weakness occur and these are discussed below. In patients with focal weakness with or without focal sensory loss, suggesting a LMN problem, it is important to examine strength by commencing in that part of the limb that the patient describes as weak. The examiner then tests every single muscle of the affected limb to establish the pattern of weakness and, from this, the anatomical basis for the weakness and the site of the pathology within the peripheral nervous system can be determined.

The following technique is recommended when examining muscle strength. The muscle/muscle group, nerve related to that muscle/muscle group, the nerve root(s) and the action of the muscle [2] are listed in each section below. Experienced neurologists have memorised the neuroanatomy; inexperienced clinicians can record the pattern of weakness and consult a textbook of neuroanatomy, the illustrations in Chapter 1, 'Clinically oriented neuroanatomy', or this chapter.

UPPER LIMBS

Muscles around the shoulder

- **Muscle**　　　Supraspinatus
  Nerve supply　Suprascapular nerve
  Nerve root　　C5–6
  Action　　　 Initial abduction of shoulder to 30°

- **Muscle**　　　Deltoid
  Nerve supply　Axillary nerve
  Nerve root　　C5–6
  Action　　　 Abduction of shoulder beyond 30°

To test the supraspinatus (Figure 3.4) the elbow should be abducted from the side of the body to approximately 30°, the examiner places a hand over the elbow and pushes the elbow towards the trunk while the patient tries to resist.

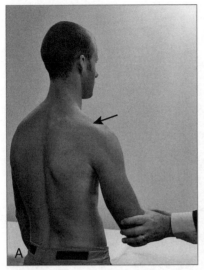

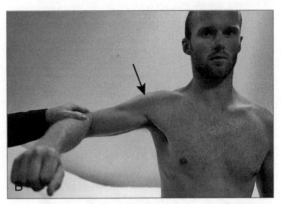

FIGURE 3.4 Testing of the **A** supraspinatus and **B** deltoid muscles (abduction of the shoulder)

To test the deltoid muscle (Figure 3.4) the elbow should be abducted from the side to 90°, the examiner places a hand over the upper arm just above the elbow and pushes downwards while the patient attempts to resist.

- **Muscle**   Infraspinatus
  Nerve supply   Suprascapular nerve
  Nerve root   C5–6
  Action   External rotation of the shoulder

The elbow is kept by the side, the forearm is flexed at 90° and the hand is semi-pronated (Figure 3.5). The examiner places a hand over the middle of the back of the forearm and attempts to internally rotate the forearm towards the body as the patient resists.

- **Muscle**   Subscapularis
  Nerve supply   Nerve to subscapularis
  Nerve root   C5–7
  Action   Internal rotation of the shoulder

The elbow is kept by the side, the forearm is flexed at 90° and the hand is semi-pronated (Figure 3.6). The examiner places a hand on the middle of the forearm and attempts to prevent internal rotation of the forearm.

- **Muscle**   Serratus anterior
  Nerve supply   Nerve to serratus anterior
  Nerve root   C5–7
  Action   Anchoring the scapular to the chest wall

There is a rare entity of winging of the scapular that is the result of damage to the nerve to the serratus anterior (see Chapter 11, 'Common neck, arm and upper back problems'). The patient is instructed to stand in front of a wall, with the elbows slightly flexed and the palms on the wall (Figure 3.7). They are then instructed to push as hard as they can and the scapular should not lift off the chest wall. If it does the muscle is weak, resulting in 'winging of the scapula'.

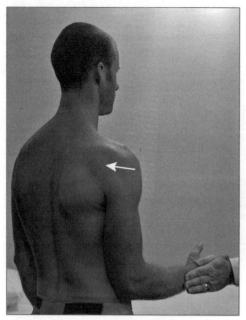

FIGURE 3.5 Testing of the infraspinatus (external rotation of the shoulder)

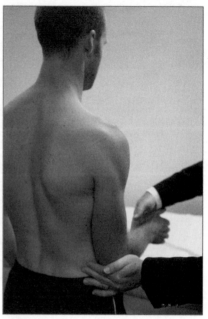

FIGURE 3.6   Testing of the subscapularis (internal rotation of the shoulder)

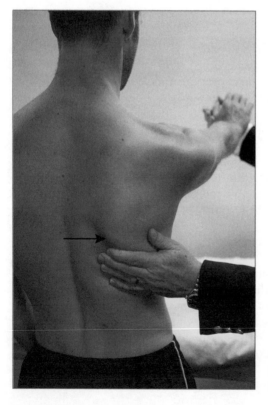

FIGURE 3.7   Testing of the serratus anterior

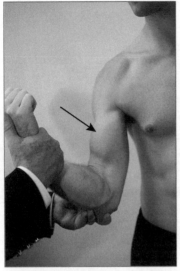

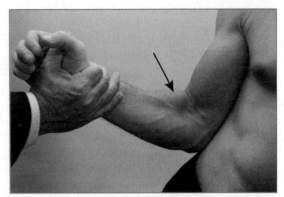

FIGURE 3.8 Testing elbow flexion with the forearm supinated

FIGURE 3.9 Testing elbow flexion with the forearm semi-pronated

Muscles around the elbow

- **Muscle**   Biceps and brachialis
  Nerve supply   Musculocutaneous nerve
  Nerve root   C5–6
  Action   Elbow flexion with arm supinated

The elbow is bent at 90° with the palm pointing towards the ceiling (Figure 3.8). The examiner grasps the elbow with the left hand and the wrist with the right hand and attempts to prevent further flexion of the elbow.

- **Muscle**   Brachioradialis
  Nerve supply   Radial nerve
  Nerve root   C6
  Action   Elbow flexion with forearm semi-pronated

The elbow is flexed at 90° with the forearm semi-pronated (Figure 3.9). The examiner places the left hand under the elbow and the right hand on the wrist and attempts to prevent further flexion of the elbow.

- **Muscle**   Triceps
  Nerve supply   Radial nerve
  Nerve root   C5–7
  Action   Elbow extension

It is very important that the elbow is only slightly flexed (as little as 20–30° from the fully extended position) when testing extension (Figure 3.10). If the elbow is fully flexed, this will result in an apparent weakness of the triceps when it is strong and, if it is fully extended, subtle degrees of weakness may be missed. The examiner places the left hand over the anterior aspect of the elbow and the right hand over the dorsal aspect of the wrist and attempts to prevent the patient from straightening their elbow.

- **Muscle**   Supinator
  Nerve supply   Posterior interosseous nerve
  Nerve root   C7–8
  Action   Supination of the forearm at the elbow

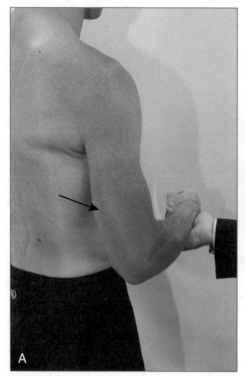
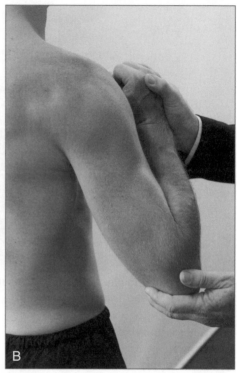

FIGURE 3.10 Testing of the triceps (elbow extension): **A** correct method; **B** incorrect method

The arm is fully extended with the palm pointing downwards. The examiner stabilises the arm with the left hand over the upper arm and then holds the patient's hand with their right hand. The patient is then asked to turn the palm upwards towards the ceiling, and the examiner turns the hand in the opposite direction.

Muscles in the forearm
- **Muscles**   Extensor digitorum longus, extensor pollicis longus, extensor carpi radialis, extensor carpi ulnaris
  Nerve supply   Posterior interosseous branch of the radial nerve
  Nerve root   C7
  Action   Finger and wrist extension

The patient is instructed to extend their wrist and the examiner places the back of their hand on the back of the patient's hand and attempts to flex the wrist while the patient resists (Figure 3.11). Similarly, the patient is asked to extend their fingers and the examiner places the back of their fingers across the patient's fingers. The 5th digit of the examiner's hand lies over the patient's metacarpophalangeal joints while the second digit of the patient's hand is beneath the metacarpophalangeal joints of the examiner.

- **Muscle**   Interossei and lumbricals
  Nerve supply   Ulnar nerve
  Nerve root   C8–T1
  Action   Finger abduction

The patient is instructed to spread the fingers apart and the examiner attempts to push them together by pressing on the base of the fingers close to the metacarpophalangeal

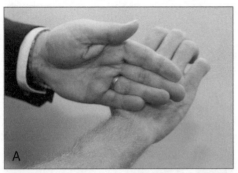 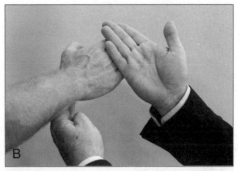

FIGURE 3.11 Testing wrist (**A**) and finger (**B**) extension (the extensor digitorum longus, extensor pollicis longus, extensor carpi radialis and extensor carpi ulnaris)

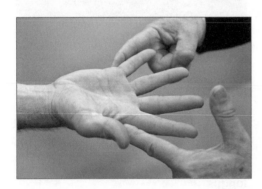

FIGURE 3.12 Testing finger abduction (interossei and lumbricals)

joints (Figure 3.12). Using this technique the patient should be able to resist very firm pressure whereas, if the examiner pushes against the tips of the fingers, even patients with normal strength cannot resist.

- **Muscle**   Abductor pollicis brevis
  Nerve supply   Median nerve
  Nerve root   C7–8
  Action   Abduction of the thumb

The patient's palm is supinated and the patient is instructed to point the thumb up towards the ceiling (Figure 3.13) while the examiner pushes down on either the base or the proximal phalanx of the thumb.

- **Muscle**   Flexor pollicis longus
  Nerve supply   Median nerve
  Nerve root   C8–T1
  Action   Flexion of the distal phalanx of the thumb

The patient is instructed to bend the tip of the thumb while the examiner uses the tip of their thumb to try and straighten the patient's thumb (Figure 3.14). Normal patients should be able to resist very firm pressure.

- **Muscle**   Flexor digitorum profundus
  Nerve supply   Median nerve
  Nerve root   C8–T1
  Action   Flexion of distal interphalangeal joints of the 2nd and 3rd digits

The examiner places the left hand over the palm and palmar surfaces of the patient's 2nd and 3rd fingers to prevent flexion at the metacarpophalangeal and proximal

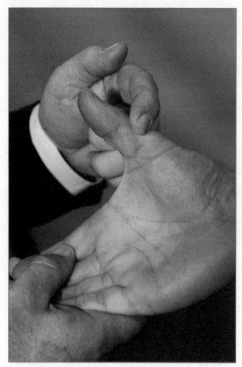

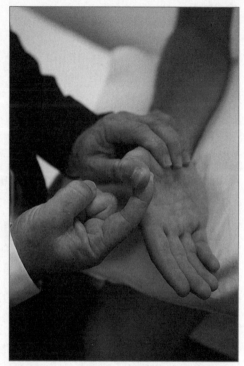

FIGURE 3.13 Testing of abduction of the thumb (abductor pollicis brevis)

FIGURE 3.14 Testing of the flexor pollicis longus

interphalangeal joints (Figure 3.15). The patient is instructed to bend the tips of the 2nd and 3rd digits while the examiner tries to straighten them using the tips of the 2nd and 3rd digits of the right hand. Normal patients can resist very firm pressure.

- **Muscle**   Flexor digitorum profundus
  Nerve supply   Ulnar nerve
  Nerve root   C8–T1
  Action   Flexion of distal interphalangeal joints the 3rd and 4th digits

The examiner places the left hand over the palm and palmar surfaces of the patient's 4th and 5th fingers to prevent flexion at the metacarpophalangeal and proximal interphalangeal joints (Figure 3.16). The patient is instructed to bend the tips of the 4th and 5th digits while the examiner tries to straighten them using the tips of the 2nd and 3rd digits of the right hand. Normal patients can resist very firm pressure.

Table 3.2 summarises the muscles/muscle groups, nerves and nerve roots of the upper limbs.

LOWER LIMBS

Muscles around the hip and knee
- **Muscle**   Iliopsoas and quadriceps
  Nerve supply   Iliopsoas and femoral nerve
  Nerve root   L2–4
  Action   Hip flexion and knee extension

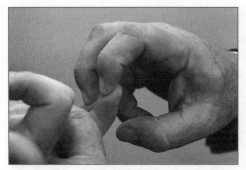

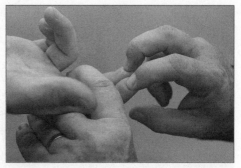

FIGURE 3.15 Testing flexion of the 2nd and 3rd digits

FIGURE 3.16 Testing flexion of the 4th and 5th digits

TABLE 3.2 Muscles, muscle groups, nerve supply and nerve root innervation in the upper limbs

Muscle/muscle group	Nerve	Nerve root
Supraspinatus	Suprascapular	C4–6
Infraspinatus	Suprascapular	C5–6
Subscapularis	Nerve to subscapularis	C 5–7
Deltoid	Axillary	C5–6
Serratus anterior	Nerve to serratus anterior	C5–7
Biceps	Musculocutaneous	C5–6
Triceps	Radial	C6–8
Brachioradialis	Radial	C5–7
Extensor carpi radialis	Radial	C6–7
Extensor carpi ulnaris	Posterior interosseous	C7–8
Extensor digitorum	Posterior interosseous	C7–8
Extensor pollicus longus	Posterior interosseous	C7–8
Abductor pollicus brevis	Median	C8–T1
Abductor digiti minimi	Ulnar	C8–T1
Flexor digitorum profundus	Median (2nd and 3rd digits) Ulnar (4th and 5th digits)	C8–T1

Note: The nerve roots reflect the main nerve root supply to that muscle. Not all muscles are listed. More detailed information is available in textbooks [2], [3]. The method of testing these individual muscles is discussed in the text and demonstrated on the DVD.

The patient is instructed to lift their leg straight up off the bed to approximately 30–40° and keep it elevated (Figure 3.17). The examiner then places their hand over the thigh just above the knee and pushes down as hard as they can while instructing the patient to resist. Patients of all ages, except perhaps the very elderly and frail, can prevent the examiner from pushing the leg downwards.

- **Muscle** Quadriceps
  Nerve supply Femoral nerve
  Nerve root L2–4
  Action Knee extension

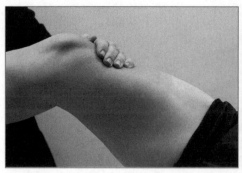
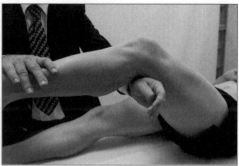

FIGURE 3.17 Testing of hip flexion   **FIGURE 3.18** Testing of knee extension

The patient's leg is elevated with the knee is slightly bent (Figure 3.18). The examiner places the left arm behind the knee and the right hand on the shin, and the patient is instructed to straighten the leg and not allow it to be bent.

- **Muscle**   Gluteus maximus
  Nerve supply   Inferior Gluteal nerve
  Nerve root   L5–S1
  Action   Hip extension

The patient is instructed to keep the leg and the heel on the surface of the bed (Figure 3.19). The examiner places a hand under the leg, just below the calf, and attempts to lift the leg up off the bed instructing the patient to keep the heel on the bed to prevent the leg from being elevated.

Testing of hip abduction is not particularly useful because it tests more than one muscle and one nerve and multiple nerve roots at the same time. It is never affected in isolation. On the other hand, hip adduction can be weak with damage to the obturator nerve (L2–4), for example, occurring during obstetric procedures.

- **Muscle**   Biceps femoris, semimembranosus, semitendinosus
  Nerve supply   Sciatic nerve
  Nerve root   L5–S1
  Action   Knee flexion

The patient is instructed to bend the knee to approximately 90° with the heel just off the bed (Figure 3.20). The examiner places the left hand on the kneecap and the right hand just below the calf. The patient is instructed to bend the knee and not allow it to be straightened.

Muscles around the ankle

- **Muscle**   Tibialis anterior, extensor hallucis longus
  Nerve supply   Deep branch of the common peroneal nerve
  Nerve root   L5–S1
  Action   Dorsiflexion of the foot

The patient is instructed to bring the foot up towards the nose (Figure 3.21B). The examiner places a hand over the dorsal aspect of the foot and pushes downwards while the patient attempts to prevent the foot from being pushed downwards. Subtle degrees of weakness may be missed using this test. A more sensitive technique is for the patient to have the ankle in a neutral position, neither plantar flexed or dorsiflexed (Figure 3.21A). The examiner places a hand over the dorsal aspect of the foot and asks the patient to lift the foot up towards the nose while the examiner pushes down firmly on the foot. An even more sensitive technique is to have the patient bend the big toe up

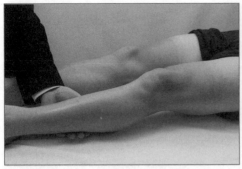
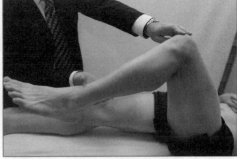

FIGURE 3.19 Testing of hip extension

FIGURE 3.20 Testing of flexion of the knee

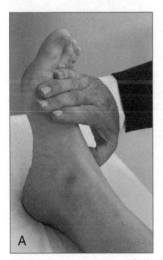
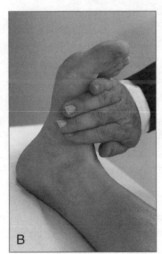
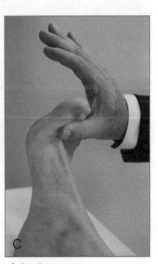

A

B

C

FIGURE 3.21 Testing of dorsiflexion of the foot: **A** and **B**; **C** of the big toe

towards their nose while the examiner pushes on the toe at the level of the metatarso-phalangeal joint (Figure 3.21C). Remember, however, as the sensitivity of testing is increased the specificity decreases, and a mild degree of weakness may be interpreted as abnormal when in fact it is a normal finding for a patient of that age.

- **Muscle** Medial and lateral gastrocnemii, soleus
  Nerve supply Posterior tibial nerve
  Nerve root L5–S1
  Action Plantar flexion of the foot

The examiner places the palm of the hand over the ball of the foot and the patient is instructed to push down as hard as they can while the examiner attempts to push the foot upwards (Figure 3.22).

- **Muscle** Tibialis anterior and tibialis posterior
  Nerve supply Deep branch common peroneal and posterior tibial nerve
  Nerve root L5
  Action Inversion of the ankle

The examiner places the palm of a hand on the medial aspect of the foot and instructs the patient to turn the foot inwards and not to allow it to be turned outwards while the examiner attempts to turn the foot out laterally and observes the tibialis anterior and

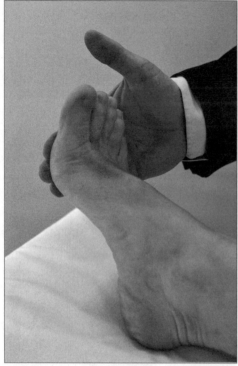 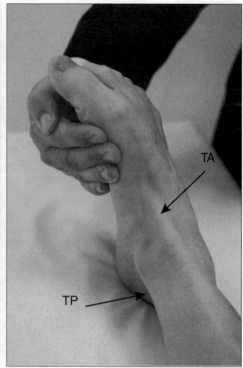

FIGURE 3.22 Testing of plantar flexion of the foot

FIGURE 3.23 Testing of inversion of the ankle

tibialis posterior tendons in front and behind the medial malleolus, respectively. These tendons can be palpated if they are not visible (Figure 3.23).

- **Muscle**   Peroneus longus and brevis
  Nerve supply   Deep branch of the common peroneal nerve
  Nerve root   L5
  Action   Eversion of the ankle

The examiner places the palm of a hand on the lateral aspect of the foot and instructs the patient to turn the foot outwards and not to allow it to be turned inwards while the examiner attempts to push the foot in medially (Figure 3.24).

It is very important to test inversion and eversion of the ankle in a patient who has a foot drop, and this is discussed further in Chapter 11, 'Common neck, arm and upper back problems'. In essence, testing these two muscles helps to differentiate between a deep branch common peroneal nerve lesion, a peripheral neuropathy and an L5 radiculopathy.

Table 3.3 summarises the muscles/muscle groups, nerves and nerve roots of the lower limbs.

Looking for changes in reflexes

Testing the reflexes should be easy, but in reality there are many factors that can influence the reflexes:

- If the patient is anxious the reflexes can give the appearance of being abnormally brisk.
- Reduced or absent ankle reflexes are almost the norm in the elderly patient.

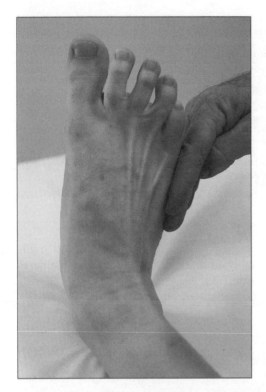

FIGURE 3.24 Testing of eversion of the ankle

TABLE 3.3 Muscle groups, nerve supply and nerve root innervation in the lower limbs

Muscle group	Nerve	Nerve root
Hip flexion	Femoral	L2–4
Hip extension	Superior and inferior gluteal	L5–S1
Knee extension	Femoral	L2–4
Knee flexion	Sciatic	L5–S1
Dorsiflexion of foot	Deep branch of common peroneal	L4–5, S1
Plantar flexion	Posterior tibial	L5–S1
Eversion of foot	Superficial peroneal	L5–S1
Inversion of foot	Posterior tibial and deep branch of common peroneal	L4–5

Note: The nerve roots reflect the main nerve root supply to that muscle. Not all muscles are listed. More detailed information is available in textbooks [2], [3]. The method of testing these individual muscles is discussed in the text above.

- Sometimes in teenagers it can be difficult to elicit the upper limb reflexes.
- If the limb is not in the correct position and the joint is not relaxed, this can give the impression of reduced reflexes.

As with all aspects of the neurological examination, one needs to interpret the findings in the context of the history and other neurological signs.

TABLE 3.4 The limb reflexes and the nerve root supply

Reflex	Nerve root supply
Biceps	C5(6)
Brachioradialis	C(5)6
Triceps	C(5,6)7
Knee jerk	L2,3,4
Ankle reflex	S1

Note: A simple way to remember is to count 1 at the ankle, 2, 3, 4 at the knee, 5 at the biceps, 6 at the brachioradialis and 7 at the triceps.

The upper limb reflexes are best tested with the patient sitting, if possible, with a pillow on their lap and the arms resting comfortably on that pillow. The lower limb reflexes are best tested with the patient lying flat (Figure 3.25).

Table 3.4 summarises the limb reflexes and nerve root supply.

THE SENSORY EXAMINATION

The primary sensory modalities tested in the clinical setting include:
- vibration
- proprioception
- pain
- temperature
- light touch.

Sensory testing can be difficult and at times confusing because inconsistent results may be obtained. Some simple techniques that can help reduce this problem are described below and demonstrated on the DVD.

It is probably irrelevant whether sensory testing commences with vibration, proprioception, pain or temperature. Vibration and proprioception can be tested quickly whereas pain and temperature sensation are more difficult to examine.

Anticipating what sensory abnormalities will be found based on the *nature and distribution of symptoms* described in the history influences the method of examination, in particular where to start looking for the sensory signs. If the patient complains of altered sensation in a particular part of the body, it is appropriate and sensible to begin to examine sensation in that region. If there were no sensory symptoms in the history, the most appropriate technique for testing sensation will depend on whether the history and motor examination suggest a central nervous system or a peripheral nervous system problem.

Vibration and proprioception

A 128-Hz tuning fork is used to test vibration sense. The tuning fork should be vibrating strongly and placed over the patient's big toe or index finger (Figure 3.26). The intensity of the vibration is gradually reduced by running the examiner's fingers slowly up the tuning fork until it stops vibrating or until the patient states they can no longer feel any vibration. This gradual reduction in the intensity of vibration increases the sensitivity of the testing, but it is important to remember that elderly patients often have

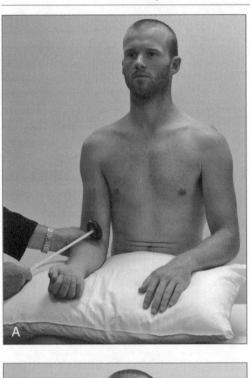
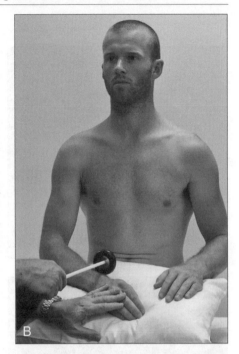
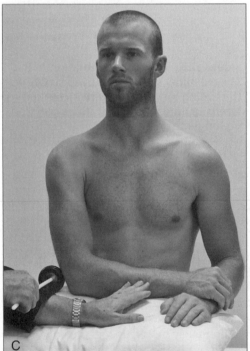
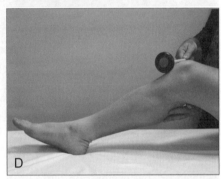
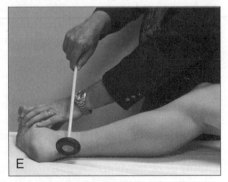

FIGURE 3.25 How to test the reflexes in the upper and lower limbs. **A** Biceps: The thumb or fingers of one hand are placed over the biceps tendon and the examiner's own fingers are struck with the tendon hammer. **B** Brachioradialis: The brachioradialis tendon can be struck directly or else the examiner can place a finger or two over the tendon and strike **C** Triceps: This is best tested with the patient's arm folded across their body and the triceps tendon struck directly. **D** Knee reflex: The knee should be at approximately 45° and the patella tendon struck directly. **E** Ankle reflex: Externally rotate the leg and have the ankle slightly plantar flexed and strike the Achilles tendon directly.

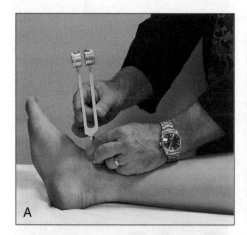

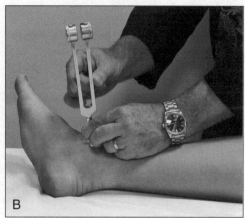

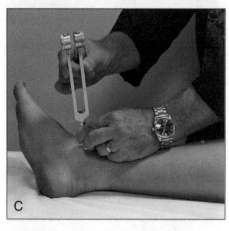

FIGURE 3.26 How to test vibration **A, B, C**: The examiner's finger is moved slowly up the tuning fork, gradually reducing the intensity until the patient states they can no longer feel vibration.

reduced or absent vibration sense in the feet and ankles. In younger patients vibration can be detected in the toes almost to the point where the tuning fork stops vibrating. In the hands, patients of all ages can appreciate vibration over the dorsal aspect of the distal phalanx of the finger, although once again older patients may have a very slight reduction in vibration sense.

Proprioception is tested by moving the index finger or big toe up or down while holding the digit on its side, initially showing the patient which way is up and which way is down and then asking the patient to close the eyes and say which way the toe or finger is being moved (Figure 3.27). It is recommended that the digit be moved two or three times in the same direction because some patients guess, and guesses may coincide with the direction of movement if the digit is alternately moved up and then down. The amplitude of movement will again depend on the age of the patient, with older patients normally losing appreciation of small degrees of movement. Very slight movement in the range of 1 or 2 mm can be detected in the index finger although the range may be slightly greater for older patients. The range of movement that can be detected in the big toe is 3 or 4 mm.

If the impairment of proprioception is very severe (and this is rare), there may be impairment at the ankle and wrist or even the knee and elbow. This assessment of the severity of proprioceptive and vibration loss adds nothing to localising the pathology.

Once there is impairment of these modalities in a limb, one is dealing with either a peripheral neuropathy (abnormalities in these modalities rarely occur with single nerve or nerve root lesions) or a central nervous system problem on the ipsilateral side of the spinal cord or the contralateral side of the brain.

As the sensitivity of testing is increased (by moving the digit only very tiny amounts), the specificity is decreased. In these circumstances, the patient may appear to have a sensory impairment when in fact it is a normal finding in a patient of that age.

Although proprioception can be tested on the face by pulling the cheek or earlobe up or down while the patient's eyes are closed, this is rarely done.

Abnormalities of vibration and proprioception virtually never occur proximally in a limb if they are not present distally.

Pain, temperature and light touch
The pain, temperature and light touch sensations are particularly useful for mapping areas of sensory loss.
- *Temperature sensation* is tested using a cold object such as the tuning fork. Patients with cold feet may not be able to appreciate that the object is cold, and this can produce an 'apparent alteration' of temperature sensation confined to the feet up to

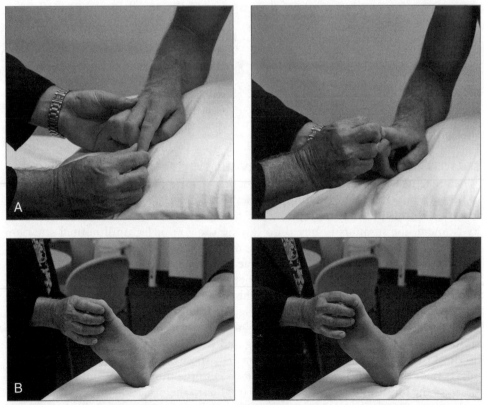

FIGURE 3.27 How to test proprioception in the hand (**A**) and foot (**B**) (Here the examiner has grasped the top and bottom of the big toe rather than grasping the sides of the toe, as is traditionally taught.)

where the limb becomes warm when in fact sensation is normal. The feet should be felt first to see if they are cold or warm. If the feet are very cold, temperature sensation should be tested using a warm object. Pain sensation will be normal in this area of 'apparently altered' temperature sensation.

- *Pain sensation* is tested using a sharp object. Hypodermic needles are too sharp, often cause bleeding and should not be used. Pain sensation is probably the most difficult modality to test. It is subjective and very dependent on how hard the sharp object is pressed into the skin. Repeated rapid stimuli (2–3) in the one spot, initially with a blunt object such as the tip of the finger and then with a sharp object, help to reduce this variability. This technique is demonstrated on the accompanying DVD.

- Testing *light touch* does not help differentiate whether the pathology is affecting a particular pathway, as both the spinothalamic tract and the pathways carrying vibration and proprioception transmit light touch sensation. Testing light touch can be very helpful when the other sensory signs are confusing. A useful technique is to gently stroke with the fingers of one hand the skin in an area of normal sensation on the same limb while using the fingers of the other hand to stroke the skin in the area of suspected abnormal sensation, moving slowly from the area of abnormal sensation until the patient says the feeling is the same. It may be necessary to do this repeatedly to confirm the findings.

If when testing pain, temperature or light touch an altered sensation is confirmed, the examination continues to test that same modality in all four directions away from the original area of abnormal sensation until the full extent of sensory loss is established. The pattern of sensory loss is then compared with the figures in Chapter 1, 'Clinically oriented neuroanatomy', to determine what part of the nervous system is affected.

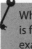 When an area of abnormal sensation is found, it is imperative to extend the examination in all four directions from where the initial sensory loss is detected until the exact extent of the sensory loss is determined.

SENSORY LOSS DUE TO A CENTRAL NERVOUS SYSTEM LESION

When the history suggests that the problem may involve the central nervous system or spinothalamic tract, the most appropriate way to test pain, temperature and light touch sensation is to commence testing over the tips of the fingers or toes. If an abnormality is found, the stimulus is moved quickly up the arm or leg until normal sensation is found. The anterior and posterior aspect of the limb should be tested, ensuring that testing crosses the skin supplied by multiple individual nerves and multiple individual nerve roots. The sensory loss should be higher up on the back than on the front of the trunk because the area of skin supplied by the thoracic nerve roots is higher on the back than on the chest or abdomen (see Figures 1.11 and 1.12). A horizontal band of sensory abnormality around the trunk is indicative of a non-organic problem. If the sensory loss extends all the way up the leg and trunk, sensation is then tested on the inside of the upper arm (T2), down the medial aspect of the forearm (C8), across the fingers from the little finger (C8), 3rd digit (C7) to the thumb (C6) and up the lateral aspect of the forearm (C6) and upper arm (C5) onto the neck (C2–4) and if necessary to the face (trigeminal nerve) and the occipital region of the head (C2–3).

Lesions in different parts of the central nervous system will produce different patterns of loss of pain, temperature and touch sensations.

- Lesions involving the spinothalamic tract of the central nervous
system will produce abnormal
pain and/or temperature sensation
affecting:
  - the whole of the contralateral
  leg if the lesion is in or above
  the thoracic spinal cord
  - the contralateral arm and leg
  if the lesion is in or above the
  upper cervical spinal cord or brain stem below the level of the pons where the
  5th nerve nucleus is situated.

> If there is no abnormality in the fingers
> and toes in patients with UMN signs (i.e.
> a central nervous system problem) then,
> apart from the very rare suspended sensory
> loss seen with central cervical spinal cord
> problems (see below), there will not be
> abnormal sensation more proximally in the
> limb.

- If the pathology is above the 5th nerve nucleus there will be abnormal pain and
temperature sensation affecting the contralateral face, arm and leg.
- If the pathology is at the level of the pons or medulla in the brain stem, this can
result in ipsilateral impairment of pain and temperature sensation on the face with
contralateral impairment in the arm and leg.
- Alterations of pain and temperature affecting the whole of one side of the body
indicate that the lesion is above the pons but cannot determine the exact site of the
pathology, and it is the associated symptoms and signs that will localise the pathology more accurately.
- Syringomyelia (a cyst within the central region of the spinal cord) in the cervical spinal cord can result in a suspended sensory loss affecting the trunk and
upper limbs and, if the lesion extends into the lower brainstem, also involve the
trigeminal nerve causing sensory loss on the face commencing in front of the
ear and extending forward in an onion-skin pattern. This is because the syrinx
affects the nerve fibres conveying pain and temperature sensation in the centre
of the spinal cord, and these nerve fibres enter the spinal cord via the dorsal root
ganglion, cross the midline and push the nerve fibres from the lower part of the
body out laterally so that a syrinx in the centre of the cord will affect the spinothalamic tract fibres from the upper part of the body closest to the syrinx first
(see Figure 3.28).

SENSORY LOSS DUE TO A PERIPHERAL NERVOUS SYSTEM LESION

If a peripheral nervous system problem is suspected but there are no sensory symptoms,
sensory testing should commence in the area where weakness is found. If there are sensory abnormalities they will reflect whether the sensory nerve root, plexus or peripheral
nerve(s) are affected and the pattern will be different depending on what part of the
peripheral nervous system is involved. It is not uncommon for inexperienced examiners
to commence sensory testing part way up the foot or hand. If pain, temperature and a
light touch sensation are not tested on the very tips of the toes and fingers, subtle degrees
of peripheral sensory loss that can occur in patients with a peripheral neuropathy can
be missed.

EXAMINING CEREBELLAR FUNCTION

Test for coordination. The patient alternately touches their nose with their index
finger and then the examiner's finger held at arm's length from the patient. It is
important to ensure that the patient is not anchoring their upper arm against their

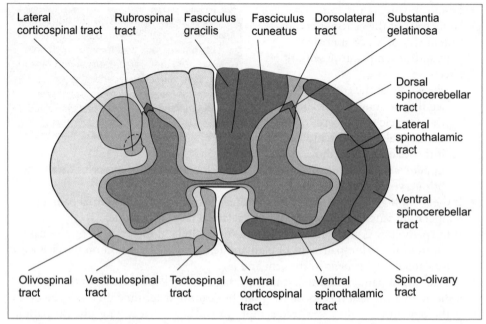

FIGURE 3.28 Cross-section of the spinal cord showing the pathways; the lateral spinothalamic tract conveys pain and temperature and the sacral nerve fibres are medial in the tract and the thoracic and cervical fibres are lateral

torso, as this can mask ataxia in the upper limb. To test the lower limbs the patient elevates their leg high up off the bed and then places the heel as accurately as possible on the opposite kneecap. This initial movement is the most important to observe, although many examiners will then test the heel sliding down the shin. This latter technique at times can obscure a subtle ataxia because the heel can be anchored against the shin. These two tests are referred to as finger-to-nose and heel-to-shin testing.

In patients with midline cerebellar disturbance, finger-to-nose and heel-to-shin testing may be normal as these largely reflect the cerebellar hemispheres. Heel-to-toe testing is performed where a patient is asked to walk in a straight line placing the heel of one foot in front of the toes of the other foot.

A third technique is rapidly alternating movements. The patient is asked to tap the back of the hand, alternating with the palm of the hand on the back of the opposite hand, repeatedly for 10 seconds. For the lower limbs rapid alternating movement is best tested by having the patient place their toes and the ball of their foot on the floor and tap their heel up and down rapidly.

Finally, patients with cerebellar disturbance may have nystagmus when the external ocular movements are tested. This is discussed in Chapter 4, 'The cranial nerves and understanding the brainstem'.

CLINICAL CASES

The following are cases illustrating how the pathways affected and the pattern of involvement can be used to localise the lesion.

Lesions within the central nervous system

CASE 3.1

The motor examination of the lower limbs reveals the patient has an UMN pattern of weakness in the leg(s), with weakness confined to hip flexion and dorsiflexion of the foot, increased tone and reflexes and extensor plantar responses, indicating involvement of the central nervous system and not the peripheral nervous system.

- On the basis of these motor findings it can be inferred that the lesion is above the level of L1 (first lumbar).
- If the weakness also involves the arm(s) with an UMN pattern of weakness affecting finger extension, finger abduction and shoulder abduction, with increased tone and reflexes, the lesion has to be above the level of C4 (4th cervical).
- The presence of an UMN facial palsy on the same side as the weakness in the arm and leg (partial weakness of the face, arm and leg on one side is referred to as a hemiparesis, total weakness is termed a hemiplegia), where the lower half of the face is weak but the forehead is not affected, indicates that the pathology is above the level of the mid pons (where the facial nerve nucleus is situated) on the contralateral side. Unless there are additional cortical signs (the meridians of latitude, see Chapter 5 for a detailed discussion), it is not possible to localise the site of the problem causing a hemiparesis or hemiplegia more accurately, other than to say that the lesion is above the mid pons.
- Similarly if there is UMN weakness confined to the leg(s), the pathology is above the level of L1 but could be either in the spinal cord, brainstem or cerebral hemispheres.

CASE 3.2

If there are UMN signs in the legs, the lesions must be above the level of L1 and, if there are lower motor signs in the arms (with wasting of muscles, absent reflexes and a pattern of weakness that fits individual myotomes), the lesion must be in the cervical region because *the pathology is always at the level of the LMN.* This assumes that the patient is suffering from a single disease entity and not multiple diseases.

CASE 3.3

If there is altered pain and temperature sensation in the entire left arm and leg, the lesion has to involve the contralateral spinothalamic pathway above the level of C4.

If the face and scalp on the same side as the limb involvement are affected, the pathology is above the contralateral nucleus of the 5th cranial nerve (which is predominantly in the pons).

In the absence of cortical signs it is not possible to localise the lesion more accurately within the central nervous system, other than to say that it is above the level of the pons in the brainstem.

CASE 3.4

If vibration and/or proprioception are abnormal in one leg, the lesion almost certainly involves the central rather than the peripheral nervous system. It must be either ipsilateral in the spinal cord or contralateral above the level of the foramen magnum where the dorsal column pathways cross the midline at the level of the gracile and cuneate nuclei.

If the abnormality of vibration and proprioception extends to the ipsilateral arm, the lesion is above C4, once again ipsilateral within the spinal cord or contralateral above the level of the foramen magnum.

It is difficult, although not impossible, to test proprioception in the head as one can use the earlobe or the skin of the cheek. However, such a technique has not been formally validated and should be used with extreme caution. Testing vibration in the head does not help in the examination of the 'dorsal column pathway'. It is therefore difficult to localise the abnormality causing this pattern of impairment of vibration and proprioception more accurately unless there are other abnormal neurological signs, for example the cortical sensory signs that are discussed in Chapter 5, 'The cerebral hemispheres and cerebellum'.

Lesions within the peripheral nervous system

CASE 3.5

The presence of distal and/or proximal weakness in both legs with reduced tone and absent reflexes indicates involvement of the peripheral nervous system, as the reduced tone and absent reflexes are LMN signs. This is the pattern of a peripheral neuropathy.

The presence of marked wasting and fasciculations also indicates that the lesion is in the peripheral nervous system, affecting the LMN and has been present for some time.

If there is sensory loss in patients with a peripheral neuropathy, it is usually in a 'glove and stocking' distribution with a circumferential loss of pain and/or temperature sensation with or without impairment of vibration and proprioception in the distal aspect of the limbs. The more severe the peripheral neuropathy the higher up the limbs the sensory abnormalities will be found.

CASE 3.6

Selective weakness of finger abduction and finger adduction without involvement of the APB muscle of the hand, plus weakness of flexion of the distal phalanges of the medial two but not the lateral two digits, is the typical pattern seen with an ulnar nerve lesion at the elbow, a common site for compression of the nerve. There is usually an associated sensory loss affecting both the palmar and dorsal surface of the medial 1½ digits and the medial aspect of the hand up to the wrist.

REFERENCES

1 Dorland's pocket medical dictionary, 21st edn. Philadelphia: WB Saunders Company; 1968.
2 Williams PL et al (eds). Gray's anatomy, 37th edn. London: Churchill Livingstone; 1989.
3 Rosenblum ML, Levy RM, Bredesen DE. AIDS and the nervous system. New York: Raven Press; 1988:410.

The Cranial Nerves and Understanding the Brainstem

THE 'RULE OF 4'

The first section of this chapter will describe the anatomy, the techniques for examining the individual cranial nerves and the more common abnormalities encountered. The second part will discuss the 'Rule of 4' to aid in localising the problem within the brainstem, in particular understanding brainstem vascular syndromes [1].

THE OLFACTORY NERVE

Anatomy
The receptors for smell are in the nasal passages. Afferent fibres pass into the skull through a multitude of small holes, called the cribriform plate, in the base of the skull situated beneath the frontal lobes in the anterior cranial fossa. The olfactory nerves thus formed pass backwards under the frontal lobes to the temporal lobes and olfactory cortex on the same side.

Method of testing
It is best to use items that are familiar to most people, such as perfume or coffee (coffee may be more suitable because some patients may have an allergy to perfume). With the eyes closed the patient is asked to recognise the odour in each nostril separately while the other is occluded.

This is not a particularly useful test because the most frequent cause of anosmia (loss of the sense of smell) is the common cold. Anosmia can also occur following severe head injuries when the olfactory nerves are torn at the floor of the anterior cranial fossa. The nerve can be compressed by a subfrontal meningioma and the loss may be unilateral. Rarely, permanent anosmia can develop without any obvious cause (idiopathic) or following an influenza-like illness.

THE OPTIC NERVE, CHIASM, RADIATION AND THE OCCIPITAL CORTEX

Anatomy
The visual pathways together, with the visual field abnormalities produced by lesions at certain sites along the pathway, are illustrated in Figure 4.1. Note that the lateral retina radiates back to the occiput on the same side via the optic nerve, chiasm and optic

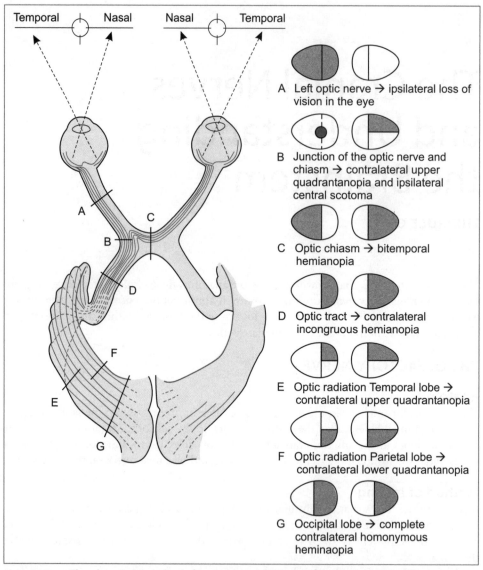

Temporal | Nasal   Nasal | Temporal

A Left optic nerve → ipsilateral loss of vision in the eye

B Junction of the optic nerve and chiasm → contralateral upper quadrantanopia and ipsilateral central scotoma

C Optic chiasm → bitemporal hemianopia

D Optic tract → contralateral incongruous hemianopia

E Optic radiation Temporal lobe → contralateral upper quadrantanopia

F Optic radiation Parietal lobe → contralateral lower quadrantanopia

G Occipital lobe → complete contralateral homonymous heminaopia

FIGURE 4.1 The drawing on the left represents the visual pathway; the drawings on the right are the visual abnormalities that occur at the relevant sites along the pathway

Reproduced from *Principles of Neurology*, 3rd edn, by RD Adams and M Victor, 1985, McGraw–Hill Book Company, Figure 12.2, p 1186 [2]

Note: Ipsilateral refers to the left and contralateral to the right.

radiation, while the fibres from the medial retina cross at the optic chiasm and radiate to the opposite occipital lobe. The left occipital lobe receives fibres from the left lateral retina and the right medial retina (i.e. the right visual field), while the opposite is the case for the right occipital lobe.

An optic nerve lesion will produce a visual field loss in one eye. The optic chiasm lies above the pituitary gland and beneath the hypothalamus and is subject to compression from pituitary and hypothalamic tumours. Lesions of the optic chiasm will produce

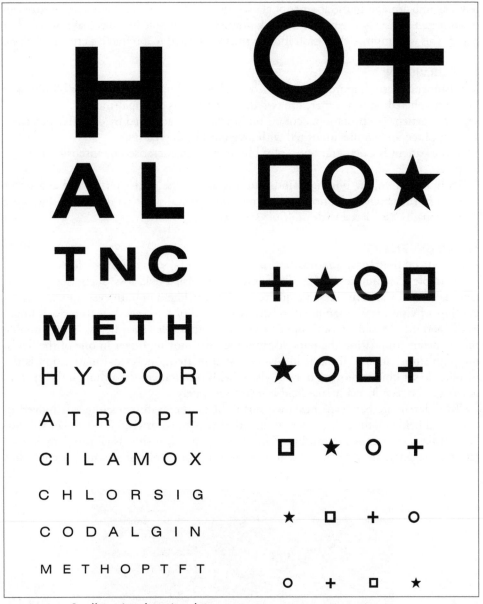

FIGURE 4.2   Snellen visual acuity chart

a bitemporal field loss. An optic radiation or occipital lobe problem will result in a contralateral visual field loss, either a hemianopia (loss of one-half of the visual field) or a quadrantanopia (loss of one-quarter of the visual field).

Methods of testing
VISUAL ACUITY
The visual acuity in each eye is assessed with glasses on (corrected) and glasses off (uncorrected) using a Snellen chart (see Figure 4.2). In patients with a neurological problem it is preferable to check the acuity corrected to remove any ocular refractive error contributing

to visual impairment. In the absence of glasses, impaired vision due to a refractive error can be corrected by asking the patient to look through a small hole in a piece of cardboard or paper. This will improve the vision if impairment is related to a refractive error in the eye.

COLOUR VISION

The Ishihara charts (Figure 4.3) are used to check colour vision. Colour blindness is most often hereditary, and there are two distinct patterns of impairment:

- If the patient is a protanope, colour blindness is characterised by defective perception of red and confusion of red with green or bluish green.
- If the patient is a deuteranope, color blindness is characterised by insensitivity to green.

  Pathological colour blindness indicates disease in the optic nerves and can occur even in the absence of prior visual symptoms, typically with a demyelinating optic neuropathy associated with multiple sclerosis.

THE VISUAL FIELDS
Severe visual field loss: quadrantanopia, hemianopia, visual inattention

A simple screening test that will detect a severe visual field loss, such as a quadrantanopia (loss of vision in the same quarter of the visual field in both eyes) or a hemianopia (loss of vision in the same half of the visual field of both eyes), is to move a finger in the peripheral vision in both upper and then both lower visual fields. If with double simultaneous stimulation the patient cannot see the moving finger in one of the fields, the problem is either a visual field loss or visual inattention. Visual inattention is the inability to see objects moving in both visual fields simultaneously, although the moving object can be seen if each visual field is tested separately.

To differentiate between these two possibilities, the examiner's finger is moved in one visual field at a time. If the visual disturbance is a loss of vision, the finger will not be seen until it reaches the midline. On the other hand, if the visual problem is inattention the single moving finger will be seen in the areas of vision where it could not

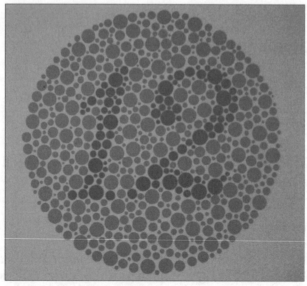

FIGURE 4.3 Ishihara sample chart

initially be seen with double simultaneous stimuli. Once again, this is the principle of testing from the area of abnormality until normality is found to define the exact pattern of impairment.

Subtle visual field defects

CENTRAL SCOTOMA

To detect more subtle defects of the visual fields at the bedside a 4-mm red pin is used. In this test the examiner holds the pin at a distance midway between himself and the patient. The visual field of the examiner is used as a normal control. The visual fields are tested with the patient covering the left eye, for example, while the examiner covers the right eye, directly opposite the patient's closed eye. The patient and the examiner look directly into each other's eye and in this way the examiner can tell if the patient's eye is moving during the test. Initially the 4-mm red pin is placed in the centre of the visual field to detect if there is a loss of central vision, a central scotoma. If there is a loss of vision in the centre, the pin is moved slowly away in each of the 4 quadrants in turn until it is visualised by the patient, establishing the size of the central scotoma. This indicates a lesion of the fovea in the eye.

ENLARGED BLIND SPOT

An enlarged blind spot occurs with a lesion of the optic discs (either optic neuritis or papilloedema). To detect an enlarged blind spot, the examiner slowly moves the 4-mm red pin out laterally from the centre at the level of the equator of the eye until the blind spot is detected. Once found, the examiner moves the pin up, down, medially and laterally until the size of the patient's blind spot is established and compared with that of the examiner.

SUBTLE HEMIANOPIA, QUADRANTANOPIA OR BITEMPORAL HEMIANOPIA

To test the visual fields for a subtle hemianopia, quadrantanopia or bi-temporal hemianopia, the examiner moves the pin slowly from the periphery to the midline in each of the 4 quadrants asking the patient to indicate when the red pin is first noticed. If a loss is detected with this technique, the pin is then moved slowly from the area of abnormal vision to normal vision to establish the exact pattern of visual loss. Testing the visual fields individually with the 4-mm red pin will NOT detect visual inattention.

A Goldman Perimeter or Bjerum Screen is used to formally test the visual fields.

EXAMINATION OF THE OPTIC FUNDI

The patient is instructed to look straight ahead, preferably at a small dot or mark on the wall. The examiner approaches from the side at about 30–45° lateral to the midline until a retinal blood vessel is visualised and this is traced back to the optic disc (Figure 4.4). The blood vessels can be traced outwards from the optic disc to detect any abnormality. To examine the fovea (central vision), the patient looks directly at the ophthalmoscope with the intensity of the light reduced.

THE 3RD, 4TH AND 6TH CRANIAL NERVES
The oculomotor (3rd) nerve

ANATOMY

The 3rd nerve nucleus is in the midbrain close to the midline, and the nerve exits the brainstem at the junction of the midbrain and pons just lateral to the midline (see Figure 1.6). It then crosses the subarachnoid space and, after traversing the cavernous sinus, it enters the orbit through the superior orbital fissure. The posterior communicating artery

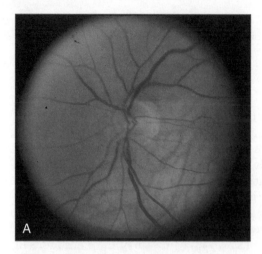

FIGURE 4.4
Normal optic disc and the more common abnormalities of the optic discs
A Normal optic disc

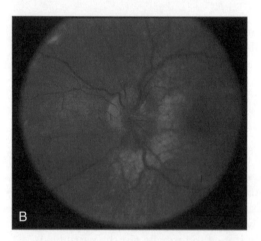

B Papilloedema

The visual acuity is normal unless the papilloedema is chronic, and the blind spot is enlarged. The visual fields are otherwise normal. The pupillary responses are normal.

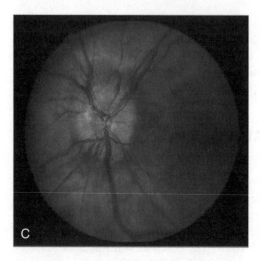

C Acute optic neuritis

The visual acuity is markedly impaired; colour vision is abnormal if the patient can read the chart (severe visual impairment will prevent the patient from seeing the numbers on the chart). The blind spot is enlarged. The direct pupillary response is slow and there is a Marcus–Gunn pupillary phenomenon (the pupil contracts promptly when the light is shone in the normal eye and when the light is shone in the abnormal eye the pupil initially dilates and then slowly contracts). Retrobulbar neuritis is the term applied to an inflammatory optic nerve lesion within the optic nerve but not affecting the optic nerve head, the part of the optic nerve that is visualised on examination of the fundus. In this situation, the visual acuity and colour vision are impaired, the visual field defect is usually a central scotoma although it may be a diffuse, lateral, superior or inferior defect. The fundus looks normal [3].

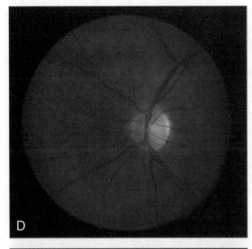

FIGURE 4.4—cont'd

D Long-standing optic neuritis with pallor of the optic disc

The visual acuity is reduced, colour vision is abnormal, and a Marcus–Gunn pupillary phenomenon is present (see 4C for an explanation of this abnormality).

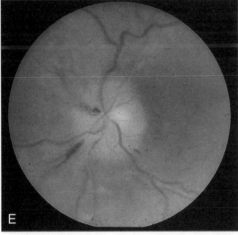

E Anterior ischaemic optic neuropathy (AION)

AION is the most common cause of acute optic neuropathy among older persons. It can be non-arteritic (nonarteritic anterior ischaemic optic neuropathy [NAION]) or arteritic, the latter being associated with giant cell arteritis. Visual loss usually occurs suddenly, or over a few days at most, and it is usually permanent. The optic disc is pale and swollen and there are flame haemorrhages.

lies close to the nerve and this artery is a common site for berry aneurysm formation which can cause a 3rd nerve palsy.

The 3rd nerve supplies the following muscles:

- levator palpebrae superioris, one of the two muscles that elevate the eyelid
- medial rectus (MR) that adducts the eye towards the nose
- superior rectus (SR) and inferior rectus (IR) that cause the eye to look up and down, respectively, when the eye is in abduction.

The trochlear (4th) nerve

ANATOMY

The 4th nerve nucleus is in the paramedian midbrain. The fibres of the 4th nerve cross the midline in the posterior aspect of the midbrain and emerge adjacent to the crus cerebri (see Figure 1.6). The 4th nerve passes through the cavernous sinus and enters the orbit via the superior orbital fissure. It supplies the superior oblique (SO) muscle that depresses the eye when it is in the adducted position and internally rotates the eye when it is looking laterally (abducted) and down. Fourth nerve palsies are commonly associated with lesions of the other oculomotor nerves due to their proximity in the cavernous sinus and orbit; an isolated 4th nerve palsy is rare but can be congenital in origin or the result of trauma.

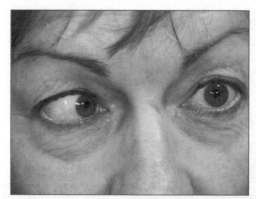

FIGURE 4.5   A left 6th nerve palsy with the patient looking to the left
The left eye cannot look laterally and is in the midline due to paralysis of the lateral rectus muscle.

METHOD OF TESTING
The trochlear nerve is tested by asking the patient to look towards the nose and then down. However, if the patient also has a 3rd nerve palsy and cannot adduct the eye towards the nose, the method of testing the 4th nerve is to ask the patient to look laterally and then down. If the 4th nerve is intact there will be internal rotation of the eye as it looks down; if the 4th nerve is impaired the eye will not internally rotate.

The abducent (6th) nerve
ANATOMY
The 6th nerve nucleus lies within the pons (encircled by the 7th cranial nerve). It exits the pons laterally at the junction of the pons and medulla (see Fig. 1.6). It crosses the subarachnoid space, passes through the cavernous sinus and enters the orbit via the superior orbital fissure to supply the lateral rectus (LR) muscle. The close proximity between the 6th nerve nucleus and the 7th nerve within the pons means it is very unusual to have an isolated 6th nerve lesion with disease within the pons. Most often a 6th nerve palsy indicates a lesion directly affecting the nerve, but occasionally it can be a false localising sign due to raised intracranial pressure. A 6th nerve palsy results in an inability to abduct (move the eye laterally within the orbit) the eye fully (see Figure 4.5).

METHOD OF TESTING
1 The patient is asked to look to the left to test the left lateral rectus.
2 The patient is asked to look to the right, testing the right lateral rectus.

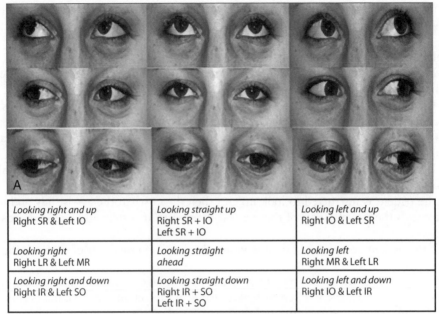

Looking right and up Right SR & Left IO	Looking straight up Right SR + IO Left SR + IO	Looking left and up Right IO & Left SR
Looking right Right LR & Left MR	Looking straight ahead	Looking left Right MR & Left LR
Looking right and down Right IR & Left SO	Looking straight down Right IR + SO Left IR + SO	Looking left and down Right IO & Left IR

FIGURE 4.6 **A** Normal full ocular movements all directions

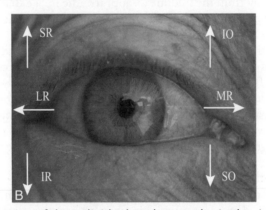

B The direction of action of the individual ocular muscles in the right eye
IO = inferior oblique, IR = inferior rectus, LR= lateral rectus, MR = medial rectus, SO = superior oblique, SR = superior rectus
Note: It is important to examine up gaze in the primary position (looking straight ahead) and also in the direction of action of each individual ocular muscle as shown.

CONTROL OF EYE MOVEMENTS, THE PUPIL AND EYELID OPENING: SYMPATHETIC AND PARASYMPATHETIC INNERVATION OF THE PUPIL AND EYELID

When a patient complains of diplopia it is important to clarify whether they actually are seeing double as some patients use the term 'double vision' to describe simple blurred vision. Once diplopia is confirmed, the next step is to enquire whether the diplopia is horizontal or vertical. Horizontal diplopia occurs with 6th nerve palsies and an internuclear ophthalmoplegia while vertical diplopia occurs with 3rd or 4th nerve palsies. An internuclear ophthalmoplegia occurs when the eye on the side of the brainstem where the pathology is fails to adduct and there is nystagmus in the contralateral eye as it looks outwards (refer to Figure 4.10).

Methods of examining eye movement

1 The examiner stands in front of the patient and observes the eye movements carefully.
2 The patient is requested to look up as a check for impairment of up gaze. This is a common finding in older patients but it may also represent a supranuclear gaze palsy, which refers to impairment of eye movements due to pathology above the cranial nerve nuclei that innervate the extraocular muscles.
3 The patient is asked to look to the right and then to the left while the examiner observes the eyes to see that there is a full range of horizontal eye movements.
4 The patient is instructed to look up and then down when the eye is fully abducted towards the lateral aspect of the eye and then when it is fully adducted towards the nose.

If the patient complains of double vision there are two methods of determining the cause.

1 Cover testing, where the patient is asked what image disappears when each eye is covered. The patient is asked to look towards an object and, if diplopia occurs, the eyes are covered one at a time and the patient is asked to say whether the image closest or furthest away from the midline disappears. The image that is furthest from the midline is the abnormal one. It is often difficult for the patient to be certain which image disappears.
2 An easier method is to use red–green glasses (see Figure 4.7) and a torch and ask the patient to identify what colour light is furthest from and what colour light is closest to the midline. The light that is furthest from the midline is the abnormal one and reflects the muscle that is affected. For example, in Figure 4.8 showing a left 3rd nerve palsy, when the patient is looking to the right the green image would be furthest to the right indicating weakness of the left medial rectus muscle. If the patient had a left 6th nerve palsy, the green image would be furthest from the midline when they look left.

The pupillary reflex

The pupil is innervated by parasympathetic fibres that constrict and sympathetic fibres that dilate the pupil. The parasympathetic fibres are on the surface of the 3rd nerve and a dilated pupil results when these are affected. A constricted pupil occurs when the sympathetic fibres are affected by a disease process. This may occur anywhere along the

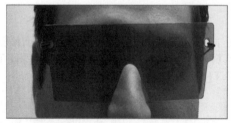

FIGURE 4.7 Red-green glasses used to test for diplopia (also reproduced in the colour section)

A light is shone into both eyes and the patient readily identifies the abnormal image by the colour of the image furthest from the midline. For example, if the patient had a left 6th nerve palsy the green image would be farthest from the midline when the patient looks to the right.

pathway from their origin in the sympathetic ganglion at the level of the 1st and 2nd thoracic nerve roots up through the neck, where the fibres are closely related to the internal carotid artery, into the cranium, where the fibres are adjacent to the carotid siphon of the internal carotid artery, into the orbit via the superior orbital fissure. Sympathetic fibres also innervate the eyelid. Impairment of the sympathetic pathway will result in mild ptosis and a constricted pupil, known as Horner's syndrome (see Figure 4.9). Other signs of a Horner's syndrome that are more subtle and more difficult to elicit are enophthalmos (the eye is partially withdrawn into the eye socket) and reduced or absent sweating (anhydrosis) on that side of the face.

Abnormalities of ocular movements and pupils

Figures 4.5, 4.7, 4.9 and 4.10 illustrate the common abnormalities of ocular movements: a 6th and 3rd nerve palsy, a Horner's syndrome and an internuclear ophthalmoplegia respectively.

THE TRIGEMINAL (5TH) NERVE

Anatomy

The trigeminal nerve has motor fibres that supply the ipsilateral pterygoid and masseter muscles (the muscles that push open and pull closed the jaw, respectively) and sensory fibres that supply sensation to the anterior one-third to two-thirds of the scalp, forehead,

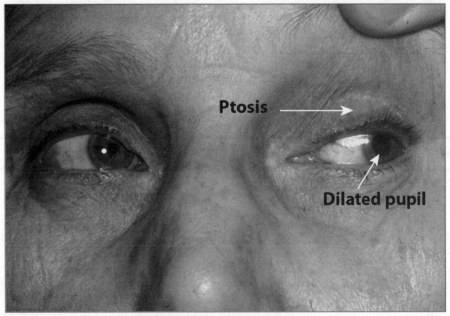

FIGURE 4.8 A left 3rd nerve palsy affecting the pupil

The pupil is dilated due to involvement of the parasympathetic fibres that constrict the pupil. The left eye cannot be elevated due to weakness of the superior oblique muscle. The other muscles that are affected but not illustrated are the medial and inferior rectus muscles and the inferior oblique. The left eyelid is being elevated to show the eye. In a 3rd nerve palsy the ptosis is severe and usually covers the entire eye. If the pupil is not affected this is referred to as a 'pupil-sparing 3rd nerve palsy' and is most often related to infarction of the 3rd nerve in patients with diabetes.

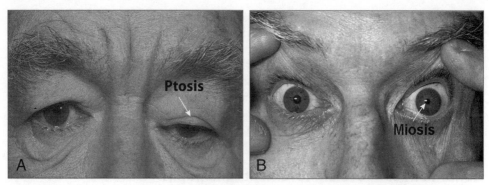

FIGURE 4.9 **A** Horner's syndrome with partial ptosis (drooping of the eyelid).
B Left Horner's syndrome with a small pupil (miosis) and the eyelid elevated to show
the pupil

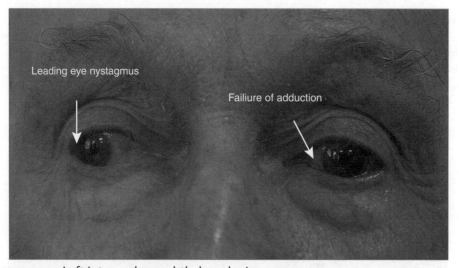

FIGURE 4.10 Left internuclear ophthalmoplegia

Note the failure of adduction of the left eye. There is often but not always nystagmus in the other (on this occasion the right) eye, termed leading eye nystagmus.

cheek and jaw on the same side, but not the angle of the jaw (see Figure 4.11). The motor fibres are only rarely affected by disease whereas there are many causes of sensory loss on the face. It is important to differentiate between altered sensation on the face due to a trigeminal nerve lesion and a quintothalamic tract lesion (the pathway between the 5th cranial nerve nucleus and the thalamus). The angle of the jaw is spared and the sensory loss affects only the anterior one-third to two-thirds of the scalp with a trigeminal nerve (peripheral nervous system) sensory problem whereas, with a quintothalamic tract (central nervous system) lesion, the sensory loss will extend over the entire (contralateral) scalp and face including the angle of the jaw. As this is almost invariably associated with spinothalamic tract involvement, the sensory loss will also affect the neck, arm and leg on the same side.

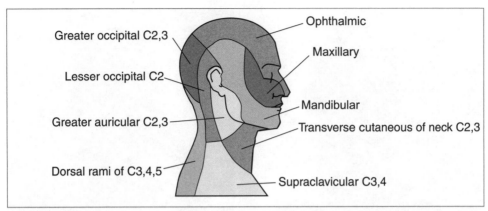

Greater occipital C2,3

Ophthalmic

Lesser occipital C2

Maxillary

Greater auricular C2,3

Mandibular

Dorsal rami of C3,4,5

Transverse cutaneous of neck C2,3

Supraclavicular C3,4

FIGURE 4.11 The sensory areas opthalmic, maxillary and mandibular supplied by the 5th cranial nerve

Reproduced from *Gray's Anatomy*, 37th edn, edited by PL Williams et al, 1989, Churchill Livingstone, Figure 7.242 [4]

Method of testing

Whether testing pain, light touch or temperature sensation, test the forehead, cheek and jaw on each side. If an area of abnormality is found, continue to test up over the forehead, across to the midline, back towards the ear and down to below the jaw until you find normal sensation, and the precise distribution of the sensory loss will be determined.

The corneal reflex is tested with cotton wool (not paper as it may abrade the cornea). Approach the eye from the side in order to avoid blinking due to the visual stimulus and touch the lateral aspect of the cornea (not the sclera) gently. The afferent pathway is the 1st division of the trigeminal nerve; the efferent pathway is the facial nerve resulting in eye closure. A similar reflex is the nasal tickle reflex. Tickle the inside of the nose with cotton wool: the afferent pathway is the 2nd division of the trigeminal nerve; the efferent pathway is the facial nerve. A normal corneal and nasal tickle response evokes forced eye closure bilaterally.

The motor component is tested by asking the patient to protrude the jaw (pterygoid muscles). If it is normal it will protrude in the midline; if there is an abnormal 5th motor nerve the jaw will deviate towards the side of the weak muscle – the side of the lesion. Another technique is to gently push the jaw to the right and then to the left; an inability to resist indicates a contralateral 5th motor nerve lesion. To test the masseter muscles the patient is requested to clench the jaw while the examiner places both hands over the muscles to feel for the contraction (see Figure 4.12). If there is an abnormality the muscle cannot be felt to contract beneath the fingers.

THE FACIAL (7TH) NERVE

Anatomy

The facial nerve nucleus is in the lateral pons of the brainstem. The nerve fibres hook around the 6th nerve nucleus and exit the pons laterally close to the 8th nerve (see Figure 1.6). The nerve then passes across the subarachnoid space and exits the skull through the facial canal and passes through the parotid gland to supply the facial muscles of the forehead, around the eyes (orbicularis oculi), the cheek and around the mouth (orbicularis oris). A branch leaves the nerve before the canal and supplies the stapedius muscle in the middle ear (the nerve to stapedius); if it is affected, for example in a patient with a Bell's palsy, it causes hyperacusis (increased sensitivity to noise) in the ear. Another

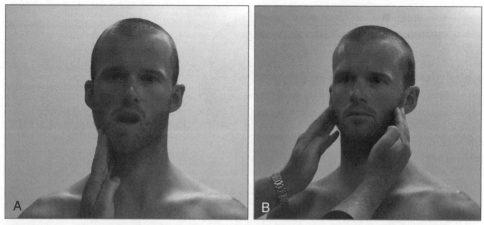

FIGURE 4.12 The technique for testing the **A** pterygoid and **B** masseter muscles

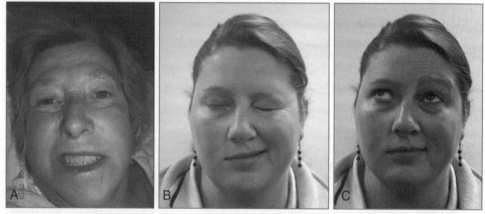

FIGURE 4.13 **A** Upper motor neuron facial weakness (note the patient can elevate both sides of the forehead)
B, C Lower motor neuron 7th nerve palsy with an inability to smile, close the eye fully and wrinkle the ipsilateral forehead

branch, the lingual nerve, supplies the sensation of taste to the anterior two-thirds of the tongue; if affected it causes altered taste on the ipsilateral side of the tongue.

Method of testing

Facial movements are tested by asking the patient to show their teeth, close their eyes tightly and then open them wide. This latter command will cause elevation of the eyebrows and differentiates a lower motor from an upper motor facial weakness. The frontalis muscle controls movement of the forehead and has bilateral innervation from the facial nerve. Thus, with an upper motor problem, the patient can still wrinkle the forehead and raise the eyebrows whereas, with a lower motor problem, they cannot (Figure 4.13 shows the difference between upper and lower motor problems).

The most common lesion affecting the facial nerve is a Bell's palsy. This typically produces a LMN weakness on the same side of the face and is often, but not invariably, associated with ipsilateral hyperacusis (increased hearing in that ear) and altered taste.

THE AUDITORY/VESTIBULAR (8TH) NERVE

Anatomy

The 8th cranial nerve has two components, the auditory or cochlear (hearing) nerve and the vestibular (balance) nerve (see Figure 4.15). The nerve emerges from the ear canal in the cerebellar–pontine angle, pierces the dura mata (the thick membrane surrounding the brain, just beneath the bone) and transverses the subarachnoid space. It enters the brainstem in the lateral pons where the vestibular and auditory nuclei are situated.

Methods of testing

The external ear canal is examined first to ensure it is not occluded by wax, and to assess the eardrum. There are many ways to test hearing, including:

1 Rustle the patient's hair that is just above the ear between your fingers.
2 Hold a mechanical watch close to the ear.
3 Whisper numbers in one ear while occluding the opposite ear.

If there is hearing impairment, then it is useful to perform the Weber test and Rinne test using a 256-Hz tuning fork. In the Weber test, the ringing tuning fork is placed in the midline of the forehead. If there is a conduction defect (middle ear problem), the noise will be heard in that ear; on the other hand, if there is an 8th nerve deafness, the noise will be heard in the opposite ear. In the Rinne test, the tuning fork is placed next to the ear and subsequently on the mastoid process. Bone conduction (on the mastoid) is louder than air conduction (next to the ear) when deafness is due to a conduction problem. An easy way to remember the features of these two tests is for examiners to occlude their own external canal and test themselves. Occluding the external canal simulates a conduction defect (see Figure 4.14).

The vestibular pathway

If a patient has the sensation that the head or room is spinning (vertigo), the problem must affect the vestibular pathway (see Figure 4.15), which runs from the ear to the cerebellum or vestibular nuclei in the brainstem and up to the vestibular cortex in the temporal lobe. Practically speaking, most cases of vertigo relate to inner ear problems and, to a lesser extent, cerebellar or brainstem lesions; they are very rarely due to more central pathology. Associated deafness and tinnitus coinciding with the vertigo (and not preexisting, unrelated problems) indicate a problem in the ear while other neurological symptoms such as diplopia, dysarthria, dysphagia, weakness or sensory disturbance point to a problem in the brainstem. Vertigo due to problems in the ear or vestibular nerve is referred to as peripheral vertigo while vertigo related to brainstem or cerebellar problems is referred to as central vertigo. Vertigo is discussed in Chapter 7, 'Episodic disturbances of neurological function'.

THE GLOSSOPHARYNGEAL (9TH) NERVE

Anatomy

The glossopharyngeal nerve nucleus lies in the lateral part of the medulla; the nerve emerges from the medulla, traverses the subarachnoid space and exits through the jugular foramen in the base of the skull. It supplies sensation to the soft palate and pharynx, together with taste to the posterior two-thirds of the tongue.

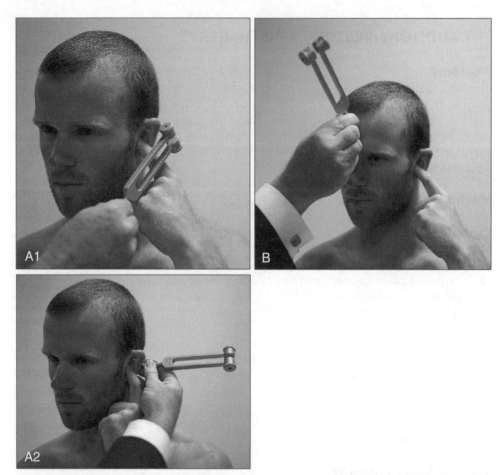

FIGURE 4.14   **A** Tuning fork Rinne's test and simulation with the ear occluded
B Tuning fork Weber's test and simulation with the ear occluded

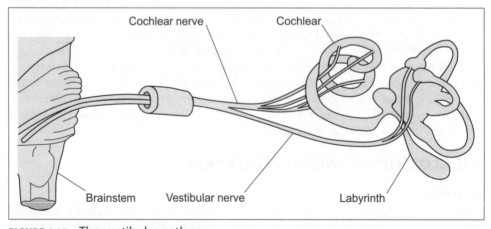

FIGURE 4.15   The vestibular pathway

Reproduced and modified from *Clinically Oriented Anatomy*, 4th edn, by KL Moore and AF Dalley, 1999, Lippincott Williams & Wilkins, Figure 7.82, p 975 [5]

Method of testing

The gag reflex is an unpleasant test and is only recommended as part of the examination when the patient complains of dysphagia. The phayrnx is touched with a blunt object such as a spatula. The patient experiences a choking sensation. The soft palate will rise to the opposite side if there is a 10th cranial nerve (the efferent arc of the gag reflex) problem. The reflex will be absent if there is a 9th cranial nerve (the afferent arc of the gag reflex) problem.

THE VAGUS (10TH) NERVE

Anatomy

The vagus nerve nucleus lies in the lateral aspect of the medulla; the nerve emerges laterally and traverses the subarachnoid space to exit through the jugular foramen at the base of the skull. It then descends in the neck to the thorax and abdomen.

Method of testing

The patient is requested to say 'ah' and movement of the soft palate is observed. If there is a problem with the vagas nerve, the palate will deviate to the opposite side as it is pulled upwards by the normal muscle (see Figure 4.16). This can also be observed with the gag reflex, described above.

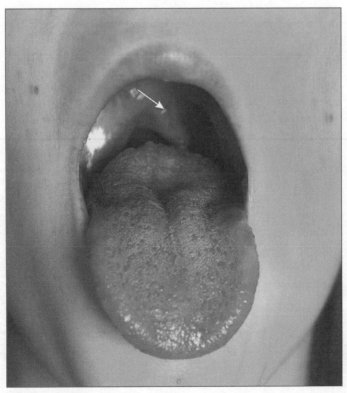

FIGURE 4.16 Deviated palate

THE ACCESSORY (11TH) NERVE

Anatomy
The accessory nerve nucleus also lies in the lateral medulla and the nerve exits adjacent to the lateral aspect of the pyramids of the motor pathway or corticospinal tract and traverses the subarachnoid space to exit through the jugular foramen in the base of the skull. After it exits the jugular foramen it is joined by the spinal nerve component that derives fibres from the C2–4 nerve roots to innervate the sternocleidomastoid and trapezius muscles. The spinal accessory nerve is prone to iatrogenic injury with posterior dissection of the neck.

Method of testing
The patient turns the head to one side and the examiner observes the sternocleidomastoid muscle on the opposite side (as the muscle pulls the sternum and mastoid closer together). To test the trapezius, the patient shrugs the shoulders against resistance (see Figure 4.17).

THE HYPOGLOSSAL (12TH) NERVE

Anatomy
The hypoglossal nerve nucleus lies adjacent to the midline of the medulla and the nerve emerges from the anterior aspect of the medulla just laterally to the pyramids of the medulla and traverses the subarachnoid space to exit through the hypoglossal canal in the base of the skull to supply the muscle of the ipsilateral half of the tongue.

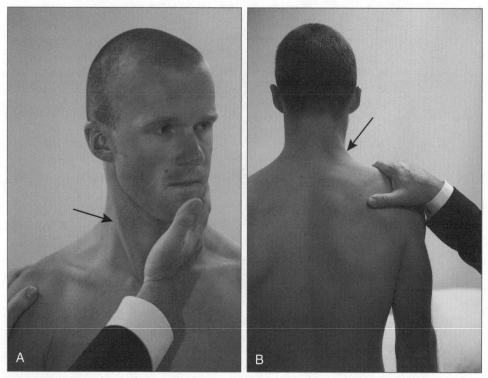

FIGURE 4.17 Method of testing the **A** sternocleidomastoid and **B** trapezius muscles

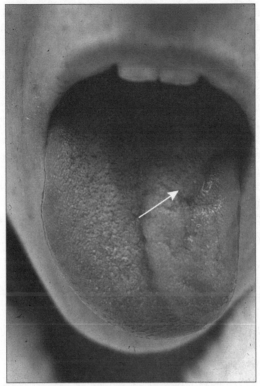

FIGURE 4.18 Wasting and deviation of the protruded tongue to the left due to a left 12th (hypoglossal) nerve palsy

Method of testing

The patient is asked to protrude the tongue and, as the muscle pushes the tongue forward, the tongue will deviate towards the paralysed side (see Figure 4.18).

The accompanying DVD demonstrates the techniques for examination of the cranial nerves.

The most common disorder to affect the brainstem is cerebrovascular disease. The following discussion entitled the 'Rule of 4' is a simplified method for understanding the brainstem and the various vascular syndromes. This has been previously published in the *Internal Medicine Journal* [1].

THE 'RULE OF 4' OF THE BRAINSTEM

Medical students are taught detailed anatomy of the brainstem containing a bewildering number of structures with curious names such as superior colliculi, inferior olives, various cranial nerve nuclei and the median longitudinal fasciculus. In reality a neurological examination can only test a few of these structures. The 'Rule of 4' recognises this and describes only those parts of the brainstem that can be examined clinically. The blood supply of the brainstem is such that there are long circumferential branches (the anterior inferior cerebellar artery 'AICA', the posterior inferior cerebellar artery 'PICA' and the superior cerebellar artery 'SCA') and paramedian branches. Involvement of the paramedian branches results in paramedian brainstem syndromes and involvement of the circumferential branches results in lateral brainstem syndromes. Occasionally, medial or lateral brainstem syndromes occur with ipsilateral vertebral occlusion.

The 4 rules of the 'Rule of 4'

1 There are 4 structures in the 'midline' (the paramedian aspect of the midbrain adjacent to the midline) beginning with **M:**
   - Motor nucleus
   - Median longitudinal fasciculus
   - Medial lemniscus
   - Motor pathway (corticospinal tract)
2 There are 4 structures to the side (lateral) beginning with **S:**
   - Spinocerebellar pathway
   - Spinothalamic pathway
   - Sensory nucleus of the 5th cranial nerve
   - Sympathetic pathway
3 There are
   - 4 cranial nerves in the medulla:
     - 12th hypoglossal nerve
     - 11th accessory nerve
     - 10th vagus nerve
     - 9th glossopharyngeal nerve
   - 4 in the pons:
     - 8th auditory and vestibular nerve
     - 7th facial nerve
     - 6th abducent nerve
     - 5th trigeminal nerve
   - 4 above the pons:
     - 4th trochlear nerve
     - 3rd oculomotor nerve
     - These two nerves are in the midbrain, the 2nd or ocular nerve and the 1st olfactory nerve are outside the midbrain
4 The 4 motor nuclei that are in the midline (actually paramedian) are those that divide (numerically) equally into 12, except for 1 and 2, (5, 7, 9, 10 and 11 are the cranial nerves that are in the lateral brainstem):
   - 3rd oculomotor nerve
   - 4th trochlear nerve
   - 6th abducent nerve
   - 12th hypoglossal nerve

Figure 4.19 depicts a cross-section of the brainstem at the level of the medulla, but the concept of 4 lateral and 4 medial structures also applies to the pons; only the 4 medial structures relate to the midbrain. Figure 4.20 shows the ventral aspect of the brainstem showing the emerging cranial nerves from the midbrain, pons and medulla.

The 4 medial structures and the associated deficit

1 The motor pathway (corticospinal tract): contralateral weakness of the arm and leg
2 The medial lemniscus: contralateral loss of vibration and proprioception affecting the arm and leg

3 The medial longitudinal fasciculus: ipsilateral internuclear ophthalmoplegia (failure of adduction of the ipsilateral eye towards the nose and nystagmus in the opposite eye as it looks laterally)

4 The motor nucleus and nerve: ipsilateral loss of the cranial nerve that is affected (3rd, 4th, 6th or 12th)

The 4 lateral structures and the associated deficit

1 The spinocerebellar pathways: ipsilateral ataxia of the arm and leg

2 The spinothalamic pathway: contralateral alteration of pain and temperature affecting the arm, leg and often the trunk

3 The sensory nucleus of the 5th cranial nerve (a long vertical structure that extends in the lateral aspect of the pons down into the medulla): ipsilateral alteration of pain and temperature on the face in the distribution of the 5th cranial nerve (see Figure 4.11)

4 The sympathetic pathway: ipsilateral Horner's syndrome, i.e. partial ptosis and a small pupil (miosis)

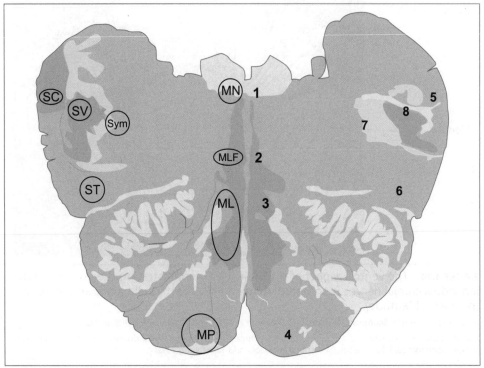

FIGURE 4.19 Cross-section of the brainstem (in this case the medulla, but the same 'Rule of 4' applies to the pons) showing the 4 midline structures and the 4 structures in the lateral (side) aspect of the brainstem.

Adapted from *Gray's Anatomy*, 34th edn, by E Davies et al, 1967, Longmans, Figure 813, p 1011 [6]

The sizes of the coloured areas do not represent the actual anatomical sizes, but have been made large enough to see and label.

1 MN = motor nucleus (3, 4, 6 or 12), 2 MLF = median longitudinal fasciculus, 3 ML = medial lemniscus, 4 MP = motor pathway (corticospinal tract), 5 SC = spinocerebellar, 6 ST = spinothalamic, 7 SY = sympathetic, 8 SV = sensory nucleus of Vth cranial nerve

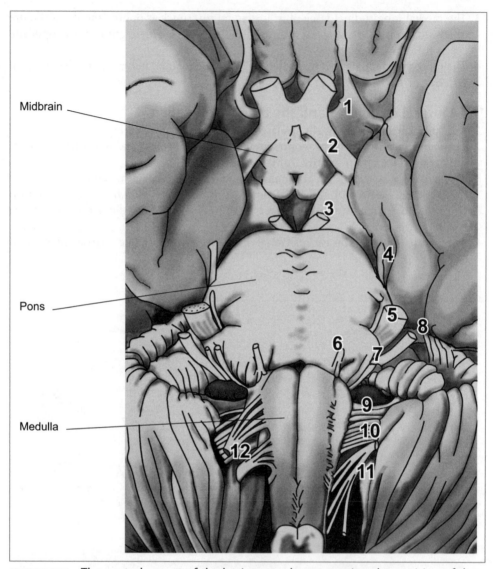

Midbrain

Pons

Medulla

FIGURE 4.20   The ventral aspect of the brainstem, demonstrating the position of the individual cranial nerves (numbered) in relation to the medulla, pons and midbrain (parallels of latitude)

Adapted from *Gray's Anatomy*, 34th edn, by E Davies et al, 1967, Longmans, Figure 806, p 1003

1 = olfactory, 2 = ophthalmic, 3 = oculomotor, 4 = trochlear, 5 = trigeminal, 6 = abducent, 7 = facial, 8 = auditory, 9 = glossopharyngeal, 10 = vagus, 11 = spinal accessory and 12 = hypoglossal

The 4 cranial nerves in the medulla and the associated deficit

1 9th (glossopharyngeal): ipsilateral loss of pharyngeal sensation
2 10th (vagus): ipsilateral palatal weakness
3 11th (spinal accessory): ipsilateral weakness of the trapezius and sternocleidomastoid muscles
4 12th (hypoglossal): ipsilateral weakness of the tongue

The 12th cranial nerve is the motor nerve in the midline of the medulla. Although the 9th, 10th and 11th cranial nerves have motor components, using the simple rule that they do not divide evenly into 12, they are thus not motor nerves in the midline.

The 4 cranial nerves in the pons and the associated deficit
1 5th (trigeminal): ipsilateral alteration of pain, temperature and light touch on the face back as far as the anterior 2/3 of the scalp and sparing the angle of the jaw
2 6th (abducent): ipsilateral weakness of abduction (lateral movement) of the eye
3 7th (facial): ipsilateral facial weakness
4 8th (auditory): ipsilateral deafness

The 6th cranial nerve is the motor nerve in the pons. The 7th is a motor nerve but it also carries pathways of taste and, using the Rule of 4, it does not divide equally into 12 and thus it is not a motor nerve that is in the midline. The vestibular portion of the 8th nerve is not included in order to keep the concept simple and to avoid confusion. Nausea, vomiting and vertigo occur with involvement of the vestibular connections in the lateral medulla.

The 4 cranial nerves above the pons and the associated deficit
1 1st (olfactory): not in midbrain
2 2nd (optic): not in midbrain
3 3rd (oculomotor): impaired adduction, elevation and depression of the ipsilateral eye with or without a dilated pupil; the eye is turned out and slightly down
4 4th (trochlear): eye unable to look down when looking in towards the nose

The 3rd and 4th cranial nerves are the motor nerves in the midbrain.

The motor and sensory pathways pass through the entire length of the brainstem and can be likened to 'meridians of longitude' while the various cranial nerves can be regarded as 'parallels of latitude'. If you can establish where the meridians of longitude and parallels of latitude intersect, you have established the site of the lesion.

Thus a medial brainstem syndrome will consist of the **4 Ms** + the relevant motor cranial nerve (3rd, 6th or 12th) and a lateral brainstem syndrome will consist of the **4 Ss** + either the 9th, 10th and11th cranial nerves if in the medulla or the 5th, 7th and 8th cranial nerves if in the pons.

Medial (paramedian) brainstem syndromes
Let us assume that the patient you are examining has a brainstem problem (most often a stroke). If you find UMN signs in the arm and the leg on one side then you know the patient has a contralateral medial brainstem syndrome because the motor pathway is paramedian and crosses at the level of the foramen magnum (at the decussation of the pyramids, where the brainstem meets the spinal cord). The involvement of the motor pathway is the 'meridian of longitude'. Refer to Figure 4.21 for a summary of the signs. So far the lesion could be anywhere in the medial aspect of the brainstem although, if the face is also affected, it has to be above the mid pons, the level of the 7th nerve nucleus.

The motor cranial nerve, 'the parallel of latitude', indicates whether the lesion is in the medulla (12th), pons (6th) or midbrain (3rd). Remember that cranial nerve palsy will be ipsilateral to the side of the lesion and contralateral to the hemiparesis. If the medial lemniscus is also affected, you will find a contralateral (the same side affected by the hemiparesis) loss of vibration and proprioception in the arm and leg as the posterior columns also cross at or just above the level of the foramen magnum.

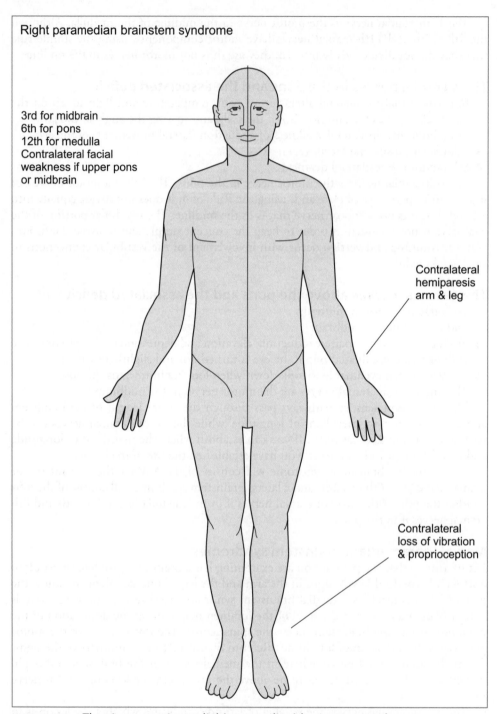

Right paramedian brainstem syndrome

3rd for midbrain
6th for pons
12th for medulla
Contralateral facial
weakness if upper pons
or midbrain

Contralateral
hemiparesis
arm & leg

Contralateral
loss of vibration
& proprioception

FIGURE 4.21 The signs seen in medial (paramedian) brainstem syndromes

The median longitudinal fasciculus (MLF) is usually not affected when there is a hemiparesis as the MLF is further back in the brainstem. The MLF can be affected in isolation, a 'lacunar infarct', and this results in an ipsilateral internuclear ophthalmoplegia, with failure of adduction (movement towards the nose) of the ipsilateral eye and leading eye nystagmus on looking laterally to the opposite side of the lesion in the contralateral eye. If the patient has involvement of the left MLF, when asked to look to the left the eye movements would be normal, but on looking to the right the left eye would not go past the midline while there would be nystagmus in the right eye as it looked to the right.

Lateral brainstem syndromes

Once again we are assuming that the patient you are seeing has a brainstem problem, most likely a vascular lesion. The 4 Ss or 'meridians of longitude' will indicate that you are dealing with a lateral brainstem problem, and the cranial nerves or 'parallels of latitude' will indicate whether the problem is in the lateral medulla or lateral pons. Refer to Figure 4.22 for a summary of the signs.

A lateral brainstem infarct will result in:

- ipsilateral ataxia of the arm and leg due to involvement of the spinocerebellar pathways
- contralateral alteration of pain and temperature sensation due to involvement of the spinothalamic pathway
- ipsilateral loss of pain and temperature sensation affecting the face within the distribution of the sensory nucleus of the trigeminal nerve (light touch may also be affected with involvement of the spinothalamic pathway and/or sensory nucleus of the trigeminal nerve).

An ipsilateral Horner's syndrome with partial ptosis and a small pupil (miosis) is due to involvement of the sympathetic pathway. The power, tone and reflexes should all be normal. So far all we have done is localise the problem to the lateral aspect of the brainstem. By adding the relevant 3 cranial nerves in the medulla or the pons we can localise the lesion to one of these regions of the brain.

The lowest 4 cranial nerves are in the medulla and the 12th nerve is in the midline so that the 9th, 10th and 11th will be in the lateral aspect of the medulla. When these are affected the result is dysarthria and dysphagia with an ipsilateral impairment of the gag reflex so that the palate will pull up to the opposite side. Occasionally, there may be weakness of the ipsilateral trapezius and/or sternocleidomastoid muscle. This is lateral medullary syndrome, usually due to occlusion of the ipsilateral vertebral or posterior inferior cerebellar arteries.

The next 4 cranial nerves are in the pons and the 6th nerve is the motor nerve in the midline, so that the 5th, 7th and 8th are in the lateral aspect of the pons. When these are affected there will be ipsilateral facial weakness, weakness of the ipsilateral masseter and pterygoid muscles (muscles that open and close the mouth) and occasionally ipsilateral deafness. A tumor such as an acoustic neuroma in the cerebellopontine angle will result in ipsilateral deafness, facial weakness and impairment of facial sensation; there may also be ipsilateral limb ataxia if it compresses the ipsilateral cerebellum or brainstem. The sympathetic pathway is usually too deep to be affected.

If there are signs of both a lateral and a medial brainstem syndrome, one needs to consider a basilar artery problem, possibly an occlusion.

In summary, if one can remember that:

- there are 4 structures in the midline commencing with the letter M

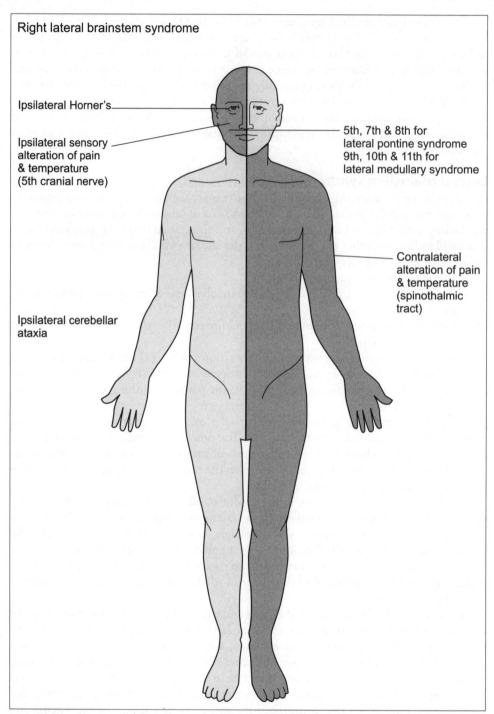

FIGURE 4.22   The signs seen in lateral brainstem syndromes

Note: Trapezius weakness is rarely seen in lateral medullary lesions.

- there are 4 structures in the lateral aspect of the brainstem commencing with the letter S
- the lower 4 cranial nerves are in the medulla
- the middle 4 cranial nerves are in the pons
- the first 4 cranial nerves are above the pons, with the 3rd and 4th in the midbrain
- the 4 motor nerves that are in the midline are the 4 that divide evenly into 12 (except for 1 and 2), i.e. the 3rd, 4th, 6th and 12th

  it will be possible to diagnose with pinpoint accuracy brainstem vascular syndromes.

REFERENCES

1 Gates P. The rule of 4 of the brainstem: A simplified method for understanding brainstem anatomy and brainstem vascular syndromes for the non-neurologist. Intern Med J 2005; 35(4):263–266.
2 Adams RD, Victor M. Principles of neurology. New York: McGraw–Hill Book Company; 1985:1186.
3 Gerling J, Meyer JH, Kommerell G. Visual field defects in optic neuritis and anterior ischemic optic neuropathy: Distinctive features. Graefes Arch Clin Exp Ophthalmol 1998; 236(3):188–192.
4 Williams PL et al (eds). Gray's anatomy, 37th edn. London: Churchill Livingstone; 1989.
5 Moore KL, Dalley AF. Clinically oriented anatomy, 4th edn. Maryland: Lippincott Williams & Wilkins; 1999.
6 Davies E et al. Gray's anatomy, 34th edn. Longmans; 1967:1011, Figure 813.

chapter 5

The Cerebral Hemispheres and Cerebellum

ASSESSMENT OF HIGHER COGNITIVE FUNCTION

Although subtitled 'Assessment of higher cognitive function', this chapter will not deal with the very complex neuropsychological testing that can be performed in patients with impairment of cognitive function. Rather, this chapter discusses a simplistic assessment of language disturbances and some very basic higher cortical functions, in particular of the parietal lobes, which can be used while taking the neurological history and examining the patient to localise the site of the pathology within the nervous system. This involves the usage of terms such as the primary pathways and secondary association areas. These terms are an aid to understanding and there is no evidence that the parietal lobes are 'hard-wired' in such a manner. In fact, symptoms from lesions in a part of the nervous system do not necessarily reflect the function of that part; the symptoms may arise from either a loss of certain functions or functional overactivity of the portions of the brain that remain intact [1]. The higher cortical functions represent the parallels of latitude within the cerebral hemisphere and, as already stated, 'the pathology is ALWAYS at the level of the parallel of latitude'. More comprehensive discussions of higher cortical function can be found in the major textbooks [1–3]. Figure 5.1 gives a lateral view of the cerebral hemispheres and the cerebellum. The frontal, parietal, occipital and temporal lobes and the various functions pertaining to those lobes are shown.

THE FRONTAL LOBES

Patients should be suspected of having a problem in a frontal lobe if they present with one of the following:
- contralateral weakness
- changes in personality or behaviour
- difficulty walking in the absence of any weakness or sensory symptoms in the legs (a condition referred to as an apraxia of gait)
- non-fluent dysphasia (dominant hemisphere only).

Contralateral weakness
The area just in front of the central sulcus, referred to as the pre-central gyrus (see Figure 5.1), is the origin of the motor fibres that innervate the muscles on the opposite side of the body. This pathway is referred to as the corticospinal tract and it crosses the midline at the level of the foramen magnum, the junction of the lower end of the brainstem and the upper end of the cervical spinal cord. Lesions affecting the pre-central gyrus will result in a contralateral hemiparesis affecting the face, arm and leg although, one limb

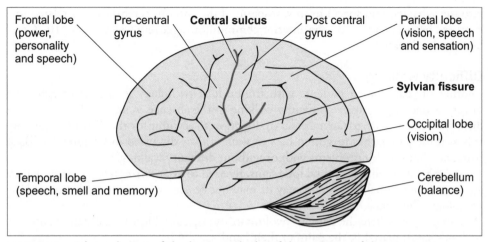

Frontal lobe (power, personality and speech)
Pre-central gyrus
Central sulcus
Post central gyrus
Parietal lobe (vision, speech and sensation)
Sylvian fissure
Occipital lobe (vision)
Temporal lobe (speech, smell and memory)
Cerebellum (balance)

FIGURE 5.1 A lateral view of the brain and a brief description of the common functions associated with the specific lobes of the brain

Note: The central sulcus separates the frontal and parietal lobes.

may be weaker than the other and the face may be affected to a variable degree (partial weakness) or with hemiplegia (total weakness).

The clues that the hemiparesis is derived from a lesion in the frontal lobe are:

- conjugate eye deviation, in which the eyes look away from the side of the weakness and towards the side of the lesion due to involvement of the area of the frontal lobe that controls conjugate deviation of the eyes to the opposite side
- cortical sensory signs due to associated involvement of the parietal lobe on that side
- non-fluent dysphasia with dominant hemisphere lesions.

Very rarely, an irritative lesion can result in a contralateral hemiparesis with the eyes deviated to the side of the weakness and away from the side of the pathology, mimicking a pontine lesion in the brainstem where there is an area responsible for conjugate deviation of the eyes to the same side. When this area of the brainstem is affected the eyes deviate away from the side of the lesion and towards the side of the paralysis.

Changes to personality or behaviour

The pre-frontal region is that part of the frontal lobes anterior to the motor cortex and the motor speech area. Diseases affecting this region of the frontal lobe result in changes to personality or behaviour best summarised by the phrase 'he/she is not him/herself'.

These patients can lose spontaneity and initiative and appear apathetic and depressed or, at the other end of the spectrum, patients can appear to 'have a short fuse'. In this situation patients can become aggressive and violent, even after a trivial incident. This is seen following some head injuries. Patients with frontal lobe pathology can develop an elevated mood and behave inappropriately, such as the vicar's wife who begins to tell dirty jokes and who was subsequently diagnosed with a meningioma (a benign tumour) in the frontal lobe.

If the olfactory tracts that lie beneath the frontal lobe are also affected, there can be an associated unilateral or bilateral anosmia (loss of the sense of smell).

An inability to perform acts voluntarily or to make decisions is seen in patients with pre-frontal problems and is termed abulia, reflecting pathology in the medial aspect of the frontal lobes. Abulia sometimes occurs with a subarachnoid haemorrhage (bleeding into the subarachnoid space) from vasospasm of the anterior cerebral artery related to a ruptured berry aneurysm on the anterior communicating artery (see Chapter 10, 'Cerebrovascular disease').

Difficulty walking

Another presentation of patients with frontal lobe pathology is apraxia of gait. The history is one of progressive difficulty walking in the absence of any weakness, sensory disturbance, ataxia or extrapyramidal dysfunction to account for the difficulty walking. It is as if the patient has forgotten how to walk. This is discussed in Chapter 12, 'Back pain and common leg problems with or without difficulty walking'.

There are a number of frontal lobe signs, referred to as *primitive reflexes*, because they are present in normal babies and may or may not be seen in patients with frontal lobe pathology. These include:

- a *grasp reflex*, where the patient involuntarily grasps an object (usually the examiner's hand) placed in the palm of their hand
- a *positive palmo-mental reflex*, where the palm of the hand is stroked and there is retraction of the ipsilateral chin beneath the lips
- a pout reflex, where the patient purses the lips when a stimulus is applied to them.

Although changes in personality and behaviour may be one of the presenting symptoms of dementia, severe depression can produce a similar clinical picture termed 'pseudo-dementia'.

THE PARIETAL LOBES

Patients with parietal lobe problems may present in a number of ways:

- speech disturbance such as fluent dysphasia and, if Wernicke's area in the posterior temporal lobe is also affected, the patient may also present with confusion (discussed in the section 'Disturbances of speech' below)
- disturbances of vision in the contralateral visual field
- lost and disoriented patients who appear to be lost or disorientated even in a familiar environment
- a concerned relative brings the patient for assessment, as some patients are not even aware of any problem at all and the problem is only detected when another person observes that there is something wrong.

Visual disturbances can occur in both dominant and non-dominant hemisphere problems; dysphasia is a feature of dominant hemisphere problems; being lost, disoriented and unaware that anything is amiss are very typical features of problems in the non-dominant hemisphere.

In both the dominant and non-dominant hemispheres, there are visual pathways that pass through and sensory pathways that terminate in the parietal lobe. If the so-called 'primary pathway' is affected, there will be a contralateral loss of function. If the 'primary pathway' is intact but the so-called 'secondary association areas' are affected, there will be a contralateral inattention with double simultaneous stimuli where the patient is not aware of the stimulus on one side when the other side is stimulated in the same manner simultaneously.

Speech disturbance (dysphasia) and the term RAAF (an abbreviation for the Royal Australian Air Force) best describe the features of problems in the dominant hemisphere, while the term 'lost in space' is the easy way to remember the characteristics of non-dominant parietal lobe problems (see Table 5.1). RAAF refers to the clinical findings

TABLE 5.1 Summary of the clinical features with lesions of the dominant and non-dominant parietal lobes

	Dominant	Non-dominant
Primary sensory pathway*	Contralateral sensory loss	Contralateral sensory loss
Secondary association area for sensation*	Contralateral sensory inattention	Contralateral sensory inattention
Primary visual pathway*	Contralateral loss of vision **	Contralateral loss of vision**
Secondary association area for vision*	Contralateral visual inattention	Contralateral visual inattention
Cortical signs*	Graphaesthesia, 2-point discrimination and stereognosis	Graphaesthesia, 2-point discrimination and stereognosis
Speech	Fluent dysphasia	Dysarthria
Other	RAAF Gerstmann's syndrome	Lost in space

*It can be seen that sensory and visual symptoms together with the unique parietal cortical signs are common to both the dominant and non-dominant parietal lobes. It is the speech disturbance and the parietal lobe abnormalities associated with Gerstmann's syndrome in the dominant hemisphere and the characteristic abnormalities seen in the non-dominant hemisphere (referred to as 'lost in space') that differentiate between the two hemispheres.

**Either loss of vision in the opposite visual field (hemianopia) or loss of vision in the upper or lower aspect of the visual field on the opposite side (quadrantanopia).

seen in dominant parietal lobe problems and, in its pure form, is referred to as Gerstmann's syndrome (for an explanation of RAAF, see 'Gerstmann's syndrome' below).

Abnormalities of vision
- Contralateral loss of vision. The optic radiation from the contralateral visual field passes through the parietal lobes to the occipital lobe (see Figure 5.1). If the 'primary pathways' are affected, there will be a loss of vision on the contralateral side resulting in a lower quadrantanopia if only the parietal lobe is affected, but often the optic radiation fibres in the temporal lobe are also affected and the resulting deficit is a contralateral homonymous (the visual field disturbance is identical when each eye is tested separately) hemianopia.
- Contralateral visual inattention. If the 'primary visual pathways' are preserved, but the so-called 'secondary association areas' are affected, there will be visual inattention elicited with double simultaneous stimuli. The patient is unable to appreciate the visual stimulus in one visual field, usually a moving finger applied simultaneously to both visual fields, but can if only one visual field is stimulated at a time.

Abnormalities of sensation
Although abnormalities of sensation are commonly detected on examination of patients with parietal lobe problems, they are only occasionally the presenting symptom.
- Contralateral loss of sensation affecting the primary sensory modalities of vibration and proprioception, pain and temperature
- Contralateral sensory inattention where the patient cannot appreciate sensation on one side of the body when the stimulus is applied simultaneously to both sides

- Unique parietal sensory phenomena
  - Impairment of 2-point discrimination
  - Impaired stereognosis
  - Impaired graphaesthesia

The sensory pathways from the body terminate in the contralateral post-central gyrus of the parietal lobes. If the so-called 'primary sensory pathways' in the parietal lobes are affected there will be abnormal sensation on the opposite side of the body, resulting in loss or impairment of vibration and proprioception with either cortical or deep hemisphere parietal lobe problems and/or loss or impairment of pain and temperature sensation with deep hemisphere but not cortical parietal lobe problems.

If the 'primary pathways' are not affected, but the area of the parietal lobe that interprets these sensory stimuli (referred to in this chapter as the 'secondary association areas') is involved in the pathological process, the resulting abnormality will be a loss of appreciation of sensation elicited with double simultaneous stimulation termed sensory inattention. Here, the examiner applies the same stimulus to both sides of the body simultaneously. This is usually performed by stroking the skin with a finger. Patients with sensory inattention do not notice the sensory stimulus on the contralateral side of the body to the pathology when both sides are stimulated simultaneously but can appreciate the sensory stimulus when only one side is stimulated.

Although abnormalities of vibration and proprioception can occur in cortical lesions, the detection of impaired vibration and proprioception cannot localise the problem to the cortex. If the primary sensory modalities of pain, temperature, vibration and proprioception are normal or only mildly affected, it is possible to perform more detailed sensory testing looking for abnormalities seen with contralateral parietal cortical lesions. The three cortical signs consist of:

1 Impairment of stereognosis: the patient is unable to appreciate the shape and size of an object, for example a pen or a coin, placed in the affected hand. Proprioception must not be affected, otherwise the inability to identify the object would reflect impairment of the proprioceptive pathway and not necessarily the contralateral parietal cortex as the site of abnormality.

2 Impairment of graphaesthesia: the patient is unable to identify a number drawn on the palm of the contralateral affected hand. The drawing must be greater than 4 cm in size and initially a number is drawn on the palm of the hand while the patient watches. The patient is then instructed to close their eyes and identify another number drawn on the palm. It is easier for patients to identify numbers if their palm is facing towards them and not the examiner. If light touch is severely impaired, abnormal graphaesthesia may occur and not indicate a cortical problem.

3 Impairment of 2-point discrimination: an inability to distinguish two points from one. This can be tested on any part of the body but the distance between the two points varies greatly from 1 mm on the tip of the tongue to 20–30 mm on the dorsum of the hands and feet [1]. The most useful site to test 2-point discrimination is on the fingertips where the normal distance is 3–5 mm. It is recommended to test the opposite hand (if it is normal) to determine the distance between the two points in this particular patient as this can vary from patient to patient depending on the age of the patient.

The above sensory and visual abnormalities occur with pathology in either the dominant (usually left) or non-dominant hemisphere with the three cortical signs contralateral to the side of the pathology.

The dominant hemisphere

In addition to the sensory and/or visual abnormalities with or without the three cortical sensory signs described above, patients with dominant hemisphere lesions may have a speech disturbance termed dysphasia and some or all of the signs of what has been referred to as Gerstmann's syndrome.

DISTURBANCES OF SPEECH

Clinicians use abnormalities of speech to localise the problem within the nervous system. On the other hand, speech therapists assess abnormalities of speech in a completely different manner and more from the therapeutic point of view. A simplified approach is shown in Figure 5.2.

- Dysarthria refers to difficulty in speaking because of impairment of the organs of speech or their innervation [4]. Dysarthria occurs with problems in many areas of the brain, including the frontal lobes or parietal lobes, cortex or deep within the subcortical white matter of either the dominant or non-dominant hemisphere. Dysarthria also occurs with brainstem and cerebellar problems, disorders of the 9th, 10th and 12th cranial nerves, disorders of the neuromuscular junction or even diseases affecting the face, tongue or palatal muscles. Although experienced neurologists may be able to differentiate between the various types of dysarthria, this is difficult for non-neurologists.
- Dysphasia is an impairment of the ability to understand and use the symbols of language, both spoken and written [4]. If the speech disturbance results in a total loss of speech, it is referred to as aphasia. Dysphasia occurs with dominant hemisphere problems (see Figure 5.3): in 90% of right-handed people and 50% of left-handed people this is the left hemisphere.

The simplest classification to understand is the one that reflects the abnormality of speech encountered: non-fluent (C) or fluent with (A) or without (B) comprehension difficulties.

A If the pathology is in the posterior aspect of the dominant temporal lobe (area A, Figure 5.3), the patient has word deafness where they cannot monitor their own speech or understand what is said to them and the patient will appear to be totally

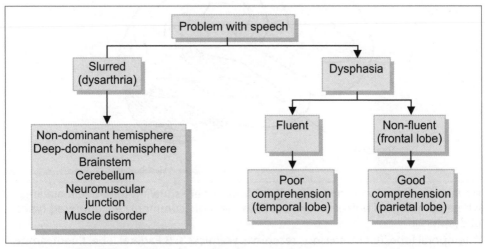

FIGURE 5.2 Simplified approach to speech disturbances

The first step is to establish whether the patient is suffering from *dysarthria*, which has poor localising value, or *dysphasia*, which localises to the dominant hemisphere:

confused. Speech is fluent with literal (letters) and verbal (words) paraphasic errors where letters of some words or entire words are replaced by other letters or words. Non-existent words, referred to as neologisms, are invented. As patients are unable to monitor their own speech the words are often said out of sequence, described as a word salad. An example of a literal paraphasic error is where the patient says 'mouse' instead of 'house', and an example of a verbal paraphasic error is where the patient says 'the sky is brown'. An example of a neologism is 'rumpstle'.

B If the temporal lobe is not affected and the pathology lies within the parietal lobe (area B, Figure 5.3), the resulting speech disturbance will be less marked. As the problem is behind the central sulcus the speech will be fluent, but the patient can understand what is being said to them and they can monitor their own speech. There are occasional literal and verbal paraphasic errors, but neologisms and word salad are not a feature. These patients have a curious deficit, where they are unable to name objects, thus the term nominal dysphasia. This type of dysphasia may be a disconnection syndrome [1]. When patients are asked to name a pen or a part of a wristwatch, for example, they struggle to find the appropriate word, but they can often but not always exhibit an understanding of how the object is used.

C As the motor cortex is very closely related to the area in the frontal lobe that is involved with the production of speech (area C, Figure 5.3), a frontal lobe disorder of speech is almost invariably associated with a contralateral hemiparesis (partial weakness) or hemiplegia (total weakness). The patient can understand what is being said; they know exactly what they want to say but are unable to produce the words. However, they are not mute, which is the inability to produce sound. They give

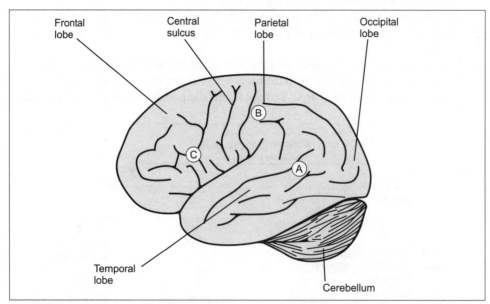

FIGURE 5.3　Lateral view of the dominant hemisphere showing the three main areas where pathological processes can produce the more commonly encountered types of dysphasia

A Temporal lobe: fluent, sensory, receptive, Wernicke's; **B** Parietal lobe: fluent, amnestic, nominal; **C** Frontal lobe: non-fluent, motor, expressive, Broca's

Note: In this illustration the sites for speech are not strictly anatomically correct, but are simply located within the relevant lobe. Various terms have been applied to the different abnormalities of speech referred to as dysphasia.

the appearance of having a stutter of variable severity reflecting the severity of the underlying speech disturbance. The patient frequently becomes very frustrated at the inability to express themselves. If the examiner shows the patient a pencil, for example, and asks them to name the object, the patient can be seen to be struggling to express the correct word. If after several attempts the examiner correctly names the object, the patient will nod in agreement.

Patients who are unable to speak are also unable to produce written language, even in the absence of paralysis of the arm.

The resulting speech disturbance that occurs if all three areas are affected is referred to as total or global dysphasia. In this situation, the patient may be able to understand or utter a few words but is unable to follow simple commands and unable to read or write.

There are a number of speech disturbances that are referred to as disconnection syndromes. These include conduction aphasia, pure word deafness and pure word blindness, to name just a few. These are believed to result from lesions affecting the association pathways joining the primary receptive areas to the language areas and not from lesions affecting the cortical language areas. A detailed discussion of these seldom encountered speech abnormalities is beyond the scope of this book, but can be found in textbooks [1–3].

GERSTMANN'S SYNDROME

Gerstmann's syndrome refers to a constellation of abnormal neurological findings reflecting involvement of the dominant parietal lobe when they occur in isolation. In clinical practice the four features that Gerstmann described almost invariably occur in association with visual and speech disturbance. A simple way to remember this is to recall the abbreviation for the Royal Australian Air Force, RAAF. The abnormalities consist of:

* **R**ight to left confusion – unable to distinguish the right from the left side
* **A**graphia – inability to write
* **A**calculia – inability to perform simple arithmetic (e.g. 13 − 7 = 6)
* **F**inger agnosia – inability to identify the correct finger.

When testing for finger agnosia the examiner asks the patient to identify the second or third digit of one hand. The side of the hand should not be tested simultaneously as this could be confused with an inability to distinguish right from left.

In most patients, many of the abnormalities described coexist. A speech disturbance is frequently associated with contralateral weakness, sensory loss or visual field disturbance.

The non-dominant hemisphere
'LOST IN SPACE'

This is the right hemisphere in 90% of right-handed patients and 50% of left-handed patients. The simple method for remembering the abnormalities that occur in lesions of the non-dominant parietal lobe is the phrase 'lost in space'. This consists of neglect of one side of the body, usually the left side because the right hemisphere is the non-dominant hemisphere in most patients. The patient may present with an inability to dress themselves, referred to as *dressing apraxia*, often only placing one arm in the sleeve of their coat, and they may neglect to shave themselves or apply makeup on one side of the face. Strictly speaking this is not true dressing apraxia, but the patient does have difficulty dressing because they are neglecting one side. Dressing apraxia where patients cannot dress themselves is a feature of dominant parietal lobe lesions. This neglect can be so severe that the patient may not be aware that their arm and leg are weak. This is referred to as *anosognosia*. Rarely, some patients may not even recognise the limb as their own, a condition that is called *autotopagnosia*. These abnormalities are often associated with visual field disturbances, visual or sensory inattention and, if the frontal lobe is involved, hemiparesis.

There are a variety of tests that can be employed to demonstrate this neglect or 'lost in space'. These include bisecting a line, drawing a map of the country and placing the capital cities on the map or drawing a house, a bicycle, a daisy or a clock face. Invariably, one side of the illustration is not completed; some examples are shown in Figure 5.4.

These patients present in a state of bewilderment, or they are reluctantly brought to medical attention by a concerned relative, who has noticed their erratic behaviour although they themselves are totally unaware that anything is the matter. These patients become lost in their own home. For example, when arising at night to go to the bathroom, as they walk down the hallway the bathroom is on the left-hand side of their body and is not 'seen'. On their way back to the bedroom, they see the bathroom because it is on the right-hand side of their body, the side that they are not neglecting. Another example is a patient who suddenly cannot find their way home despite the fact that they have driven the same way home for 20 years.

The terms *inattention* and *neglect* are often confused by students. Inattention is rarely symptomatic and is elicited with bilateral simultaneous visual or sensory stimuli, while neglect can be thought of as a more severe form of inattention that results in significant symptoms and disability.

There are a number of very rare problems referred to as *apraxia* that may be seen in patients with parietal lobe dysfunction. Apraxia is an impairment of the ability to use objects correctly in the absence of any obvious physical disability that would prevent them from doing so. Apraxia can be elicited by requesting the patient to demonstrate how to use a toothbrush, hammer or comb [1–3]. These are described more fully at the end of this chapter.

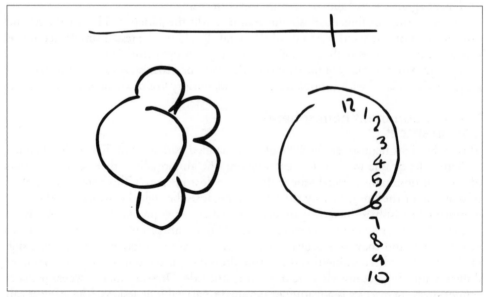

FIGURE 5.4 Diagrams that patients with left-sided neglect draw

The circles are usually incomplete, the numbers on a clock face or the petals on a daisy are missing down the left side and the left half of a line is neglected so that, when requested to divide the line in half, the patient draws a line through the right half of the line.

THE OCCIPITAL LOBES

The presenting symptoms of occipital lobe pathology include:
- Visual loss. The occipital lobes are the termination of the visual pathways and are essential for visual perception and recognition. The pathways are illustrated in Figure 4.1. The fibres from the medial half of the orbit cross in the optic chiasm, and lesions of the occipital lobe will result in a congruent contralateral visual field loss termed a homonymous hemianopia. Blindness can result from bilateral occipital lobe lesions and, in these circumstances, some patients are unaware that they are blind and behave as if they can see, a condition called Anton's syndrome or cortical blindness. The pupillary light reflexes are preserved and the eyes and fundi are normal to examination.
- Prosopagnosia. Very occasionally patients may present with prosopagnosia, which is an inability to recognise their own features in a mirror or the faces of other people. It is almost invariably associated with a visual field abnormality, usually an upper quadrantanopia.
- Visual illusions, also termed metamorphopsias, are distortions of size, form or colour. Objects may seem too small (micopsia) or too large (macropsia).
- Visual hallucinations, both unformed and formed, arise out of the occipital lobe or the junction between the occipital and temporal lobes. Formed visual hallucinations include objects, animals or people, but these may be of distorted size, either larger or smaller than normal. Unformed visual hallucinations include flashing lights, colours, stars, circles or squares and also reflect occipital lobe pathology.

THE CEREBELLUM

Disorders of the cerebellum were first characterised in the latter part of the 19th century and in the early part of the 20th century [5, 6]. Babinski recognised the impairment of rapid alternating movements and referred to this as dys- or adiadochokinesis [6].

The classic presenting features of disorders of the cerebellum include incoordination of voluntary movement (referred to as *ataxia*), a characteristic intention tremor (see Chapter 13, 'Abnormal movements and difficulty walking due to central nervous system problems') and difficulty walking due to disequilibrium and dysarthria.
- Ataxia is tested in the upper limbs by asking the patient to touch their nose and then your finger. Ensure that your finger is far enough away from the patient so that the patient has to extend their arms fully; if it is not, the patient can anchor their arm against the chest wall and disguise any ataxia. In the lower limbs ataxia is tested by asking the recumbent patient to lift their leg high up in the air and touch the examiner's finger and then place their heel on their own kneecap. One looks for unsteadiness as the patient's finger approaches the examiner's finger or their nose and as the heel approaches the finger or kneecap.
- Ataxia is often examined by watching the patient slide their heel down the shin. This, however, can disguise ataxia because the patient can stabilise their leg with the heel running along the shin. Abnormalities of cerebellar function will lead to the test being performed slowly and inaccurately.
- Cerebellar function is also tested by performing rapid alternating movements. For the upper limbs this is tested by asking the patient to tap the back and then the palm of their hand on the back of their other hand. For the lower limbs the patient taps their heel up and down on the floor.

- Patients with cerebellar disorders may also develop involuntary jerking of the eyes referred to as nystagmus. This is elicited by asking the patient to look up, down and to each side.
- The dysarthria that occurs with cerebellar dysfunction is characterised by slow slurring of the speech, or speech where the words are broken up into syllables, referred to as scanning dysarthria. This latter form of dysarthria is characteristic of cerebellar pathology. Another term that is very descriptive is *explosive speech* because the words are at times very soft and at other times very loud.
- Difficulty walking related to cerebellar dysfunction is discussed in Chapter 12, 'Back pain and common leg problems with or without difficulty walking'. In essence, lesions of the anterior of vermis of the cerebellum result in truncal ataxia while lesions affecting the cerebellar hemispheres cause ataxia of the limbs.

THE TEMPORAL LOBES

Patients presenting with symptoms related to temporal lobe pathology are less common than those with frontal, parietal or occipital lobe involvement. Symptoms include:
- fluent dysphasia
- visual field defects
- auditory, visual, olfactory and gustatory hallucinations
- memory problems.

The disorder of speech has been discussed earlier in this chapter. The visual field defect is a contralateral homonymous upper quadrantanopia. The various hallucinations are discussed in Chapter 8, 'Seizures and epilepsy'. Although the temporal lobes are involved with vestibular function, vertigo is only rarely seen with temporal lobe pathology; it may be the aura of a seizure (see Chapter 8).

Disturbances of memory

Memory includes three basic mental processes:
1 registration (the ability to perceive, recognise, and establish information in the central nervous system)
2 retention (the ability to retain registered information)
3 recall (the ability to retrieve stored information at will).

Short-term memory (which has been called immediate memory) has been defined as the reproduction, recognition or recall of perceived material within a period of up to 30 seconds after presentation.

Long-term memory can be divided into recent memory (events occurring during the past few hours or days), recent past memory (events occurring during the past few months) and remote memory (events occurring in past years).

TRANSIENT GLOBAL AMNESIA

Transient global amnesia (TGA) is one of the more commonly encountered disturbances of memory.

The diagnostic criteria include the episode being witnessed and involve anterograde amnesia. The patient must not have any evidence of neurological signs or deficits, features of epilepsy, active epilepsy or recent head injury. Finally the episode must have resolved within 24 hours [7]. These patients appear bewildered; they keep asking the same questions over and over again because they are unable to lay down new memory. Patients remain alert and attentive, and cognition is not impaired. However, they are disoriented in time and place. In all other respects they are normal. The duration of attacks is usually 1–8 hours but should be less than 24 hours. After the attack resolves, the period of amnesia shrinks with a permanent memory loss of variable duration from just a short period at the commencement of the episode to the entire episode.

The aetiology of this condition is unknown, but punctate lesions in the lateral aspect of the hippocampal formation on either side or bilaterally have been demonstrated by diffusion weighted MRI (dwMRI), not in the hyperacute phase but at 48 hours [8].

The difficulty with TGA is the lack of a gold standard test to confirm the diagnosis. There are a number of other conditions that can present with abrupt onset of a memory disturbance, including Wernicke–Korsakoff syndrome, cerebral ischaemia in the posterior circulation affecting the medial aspect of both temporal lobes, subarachnoid haemorrhage, following cerebral angiography, head injury and epilepsy. Establishing a diagnosis from the clinical features is not difficult if the episode has been witnessed, as most of the other conditions are associated with other neurological symptoms or signs.

DEMENTIA

Dementia is a global deterioration in intellectual functioning, in particular short-term memory, although remote memory is usually also significantly impaired in patients with dementia compared to that of non-demented persons of comparable age. There is also impairment of abstract thinking, judgement and other cortical functions and personality change.

There are many causes of dementia, and many are incompletely understood. The diagnosis is based on the clinical features with very few tests available to confirm the diagnosis.

A detailed discussion of dementia is beyond the scope of this chapter. A more detailed discussion can be found in Chapter 14, 'Miscellaneous neurological disorders'.

DEMENTIA VERSUS PSEUDODEMENTIA

Patients with severe depression may present with features suggesting possible dementia. This is referred to as pseudodementia. A prominent complaint is impaired memory, but during the history taking it becomes obvious that the patient can usually remember the details of the illness and that there is no other alteration in intellectual function.

TESTING HIGHER COGNITIVE FUNCTION

Higher cognitive function (HCF) consists of memory, orientation, concentration, language, stimulus recognition (examined by tests for agnosia), and performance of learned skilled movements (examined by tests for apraxia). Agnosia is the inability to recognise sensory stimuli and apraxia is the inability to use objects properly [4].

The Mini-Mental State Examination

The Mini-Mental State Examination [9] is a standardised, widely accepted test that is used to screen for cognitive impairment. It examines orientation in some detail and then briefly touches on registration and recall, attention/concentration, language and constructional abilities. It consists of 11 questions and can be administered in 5–10 minutes. This is a screening test that may indicate a need for more extensive testing. Details are given in Appendix A.

SOME RARER ABNORMALITIES OF HIGHER COGNITIVE FUNCTION

Agnosia

Agnosia is a disorder that is characterised by the inability to recognise and identify objects or persons. The more common types of agnosia are listed below.

- Auditory agnosia – the inability to recognise the significance of sounds (dominant temporal lobe)
- Finger agnosia – the loss of ability to indicate one's own or another's fingers (dominant parietal lobe)
- Tactile agnosia – the inability to recognise familiar objects by touch or feel (parieto-temporal cortices, possibly including the 2nd somatosensory cortex)
- Visual agnosia – the inability to recognise objects by sight (posterior occipital and/or temporal lobe(s) in the brain)
- Prosopagnosia – the inability to recognise faces of people well known or newly introduced to the patient (mesial cortex of occipital and temporal lobes)
- Anosognosia – the inability to recognise that a part of the body is affected by disease (non-dominant parietal lobe)

Apraxia

Apraxia is defined as a disorder of skilled movement not caused by weakness, akinesia, deafferentation, abnormal tone or posture, movement disorders such as tremors or chorea, intellectual deterioration, poor comprehension or uncooperativeness [10]. It is one of the best localising signs of the mental status examination and also predicts disability. Thus, for an experienced neurologist detection of the various forms of apraxia is very important. The more common forms of apraxia are listed below together with the most common site of the pathology.

- Sensory (ideational) apraxia – loss of the ability to make proper use of an object due to the lack of perception of its purpose (dominant posterior temporoparietal junction)
- Constructional apraxia – the individual fails to represent spatial relations correctly in drawing or construction (non-dominant parietal lobe)
- Ideomotor apraxia – simple single acts can be performed but not a sequence of acts (dominant parietal lobe and the premotor cortex)
- Dressing apraxia – difficulty in orienting articles of clothing with reference to the body; the obvious test is to ask the patient to put on an article of clothing (non-dominant parietal lobe if one side is neglected but dominant if absolutely no idea how to dress)

Wernicke–Korsakoff encephalopathy

The reason for including Wernicke–Korsakoff syndrome in this book is that although rare it is preventable and treatable by the prompt administration of parenteral thiamine. It should be regarded as a medical emergency and, as a general rule, thiamine should be given to all confused patients.

The term Wernicke encephalopathy [11, 12] is used to describe the clinical triad of confusion, ataxia and nystagmus (or ophthalmoplegia). At autopsy, punctate hemorrhages affecting the gray matter around the 3rd and 4th ventricles and aqueduct of Sylvius are seen. When persistent learning and memory deficits are present, the symptom complex is often called Wernicke–Korsakoff syndrome. Korsakoff syndrome or amnestic disorder is characterised by the inability to learn new information, while other higher cognitive functions are retained. Lack of motivation, lack of insight, a flat affect and denial of difficulties are common. Spontaneous speech is minimal. Confabulation (false memories which the patient believes to be true) may occur in the early stages but usually disappears with time. These patients are severely disabled and are usually incapable of independent living. The syndrome is due to thiamine (vitamin B_1) deficiency related to malnutrition and is very common in patients suffering from alcoholism.

The onset is over days to weeks and, although all the features can develop simultaneously, the initial manifestation is often ataxia followed later by confusion. The nystagmus is both vertical and horizontal and is usually associated with bilateral 6th nerve palsies. The truncal ataxia can be so severe it renders the patient unable to walk. Limb ataxia, dysarthria and intention tremor are rare.

REFERENCES

1 Adams RD, Victor M. Principles of neurology. New York: McGraw–Hill Book Company; 1985:1186.
2 Rowland LP (ed). Merritt's textbook of neurology. Vol 11e. Philadelphia, PA: Lippincott Williams & Wilkins; 2005.
3 Wilson JD et al (eds). Harrison's principles of internal medicine, 12th edn. New York: McGraw–Hill; 1991.
4 Dorland's pocket medical dictionary, 21st edn. Philadelphia: WB Saunders Company; 1968.
5 Holmes G. The cerebellum of man: Hughlings Jackson lecture. Brain 1939; 62:1.
6 Babinski J. De l'asynergie cerebelleuse. Rev Neurol 1899; 7:806.
7 Hodges JR, Warlow CP. Syndromes of transient amnesia: Towards a classification. A study of 153 cases. J Neurol Neurosurg Psychiatry 1990; 53(10):834–843.
8 Sedlaczek O et al. Detection of delayed focal MR changes in the lateral hippocampus in transient global amnesia. Neurology 2004; 62(12):2165–2170.
9 Folstein MF, Folstein SE, McHugh PR. "Mini-mental state". A practical method for grading the cognitive state of patients for the clinician. J Psychiatr Res 1975; 12(3):189–198.
10 Heilman KM, Rothi LJG. Apraxia. In: Heilman KM, Valenstein E (eds). Clinical neuropsychology. Oxford: Oxford University Press; 1993:141–163.
11 Thomson AD et al. Wernicke's encephalopathy revisited. [translation of the case history section of the original manuscript by Carl Wernicke 'Lehrbuch der Gehirnkrankheiten fur Aerzte and Studirende' (1881) with a commentary]. Alcohol 2008; 43(2):174–179.
12 Pearce JM. Wernicke–Korsakoff encephalopathy. Eur Neurol 2008; 59(1–2):101–104.

chapter 6

After the History and Examination, What Next?

Upon completing the history and examination, the next step is determined by the following factors:

- diagnostic certainty
- the availability of tests to confirm or exclude certain diagnoses
- the potential complications of those tests
- the severity and level of urgency in terms of the consequences of a particular illness not being diagnosed and treated promptly
- the benefit versus risk profile of any potential treatment
- the presence of any social factors or past medical history that could influence a course of action or treatment in this particular patient.

This chapter will discuss each of these aspects and how they influence the course of action.

LEVEL OF CERTAINTY OF DIAGNOSIS

There are three possible scenarios:
1 A particular diagnosis seems obvious.
2 One particular diagnosis is not apparent, and there are several possible diagnoses.
3 You have no idea what is wrong with the patient.

A particular diagnosis seems certain

In most instances the diagnosis is apparent. In the general practice setting almost 90% of diagnoses are established at the completion of the history and examination [1]. In one outpatient clinic this figure was 73% (history 56% and examination 17%) in patients with cardiovascular, neurological, respiratory, urinary and other miscellaneous problems [2]. In patients with neurological problems the initial diagnosis is less obvious and was correct in only 60% of patients presenting to an emergency department [3]. In this setting the appropriate course of action is to initiate investigations that can confirm the diagnosis, exclude alternative diagnoses with potentially more severe adverse outcomes and institute a plan of management taking into account factors in the past, social and medical drug history that would influence management in this particular patient.

A word of caution: being absolutely certain *is potentially the most dangerous scenario*. Doctors are strongly anchored by their initial diagnoses [4] (see Case 6.1) and are at risk of closing their minds to possible alternatives, often in the presence of clinical features or results from investigations that should raise doubt about the diagnosis.

CASE 6.1   An incorrect initial diagnosis

An example is a 65-year-old patient with confusion and headache who was treated for herpes zoster (HZV) meningoencephalitis because the CSF contained HZV DNA. The CSF findings of a very high white cell count and protein level and very low glucose level were most atypical for HZV meningoencephalitis. In addition, the patient was failing to respond to the appropriate treatment for HZV. The positive test for DNA related to the presence of herpes zoster ophthalmicus [5]. The patient had malignant meningitis.

Doctors recognise patterns of familiar problems with respect to critical cues [6]. Doctors who are more experienced appear to weigh their first impressions more heavily than those who are less experienced and at risk of closing their minds early on in the diagnostic process [7]. Even experienced clinicians may be unaware of the correctness of their diagnoses when they initially make them [8].

If there are tests to confirm the diagnosis, it is appropriate to perform those tests, provided the patient is informed of the risks associated with them. When ordering tests and reviewing the results, it is most important to be aware of the **sensitivity** and **specificity** and the influence of the prevalence of the disease on the **positive predictive value** and the **negative predictive value** of those tests [9] (for a discussion of these concepts, refer to the section 'Understanding and interpreting test results' below).

If there are no tests, one can proceed cautiously with management, but it is most important to review the response to therapy. A lack of response to therapy or the emergence of unexpected side effects (the latter is a personal observation) is often a clue that the diagnosis is incorrect. Conversely, *a response to a therapy does not prove the diagnosis.* This author has seen patients with vertebral artery dissection, viral meningitis and pituitary cysts 'respond' to treatment for migraine. This is discussed in more detail below.

There are several possible diagnoses

It is imperative to keep the diagnostic options open by making provisional diagnoses while keeping alternatives in mind. Be circumspect and take action to minimise the possibility of missing other critical diagnoses [10]. Once again, if there are tests that can differentiate one particular diagnosis from another, it would be most appropriate to perform those tests. If a specific diagnosis cannot be made following the investigations, the approach is similar to that discussed in the following section.

You have no idea what is wrong

In the setting of uncertainty there are several possible courses of action. A *particularly useful strategy is to start again:* take a more detailed history and repeat the examination.[1] This is the approach recommended when you have absolutely no idea what the diagnosis is. In this situation performing many tests is often misleading because of the sensitivity and specificity of tests.

If you have elicited a detailed history, but still have no idea what is wrong with the patient, there are several options including:

- wait and see
- perform investigations

---

1   Recommended to the author by Dr Arthur Schwieger in 1985 and, to this day, remains one of the most powerful clinical tools available.

- seek a second opinion
- consult a textbook
- search for an answer on the Internet.

These various approaches will be discussed in terms of their relative merits and deficiencies.

WAIT AND SEE

In resolving uncertainty, time is a very powerful diagnostic tool. The idea is to wait for a period of time in the hope that the diagnosis becomes clear or the patient gets better [10], [11]. The effective use of this approach requires considerable skill, however. Often in this situation a doctor may order unnecessary tests in the hope that a diagnosis may be established; most often it is not. If the 'wait and see' approach is adopted, it is important to:

- inform the patient that there is uncertainty
- advise them of the possible outcomes
- recommend that they report immediately should symptoms worsen or if any new symptoms develop.

Shared medical decision making is a process in which patients and providers consider outcome probabilities and patient preferences and reach a healthcare decision based on mutual agreement. Shared decision making is best employed for problems involving medical uncertainty [12]. However, it is important to consider the fact that not all patients wish to be involved in shared medical decisions [13].

UNDERTAKE INVESTIGATIONS

In most cases there are tests that can confirm or exclude a particular disease. In this situation it is important to understand the concepts of the sensitivity and specificity of tests and the importance of prevalence of the disease. The essential questions to ask when considering investigations include:

- In what way will the results, whether positive or negative, alter the management of this patient?
- What is the risk of undertaking the test?

There is a more detailed discussion of investigations later in this chapter.

There are no tests for some diseases and the diagnosis is based entirely on the clinical features. When there are several possible diagnoses or when one has absolutely no idea what the diagnosis might be, performing numerous tests in the hope of making a diagnosis is a wonderful way of giving the illusion that something useful is being done when often all that may be achieved is stalling or buying time. It is a tactic that is used by a number of clinicians in the hope that a diagnosis will be made by a test result (unlikely), the illness will progress so that the diagnosis will become apparent or the patient's problem will resolve. A reasonable approach is to think of the worst case scenario (the most serious diagnosis that the symptoms could represent, a diagnosis that if missed could result in an adverse outcome) and proceed accordingly.

OBTAIN A SECOND OPINION

Although doctors prefer to obtain information from journals and books, they often consult colleagues to get answers to clinical and research questions [14], [15]. Even for doctors whose first choice of information source was the medical literature – either books or journals – the most frequent second choice was consultations [14].

In a study of 254 referrals seen by a neurologist there was a significant change in diagnosis in 55%, and in management in nearly 70% [16].

There are several ways of obtaining a second opinion:
- the 'informal consultation with a colleague'
    - telephone advice
    - the 'curbside' conversation in the corridor without actually seeing the patient
    - presenting at meetings and seeking several opinions, often but not invariably with the patient at the meeting
- the 'formal second opinion' when a colleague is asked to see the patient.

Telephone advice
Telephoning a colleague for advice is common. The recipient of the call is in a very difficult situation as providing the correct advice very much depends on being given the correct history and examination findings. An experienced clinician often knows the particular questions to ask and can decide if and when they should actually see the patient. It is probably wiser for an inexperienced clinician to arrange to formally see the patient in consultation.

Corridor or curbside consultation
'Corridor or curbside consultation' is another approach used often [17]. Unfortunately, and sometimes with dire consequences, this is used by medical practitioners to seek informal advice about their own medical problems. The model of a good curbside consultation 'is to say what you know and what you don't know. Then you hope the person you are consulting with will treat you with respect' [17]. Requesting doctors who could not present relevant information, frame a clear question or answer consultant questions in a well-informed manner were generally asked to formally refer the patient [17]. Perley et al [17] commented that tacit rules govern curbside consultation interactions, and negative consequences result when the rules are misunderstood or not observed.

Once again, the correct advice very much depends on being given the correct information. The neurologist providing advice will want to know the mode of onset and progression of the symptoms of the current illness together with the EXACT nature and distribution of the symptoms and the abnormal neurological signs, if present. It is difficult for inexperienced clinicians to perform detailed neurological examinations but there should be no reason why, as outlined in Chapter 2, 'The neurological history', an inexperienced clinician cannot obtain a detailed history. Finally, the neurologist would want information about the social, past and drug history that may influence any subsequent course of action.

Clinical meetings
Second opinions are often sought for the purpose of diagnosis and/or treatment in clinical meetings. There is the perception that one is obtaining multiple opinions. Although this can be a valuable tool, particularly if one of the participants identifies the problem, in a more complex case often what is said in meetings is very different to what is said in a formal consultation. Thus, the advice obtained in clinical meetings should be viewed circumspectly. A brain biopsy is often recommended in clinical meetings, but not often performed despite the recommendation.[2]

The formal second opinion
The formal second opinion is probably the most effective method of dealing with diagnostic or therapeutic uncertainties. *There is no shame in asking a colleague to formally see the patient for a second opinion.* If you do, it can be a learning experience; if you do

---

2 Personal observation.

not and the patient perceives a lack of progress, they will independently seek a second opinion and you will miss out on a learning opportunity. If a patient requests a second opinion, NEVER hesitate to arrange one.

Remember a second opinion is simply that; you are the clinician caring for the patient and the 'buck stops with you'. You must decide if the second opinion is useful or not and act accordingly – this may include obtaining a third opinion!

CONSULT A TEXTBOOK

Yet another approach is to consult textbooks. This is useful if you are looking at the clinical features of a particular disease(s) or to learn what investigations would be appropriate. However, therapy is evolving so rapidly that recommended therapy in textbooks is soon out of date.

SEARCH THE INTERNET

An increasingly popular and useful strategy is to search the Internet[3] [18–20]. Patients frequently look for answers on the internet [21]. In the author's own experience many patients bring the results of their searches to the consultation. In one study [19] Google was able to make the correct diagnosis in 58% of the cases in the *New England Journal of Medicine* clinical-pathological conferences. In a comparison of PubMed, Scopus, Web of Science and Google Scholar, the keyword search function of PubMed was superior. While Google Scholar could retrieve the most obscure of information, its use was marred by inadequate and less frequently updated citation information [22]. Searching in Google Scholar can be refined by adding + emedicine to the search [23]. For example, 'trigeminal neuralgia' yields 48,000 'hits' while 'trigeminal neuralgia + emedicine' retrieves 478 references. Many remain skeptical [24] and, as recently as 2 years ago, Twisselmann stated that the jury is still out on whether searching for symptoms on the Internet is the way forward for doctors and consumers [25].

The author has adopted the practice of frequently consulting the Internet even in the midst of a formal consultation.[4] It is a useful way to look for any new advances in therapy, to provide information to the patient or referring practitioner by adding the abstracts and references to the letter or even to search for an obscure diagnosis (see Case 6.2).

CASE 6.2 A trumpet player with nasal escape

This example illustrates how this approach can be very useful. A young trumpet player developed nasal escape of air after 30 minutes of playing and could not continue to play. The symptoms took too long to develop and persisted for too long after cessation of playing to be related to myasthenia gravis. A quick search of 'trumpet player and nasal escape' revealed the diagnosis of a very rare condition termed velopharyngeal incompetence [26].

---

3 Websites with instructions for searching the Internet for medical information are at the end of this chapter. Chapter 15, 'Further reading, keeping up-to-date and retrieving information', lists many relevant websites together with their URLs.

4 It is important to inform the patient that you are looking up something that might help with their problem and not to spend too long or the patient will feel neglected. If you cannot find a ready answer, continue the search at a later time.

An online information retrieval system [27] was associated with a significant improvement in the quality of answers provided by clinicians to typical clinical problems. In a small proportion of cases, use of the system produced errors [27]. Despite ready access to the Internet many doctors do not yet use it in a just-in-time manner to immediately solve difficult patient problems but instead continue to rely on consultation with colleagues [28, 29]. One major obstacle is the time it takes to search for information. Other difficulties primary care doctors experience are related to formulating an appropriate search question, finding an optimal search strategy and interpreting the evidence found [29].

Computer programs that can be used as an aid in diagnosing multiple congenital anomaly syndromes have been used for many years and are designed to aid the paediatrician diagnose rare disorders in children [30]. Other computer-aided software systems for diagnosing neurological diseases exist [31], and it is likely that more software will be developed in the future. Such software will always be dependent upon the information provided by the user.

AVAILABILITY OF TESTS TO CONFIRM OR EXCLUDE CERTAIN DIAGNOSES

This section discusses the general principles of investigations or tests. Essentially it will cover why tests give the 'wrong' or unexpected result and what to do when this occurs. There are many excellent books that discuss the interpretation of tests in great detail [32–34].

Understanding and interpreting test results

SENSITIVITY, SPECIFICITY, POSITIVE AND NEGATIVE PREDICTIVE VALUES

In order to understand how to interpret investigations correctly, you need to understand some basic principles. All tests have an associated sensitivity, specificity and positive and negative predictive values and are very much influenced by the prior likelihood that the disease is present in a particular patient. The usefulness of a test is very dependent on the prior probability that a patient has a particular disease, i.e. the prevalence of the disease.

- **Sensitivity** refers to how good a test is at correctly identifying people who have the disease.
- **Specificity** is concerned with how good the test is at correctly excluding people who do not have the condition.
- **Positive predictive value** refers to the chance that a positive test result will be correct.
- **Negative predictive value** is concerned only with negative test results.

For any diagnostic test, the positive predictive value will fall as the prevalence of the disease falls while the negative predictive value will rise. In practice, since most diseases have a low prevalence, even when the tests we use have apparently good sensitivity and specificity, the positive predictive value may be very low.

Table 6.1 shows the results of a test with a sensitivity of 90% and a specificity of 80%. When the test is performed on 100 patients with the suspected diagnosis, 10 patients with the diagnosis will have a negative test while 20 patients who do not have that particular diagnosis will have an incorrect positive test. The ideal test would be one with 100% sensitivity and 100% specificity, but this does not occur.

The pre-test likelihood of a patient having a particular diagnosis also greatly influences how a test result should be interpreted. Using the same values for sensitivity and

TABLE 6.1 The influence of sensitivity (90%) and specificity (80%) of a test on the results for 100 patients with the suspected diagnosis

	+ve Test	−ve Test
Patient has disease	90	10
Patient does not have disease	20	80

TABLE 6.2 The effect of a 50% likelihood that the patient has a disease and the influence of the sensitivity and specificity on the number of correct diagnoses (n = 100)

	+ve Test	−ve Test
Patient has disease	45	5
Patient does not have disease	5	45

Note: An equal number of patients with the disease will have a negative test as patients without the disease will have a positive test.

TABLE 6.3 The number of positive and negative test results when the likelihood of a particular diagnosis is low (10%), i.e. doing tests to exclude rare conditions causes more problems than it solves (n = 100)

	+ve Test	−ve Test
Patient has disease	9	1
Patient does not have disease	18	72

specificity, if 100 patients are tested for a particular diagnosis when only 50 of them have that diagnosis (see Table 6.2), a positive test will detect 45 of the patients with the disease (90% of 50) but the test will also be positive in 10 (20% of 50) patients who do not have the disease!

If the prior probability of a particular diagnosis being present is even lower, the results will be even more dramatic. If the patient is very unlikely to have the disease, say a 10% chance (i.e. 10 in every 100 patients tested), with the same sensitivity and specificity of 90% and 80%, respectively, a positive result will correctly identify 9 patients with the disease but will incorrectly diagnose 18 patients without the disease (90% of 10 = 9 and 20% of 90 = 18). The rarer the problem, the more certain we can be that a negative test excludes that disease, but less certain that a positive test indicates an abnormality (see Table 6.3).

In this setting a negative test in the presence of a strong suspicion of a diagnosis may lead inexperienced clinicians to dismiss that diagnosis. The antithesis of this is a patient being incorrectly diagnosed with a particular illness because of a false positive test.

The variability in prevalence of a particular disease between one study and another means that predictive values found in one study do not apply universally [35]. A common practice of inexperienced doctors is to repeat borderline abnormal tests simply because the result is 'outside the normal range' even when the test result is irrelevant to the clinical problem. In this situation it is better to discuss the result with the relevant pathologist or radiologist.

INCIDENTAL AND IRRELEVANT FINDINGS ON TESTS: THE 'INCIDENTALOMA'

An 'incidentaloma' is the finding of an abnormality on a test, usually some form of medical imaging, which is not related to the patient's symptoms and signs. Typical examples of this include the presence of a degenerative disease in the cervical, thoracic or lumbar spine with advancing age that may be completely asymptomatic, an asymptomatic lacunar cerebral infarct or an unidentified bright object on MRI scan in a patient being investigated for headaches. Often only experience can teach and provide the confidence to ignore such incidental findings.

WHY TESTS GIVE THE WRONG RESULT AND WHAT TO DO WHEN THIS OCCURS

Although the sensitivities and specificities of investigations largely explain why tests may be negative or positive in the wrong setting, a test may also be negative for a number of other reasons. Patients with intermittent disturbances of neurological function will usually have normal tests between events; the test will only be positive if the examiner happens to capture an event and, if episodes are infrequent, this is unlikely. Symptoms can also precede the development of abnormalities that can be detected with currently available investigations, e.g. carpal tunnel syndrome, acute inflammatory demyelinating peripheral neuropathy, where the nerve conduction studies can be normal in the early stages, or patients with a cerebral infarct, where a CT scan of the brain can be normal for several hours after the onset of the infarction.

Other causes of a 'negative test' are when the test is directed to the wrong part of the body or the test that is ordered is not suitable for detecting abnormalities in that region. For example, a patient may present with difficulty walking and a normal CT scan of the lumbosacral spine when they have a problem in the cervical or thoracic spinal cord, and a CT scan of the thoracic spine is negative because it is not a sensitive enough test for detecting abnormalities in this region.

The relative 'fallibility' of tests emphasises the importance of the detailed history and examination. If you are absolutely certain that a patient has a particular diagnosis, then a negative test should not dissuade you from that diagnosis. The corollary of this is a positive test should not imply a diagnosis if the symptoms and signs are not consistent with that diagnosis.

HOW QUICKLY SHOULD TESTS BE PERFORMED?

This is discussed below in the section 'Severity and urgency: the potential consequences of a particular illness not being diagnosed and treated'.

THE POSSIBLE COMPLICATIONS OF TESTS

There are very few tests that are not associated with risk. Venesection is perfectly safe in close to 100% of patients but rarely can be associated with injury to a nerve that can result in long-term pain and dysaesthesia. Although this complication is extremely rare (<0.02% [36]), the result can be very distressing.

When ordering any investigation it is important to consider the potential complications of the test in relation to the seriousness of the illness that is being investigated. A patient with a life-threatening illness might be willing to consider a potentially life-threatening investigation if it could make a significant difference; on the other hand, a patient with symptoms without disability would be concerned about any investigation that might cause harm.

It is most important that the patient is fully informed of the risks versus benefits of the procedure beforehand.

SEVERITY AND URGENCY: THE POTENTIAL CONSEQUENCES OF A PARTICULAR ILLNESS NOT BEING DIAGNOSED AND TREATED

In everyday clinical practice if a diagnosis is clearly established, knowledge of the natural history of this condition would dictate how quickly one would investigate and treat the patient. Clearly, patients presenting comatose or with status epilepticus (a seizure that lasts more than 30 minutes, or recurrent seizures without return of consciousness between seizures) require urgent intervention.

The difficulty arises in the patient with a neurological problem when there is uncertainty as to the diagnosis. There is very little in the literature that can provide guidance in this area. Scoring tools for priority setting for general surgery and hip and knee surgery were useful but were not particularly good for MRI scanning [37]. The discussion below contains observations made by this author during many years of clinical practice and observations from colleagues who were asked specifically, 'What do you think constitutes an urgent problem?'

The overriding principle is to consider the worst case scenario. It is prudent to consider the most serious possible diagnosis that, if left untreated, could result in significant morbidity or mortality. This will dictate the 'level of urgency' and how promptly a doctor should act (see Case 6.3).

CASE 6.3 Assessing urgency in a patient with an uncertain diagnosis

An example is a patient who presents with symptoms that suggest cerebral ischaemia, but the diagnosis is far from certain. Discuss with the patient that there is uncertainty regarding the diagnosis and that, if it is not treated as cerebral ischaemia when it is (i.e. an inappropriate course of action is taken), the consequences could be potentially disastrous. On the other hand, if investigation and treatment on the basis that it may be cerebral ischaemia can be undertaken without significant risk, then often that is a reasonable approach until the diagnosis can be clarified with more certainty.

Experienced clinicians can often accurately assess the level of urgency in a particular clinical setting. Although this may well relate to their level of expertise and 'having seen it before', more often it is because they use the tempo of the illness (the rapidity of development of symptoms and signs) to dictate how quickly they should act.
- *Rapidly evolving weakness* dictates immediate action.
- Although not all patients with *symptoms related to the spinal cord* have urgent neurological problems, disorders in this region can result in devastating neurological deficits and the degree of recovery is very dependent on the severity of the spinal cord lesion [38]. The investigations should be prompt if one suspects spinal cord disease.[5] One would consider spinal cord problems with leg weakness and, particularly if there is associated sphincter disturbance, with bilateral leg weakness if the

---

5 The author was once told by a senior consultant 'the spinal cord is unforgiving'.

TABLE 6.4 Some urgent and non-urgent clinical presentations

Very urgent	Less urgent
LOC	Symptoms lasting seconds
Status epilepticus	Symptoms without functional loss
Recurrent symptoms within a short period	Isolated sensory symptoms
	Intermittent symptoms affecting multiple organ systems as well as the nervous system

LOC = loss of consciousness

lesion is in the thoracic spinal cord and four-limb weakness if the lesion is in the cervical spinal cord.

- Similarly, patients with *symptoms related to the brainstem* such as diplopia, dysphagia and vertigo, particularly if combined with ataxia or limb weakness, should be investigated as a matter of urgency.
- Patients with *recurrent symptoms within a short period of time* should also be dealt with as a matter of urgency. As a general rule, symptoms of weakness are more likely to imply significant neurological problems rather than isolated sensory symptoms.
- Similarly, *symptoms associated with loss of function* are more likely to be significant than symptoms without functional loss. Patients with multiple symptoms not associated with any loss of function, particularly if also associated with non-neurological symptoms, are less likely to have a serious illness requiring urgent intervention. Transient symptoms lasting seconds are also unlikely to be of any significance. One study found that higher numbers of physical symptoms and the complaint of pain were indicators of possible non-organic disease [39].

A summary of urgent and non-urgent presentations is given in Table 6.4. A simple rule is: 'if in doubt do not hesitate to ask for help'.

THE BENEFIT VERSUS RISK PROFILE OF ANY POTENTIAL TREATMENT

All medical interventions, whether they are pharmacological or surgical, have the potential to cause harm.

- Most patients can tolerate most drugs with few or no side effects. When a diagnosis is clearly established, the choice of the appropriate treatment would primarily be dictated by the knowledge that one particular therapy has greater efficacy than another.
- On the other hand, if there are several treatments with equal efficacy, the choice of therapy would then depend on the risk profile and the patient's willingness to consider particular side effects. For example, there may be two or three drugs that could be used to treat a patient who suffers from epilepsy; the drugs that may cause weight gain or interfere with the oral contraceptive pill would be most unacceptable to a young female patient.
- In the setting where the diagnosis is uncertain and one is instituting empirical therapy, it is important to inform the patient of the perceived benefits of the therapy prescribed but also to alert the patient to the potential risks of that therapy. More

importantly, carefully monitor the response to therapy and be willing to reconsider the diagnosis and/or choice of therapy.

SOCIAL FACTORS AND PAST MEDICAL PROBLEMS THAT MAY INFLUENCE A COURSE OF ACTION OR TREATMENT

This has already been discussed briefly in Chapter 2, 'The neurological history', where the importance of not using information about the past history, family history and social history to make a diagnosis was stressed. Once a diagnosis is established, however, the subsequent management of the patient is very much influenced by their past medical history, their social circumstances and, more importantly, the drugs that they are currently taking.

* Ten to thirty per cent of admissions to hospital are due to iatrogenic drug-related problems [40, 41]. Computer software can alert clinicians to the potential for drug interactions and should be consulted when prescribing a new medication.
* Other medical problems will have a major impact on subsequent management and may limit the therapeutic options as a choice of therapy could be contraindicated in that condition.
* Similarly, an elderly patient who has the support of spouse and family can be managed at home as opposed to the patient who has no support and who develops an illness that would prevent them from living independently.

REFERENCES

1 Crombie DL. Diagnostic process. J Coll Gen Pract 1963; 6:579–589.
2 Sandler G. Costs of unnecessary tests. BMJ 1979; 2(6181):21–24.
3 Moeller JJ et al. Diagnostic accuracy of neurological problems in the emergency department. Can J Neurol Sci 2008; 35(3):335–341.
4 Berner ES et al. Clinician performance and prominence of diagnoses displayed by a clinical diagnostic decision support system. AMIA Annu Symp Proc 2003:76–80.
5 Gregoire SM et al. Polymerase chain reaction analysis and oligoclonal antibody in the cerebrospinal fluid from 34 patients with varicella-zoster virus infection of the nervous system. J Neurol Neurosurg Psychiatry 2006; 77(8):938–942.
6 Coughlin LD, Patel VL. Processing of critical information by physicians and medical students. J Med Educ 1987; 62(10):818–828.
7 Eva KW, Cunnington JP. The difficulty with experience: Does practice increase susceptibility to premature closure? J Contin Educ Health Prof 2006; 26(3):192–198.
8 Friedman CP et al. Do physicians know when their diagnoses are correct? Implications for decision support and error reduction. J Gen Intern Med 2005; 20(4):334–339.
9 Loong TW. Understanding sensitivity and specificity with the right side of the brain. BMJ 2003; 327(7417):716–719.
10 Hewson MG et al. Strategies for managing uncertainty and complexity. J Gen Intern Med 1996; 11(8):481–485.
11 Sloane PD et al. Introduction to clinical problems. In: Essentials of family medicine. Sloane PD, Slatt LM, Ebell MH, Jacques LB, Smith MA (eds). Philadelphia: Lippincott Williams & Wilkins; 2007:126.
12 Frosch DL, Kaplan RM. Shared decision making in clinical medicine: Past research and future directions. Am J Prev Med 1999; 17(4):285–294.
13 Levinson W et al. Not all patients want to participate in decision making. A national study of public preferences. J Gen Intern Med 2005; 20(6):531–535.
14 Haug JD. Physicians' preferences for information sources: A meta-analytic study. Bull Med Libr Assoc 1997; 85(3):223–232.
15 Campbell EJ. Use of the telephone in consultant practice. BMJ 1978; 2(6154):1784–1785.
16 Roberts K et al. What difference does a neurologist make in a general hospital? Estimating the impact of neurology consultations on in-patient care. Ir J Med Sci 2007; 176(3):211–214.
17 Perley CM. Physician use of the curbside consultation to address information needs: Report on a collective case study. J Med Libr Assoc 2006; 94(2):137–144.

18 Maulden SA. Information technology, the internet, and the future of neurology. Neurologist 2003; 9(3):149–159.

19 Tang H, Ng JH. Googling for a diagnosis – use of Google as a diagnostic aid: Internet based study. BMJ 2006; 333(7579):1143–1145.

20 Yu H, Kaufman D. A cognitive evaluation of four online search engines for answering definitional questions posed by physicians. Pac Symp Biocomput 2007:328–339.

21 Shuyler KS, Knight KM. What are patients seeking when they turn to the Internet? Qualitative content analysis of questions asked by visitors to an orthopaedics web site. J Med Internet Res 2003; 5(4):e24.

22 Falagas ME et al. Comparison of PubMed, Scopus, Web of Science, and Google Scholar: Strengths and weaknesses. FASEB J 2008; 22(2):338–342.

23 Taubert M. Use of Google as a diagnostic aid: Bias your search. BMJ 2006; 333(7581):1270; author reply 1270.

24 Rapid responses. Googling for a diagnosis – use of Google as a diagnostic aid: Internet based study. 2006. Available: www.bmj.com/cgi/eletters/333/7579/1143 (1 Dec 2009).

25 Twisselmann B. Use of Google as a diagnostic aid: Summary of other responses. BMJ 2006; 333(7581):1270–1271.

26 Conley SF, Beecher RB, Marks S. Stress velopharyngeal incompetence in an adolescent trumpet player. Ann Otol Rhinol Laryngol 1995; 104(9 Pt 1):715–717.

27 Westbrook JI, Coiera EW, Gosling AS. Do online information retrieval systems help experienced clinicians answer clinical questions? J Am Med Inform Assoc 2005; 12(3):315–321.

28 Bennett NL et al. Information-seeking behaviors and reflective practice. J Contin Educ Health Prof 2006; 26(2):120–127.

29 Coumou HC, Meijman FJ. How do primary care physicians seek answers to clinical questions? A literature review. J Med Libr Assoc 2006; 94(1):55–60.

30 Pelz J, Arendt V, Kunze J. Computer assisted diagnosis of malformation syndromes: An evaluation of three databases (LDDB, POSSUM, and SYNDROC). Am J Med Genet 1996; 63(1):257–267.

31 Computer-aided diagnosis software for neurological diseases. 2007. Available: http://www.flintbox.com/technology.asp?page=3087&lID=MCU (1 Dec 2009).

32 Sackett DL et al. Evidence-based medicine. How to practice and teach EBM. Toronto: Churchill Livingsone; 2000:261.

33 Greenhalgh T. How to read a paper. The basics of evidence based medicine, 2nd edn. London: BMJ; 2001:222.

34 Sackett DL, Haynes RB, Tugwell P. Clinical epidemiology: A basic science for clinical medicine. Boston: Little, Brown; 1985:370.

35 Altman, D.G. and J.M. Bland, *Diagnostic tests 2: Predictive values.* BMJ, 1994. 309(6947): p.102.

36 Newman BH, Waxman DA. Blood donation-related neurologic needle injury: Evaluation of 2 years' worth of data from a large blood center. Transfusion 1996; 36(3):213–215.

37 Noseworthy TW, McGurran JJ, Hadorn DC. Waiting for scheduled services in Canada: Development of priority-setting scoring systems. J Eval Clin Pract 2003; 9(1):23–31.

38 Catz A et al. Recovery of neurologic function following nontraumatic spinal cord lesions in Israel. Spine 2004; 29(20):2278–2282; discussion 2283.

39 Fitzpatrick R, Hopkins A. Referrals to neurologists for headaches not due to structural disease. J Neurol Neurosurg Psychiatry 1981; 44(12):1061–1067.

40 Koh Y, Fatimah BM, Li SC. Therapy related hospital admission in patients on polypharmacy in Singapore: A pilot study. Pharm World Sci 2003; 25(4):135–137.

41 Courtman BJ, Stallings SB. Characterization of drug-related problems in elderly patients on admission to a medical ward. Can J Hosp Pharm 1995; 48(3):161–166.

WEBSITES

The following are websites that illustrate how to search the Internet for medical information:

PubMed Tutorial: http://www.nlm.nih.gov/bsd/disted/pubmed.html

Google Web Search Help Centre: http://www.google.com/support/bin/static.py?page=searchguides.html&ctx=advanced&hl=en

UC Berkeley Library Internet Searching Tutorial: http://lib.berkeley.edu/TeachingLib/Guides/Internet/FindInfo.html

chapter 7

Episodic Disturbances of Neurological Function

The assessment of patients with intermittent disturbances of neurological function is one of the most interesting and challenging aspects of clinical neurology. One needs to be an amateur detective like Sherlock Holmes, whom Arthur Conan Doyle modelled on Dr Joseph Bell, one of his teachers at the medical school of Edinburgh University. Dr Bell was a master at observation, logic, deduction and diagnosis [1]. This chapter discusses the various causes of episodic disturbance of neurological function. There is only a brief discussion of epilepsy and cerebrovascular disease as they are covered in more detail in Chapter 8, 'Seizures and epilepsy', and Chapter 10, 'Cerebrovascular disease', respectively. Vertigo is discussed in this chapter as most often it is an episodic disturbance, but mainly because it seemed to fit better in this chapter than in any other.

Patients are rarely seen by the neurologist during the episode. Therefore, the diagnosis of intermittent disturbances of neurological function is almost entirely dependent on the history. As the symptoms are episodic, these patients rarely if ever have any abnormal neurological signs and investigations only rarely yield a diagnosis.

- If you have only 30 minutes, spend 29 on the history, 1 on the examination and none on tests.
- Sometimes a diagnosis is not possible when the patient is first seen. Provided you are convinced that a delay in diagnosis would not lead to a severe adverse outcome, give the patient a list of things to observe that will help clarify the diagnosis.

Sometimes it is not possible to diagnose the problem when the patient first presents. A very useful technique is to send the patient away with a list of things to observe and record. This will often enable a diagnosis to be made at a subsequent consultation. However, this technique can only be employed if the episodes are likely to be benign and the patient is advised to avoid activities that could result in harm should an event recur during that activity. For example, where there is a suspicion of epilepsy patients should be advised not to drive, go swimming, have a bath alone etc.

THE HISTORY AND INTERMITTENT DISTURBANCES

Most inexperienced clinicians simply ascertain the nature of the symptoms. They do not determine their exact distribution, the mode of onset and progression of each and every symptom, particularly in relation to the other symptoms, nor the circumstances under which symptoms occur, which often provides the vital clue to the diagnosis.

> It is usually more rewarding to obtain a blow-by-blow description from the patient and/or any eyewitness of several individual episodes, rather than asking the patient to summarise what happens when they have a 'turn'.

The recommended method of taking a history is different from that described in Chapter 2, 'The neurological history'. It is far more useful to ask the patient to provide a detailed account of several individual episodes.

As you take the history question the patient about the symptoms:

1 immediately before (pre-ictal) the episode
2 during the event (ictus)
3 after the event (post-ictal).

Note: The strict definition of the term ictus is a stroke, blow or sudden attack, but it is used here to mean the event or episode.

A suggested method of history taking

Begin by asking the patient the following questions:

1 Tell me about the last episode you had: what were you doing at the time it commenced?
2 What was the very first symptom that you noticed?
3 From the moment you first noticed that symptom, was it at its most severe or did it become more intense or spread to involve other parts of the body?
4 If it did, how long did it take to spread or reach maximum intensity?
5 How long did it last?
6 What was the next symptom that you noticed?
7 How long after the first symptom did it commence?
8 Was the initial symptom showing signs of improving or worsening before this symptom began?
9 How long did this symptom take to develop in terms of maximum intensity or extent of involvement of the body?

Keep asking questions in this manner until the entire episode has been described and there is a clear understanding of the exact nature and distribution of each and every symptom and the time course of the episode. Then ask the patient to describe another episode(s) using the same technique.

The value of such a painstaking approach is highlighted by the following cases seen by the author over the years.

Cases involving single episodes

> **CASE 7.1**
>
> Dear Doctor,
> Thank you for seeing this young man with epilepsy. He walked into a video games parlour, noticed a strange smell and was witnessed to have an epileptic seizure with incontinence of urine.
> Dr 'Too Quick'

On the surface this does appear to be an epileptic seizure preceded by an olfactory aura (see Chapter 8, 'Seizures and epilepsy', for further discussion of the term 'aura', which is used to describe the initial symptom(s) of a seizure, often referred to as the warning symptoms). However, this doctor was too quick in jumping to the diagnosis of epilepsy and used only the nature of the symptoms to make a diagnosis, recalling that some seizures are associated with an altered smell. The correct diagnosis was apparent when a detailed history was obtained.

CASE 7.1 *cont'd*

The young man walked into the games parlour and was watching others play the video games. The room was very hot and stuffy and he began to feel light-headed, nauseated and clammy. Several minutes later he was feeling worse and his vision started to fade. Thinking he was about to faint, he began to walk outside to get fresh air when he lost consciousness. His next recollection was lying on the floor with people telling him that he had suffered an epileptic seizure. Clearly, with the prolonged symptoms typical of syncope, his seizure was a secondary phenomenon due to syncope (see below) and not a seizure due to epilepsy. When asked about the strange smell, he stated that the room stank!

CASE 7.2

A 38-year-old right-handed woman presented with the sudden onset of an inability to speak for approximately 30 seconds. She knew what she wanted to say but was unable to express any words (a non-fluent dysphasia, see Chapter 5, 'The cerebral hemispheres and cerebellum'). Despite her young age the patient was initially thought to have had an episode of cerebral ischaemia and underwent an urgent cerebral angiogram (pre-MRI and CT angiography era) that demonstrated a left frontal meningioma.

The non-fluent dysphasia indicated involvement of the frontal speech area in the dominant hemisphere. The fact that she was right-handed meant it was most likely (90% chance) it was the left hemisphere. The sudden onset suggested a vascular, mechanical or an electrical problem. A more detailed history established that, in addition to the inability to speak, the patient had noticed that the jaw had clenched shut involuntarily during the episode. This is a positive phenomenon and indicates that the problem was a focal seizure affecting the speech cortex related to the meningioma and not a transient ischaemic attack (TIA). Positive phenomena such as transient jaw clenching do not occur with cerebral ischaemia.

Cases involving recurrent episodes or transient symptoms

In patients with recurrent episodes or transient neurological symptoms, establish whether all episodes were identical and whether the symptoms varied from one episode to another by asking: 'Are all your turns the same or are some different to the others?' If the episodes varied, it is more rewarding to ask about several individual episodes. This is most relevant in some patients with epilepsy who may have multiple types of seizures (see Chapter 8, 'Seizures and epilepsy'). If the events were all identical, it is possible to use the approach of asking the patient to imagine having an episode right now in front of you and using the questioning technique described above to obtain a detailed description of each and every symptom. This approach could miss the diagnosis when the circumstances under which these episodes occurred provide the vital clue to the diagnosis. This is highlighted by the next two cases.

CASE 7.3

Dear Dr,
Thank you for seeing this 56-year-old woman who has had three episodes of vertebro-basilar insufficiency. In all three episodes there was weakness in all four limbs, true vertigo with the room spinning, double vision and slurred speech. In two of the episodes she lost consciousness.
Yours sincerely,

Note the same error: only the nature of the symptoms was obtained. The weakness in all four limbs combined with true vertigo (the room spinning), diplopia (double vision) and dysarthria (slurred speech) clearly points to involvement of the brain stem. The intermittent nature of the symptoms combined with the age of the patient suggests the diagnosis of vertebrobasilar insufficiency (VBI, transient cerebral ischaemia in the posterior circulation). To the experienced clinician the transient loss of consciousness (LOC) in two of the episodes is atypical and would raise doubts about this being primarily related to cerebral vascular disease. (LOC is extremely rare in patients with VBI. See Chapter 10, 'Cerebrovascular disease'.)

A more detailed history obtained the vital clue.

CASE 7.3 *cont'd*

On the first occasion the patient was walking up a flight of stairs and the symptoms developed as she reached the top. She kept walking and, as she walked out of the stairwell, she lost consciousness. The second episode occurred while the patient was walking up over an overpass. The symptoms subsided when she stopped walking at the top of the overpass and, on this occasion, she did not black out. The third episode was identical to the first and once again occurred after the patient climbed a flight of stairs.

The detailed description of the three individual events revealed that they all occurred with exercise, and cerebral ischaemia related to vascular disease does not occur in such a predictable manner.[1] Examination of the patient demonstrated severe aortic stenosis, and the explanation for her symptoms was exercise-induced hypotension due to poor cardiac output with initial selective involvement of the posterior circulation causing the focal symptoms and the subsequent global cerebral ischaemia resulting in LOC.

The patient described in Case 7.4 alerted this author to the importance of obtaining a blow-by-blow description of each of the episodes. She had recently been discharged from hospital without a clear diagnosis and after having undergone extensive investigation over a 2-week period. The patient was an 85-year-old woman who would be called in the trade 'a poor historian'.

---

1 Except in the very rare instance of subclavian steal syndrome where stenosis of the left subclavian artery proximal to the vertebral artery means that the left arm 'steals' blood from the brainstem when it is exercising.

CASE 7.4

Good morning, Mrs S. Could you please tell me about your funny turns?
'They are terrible, doctor, I feel awful.'
Could you be a little more specific as to what happens?
'I feel dizzy in the head and unwell and then I do not remember what happens.'
What do you mean by dizzy?
'It is awful, doctor, I feel terrible.'
Can you describe to me what you mean by dizzy?
'It's a terrible feeling in my head.'
How long have you had them for?
'6 months.'

It was evident after 10 minutes that this line of questioning was getting nowhere and that a different approach was required. The remainder of the consultation went along the following lines.

CASE 7.4 *cont'd*

Can you tell me about the last episode you had?
'Yes doctor, it was terrible, it was awful.'
I understand that it was terrible but what were you doing at the time it happened?
'I was watching television.'
What time of day?
'Just before lunch about midday.'
And then what happened?
'I stood up to change the TV channel.'
And then what happened?
'That terrible turn, doctor, where I felt awful and dizzy in the head and then I don't remember what happened after that except I was on the floor in front of the TV.'
Can you tell me how long you felt dizzy for before you blacked out?
'I don't think it was very long but I am not sure.'
How long were you out to it?
'I do not know but the same TV show was on so it could not have been very long.'
Were you aware of anything the matter with you when you came to?
'No.'
And then what happened?
'I crawled to my bed and went to sleep.'
Can you tell me about another episode? What were you doing when it started?
'I was having lunch.'
What time of day?
'About 12.30 pm.'
And then what happened?
'I stood up to go to the sink and that awful thing happened again.'

After the patient described two further episodes it became clear that every one occurred about midday and only when she stood up. Six months beforehand she had been placed on prazosin, a drug for hypertension and one that is often associated with postural hypotension. Her blood pressure fell from 170/100 lying to 110/65 on standing and her symptoms resolved upon cessation of this drug.

In each of these four cases the crucial clue(s) were missed because a very detailed history was not obtained.

GENERAL PRINCIPLES OF CLASSIFICATION OF INTERMITTENT DISTURBANCES

In patients with episodic disturbances of function, it is not only the nature and distribution of the symptoms but also the time course of the individual symptoms in relation to each other, the duration of each symptom and of the whole episode, and often the circumstances under which they occur that differentiates the various possible diagnoses.

There are many ways to classify intermittent disturbances of neurological function. The traditional approach is to classify them according to the aetiology or underlying pathological basis. On the other hand, the simplest classification from the clinical point of view depends on what can readily be observed during episodes and is shown in Figure 7.1. Patients:

* fall (or slump if seated) or do not fall
* have a 'blackout' or they do not, whether they fall or not
* may or may not experience abnormal movements under any of these circumstances
* may experience episodes that vary in duration from seconds to minutes or even hours.
  The various causes of intermittent disturbances can be differentiated along these lines. Most episodes in patients who fall with or without LOC are brief. The exceptions are:
* the very rare prolonged tonic–clonic seizure lasting many minutes
* syncope with a prolonged aura
* a secondary head injury causing LOC complicating the fall, whatever the cause.

If the head injury is more severe, retrograde (occurring prior to the LOC) amnesia may give the impression that the episode has lasted for a longer time simply because the patient cannot recall what happened.

The duration and the nature of the symptoms of episodes varies most from one episode to another in patients who have 'funny turns' where there is no fall or LOC. This is seen more commonly in patients with a psychological disturbance.

Most intermittent disturbances result from one of the mechanisms illustrated in Figure 7.2.

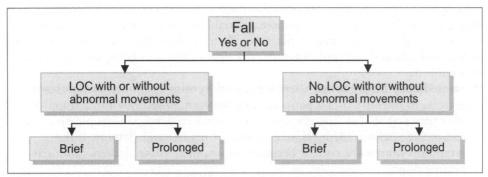

FIGURE 7.1   A suggested approach to intermittent disturbances

Brief = seconds to a few minutes, LOC = loss of consciousness, prolonged = many minutes to hours or even days

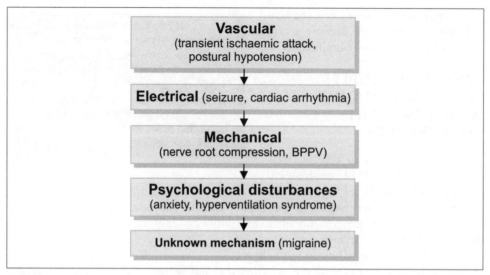

FIGURE 7.2 Basic mechanisms underlying intermittent disturbances of function
BPPV = benign paroxysmal positional vertigo

EPISODIC DISTURBANCES WITH FALLING
Falling with loss of consciousness

The four most common causes of transient LOC with falling are given in Figure 7.3. A complete summary of the numerous causes of transient LOC associated with a fall are listed in Table 7.1. Table 7.2 summarises the main clinical features of the common causes. Note that all are brief in duration.

It does not require experience, just patience and time, to obtain a detailed history in patients with episodic disturbances of function. Obtain a blow-by-blow description of episodes with particular attention to:
- the circumstances under which they occur
- the nature and distribution of the symptoms
- the time course of each and every symptom both individually and in relation to each other.

Syncope (fainting, vasovagal or neurocardiogenic syncope)

Although syncope can afflict anyone of any age it tends to occur more commonly in young adults [2]. The patient is almost invariably standing, occasionally sitting and very, very rarely in a recumbent position. There is often, but not always, a trigger such as pain, alcohol, stressful situations, the sight of blood or being in a hot crowded environment.

- **Immediately before ictus:** There are several warning (pre-ictal) symptoms that increase in intensity over a period lasting between 30 seconds and 2 minutes after they first appear. These warning symptoms are referred to as pre-syncope and include light-headedness, nausea and feeling hot and clammy. If the symptoms worsen the patient becomes sweaty, their vision darkens and their hearing dims.
- **During ictus:** The patient subsequently loses consciousness (ictus), the eyes are closed, they are very pale and there are no abnormal movements unless the patient

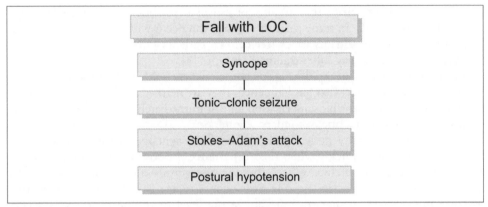

FIGURE 7.3   The four most common causes of transient loss of consciousness with falling

TABLE 7.1   Causes of transient loss of consciousness with falling

Common causes	Less common causes	Very rare causes
Syncope Tonic–clonic seizures Stokes–Adams attack or other arrhythmia Postural hypotension	Sudden and severe gastrointestinal haemorrhage Subarachnoid haemorrhage Intracerebral haemorrhage Sudden unilateral carotid occlusion Massive pulmonary embolism Aortic stenosis	Obstructive hydrocephalus Colloid cyst of the third ventricle Idiopathic hypertrophic subaortic stenosis Pulmonary hypertension

TABLE 7.2   The main pre-ictal, ictal and post-ictal features of the four most common causes of a fall with loss of consciousness

Type of event	Pre-ictal	Ictal	Post-ictal	Duration
Syncope	Seconds to minutes	LOC, no abnormal movement	No drowsiness or confusion	2–3 minutes
Tonic–clonic seizure	Aura (if present) lasting seconds	LOC + abnormal movements	Drowsy and confused	Ictus 2–3 minutes Drowsiness many minutes longer in older patients
Stokes–Adams attack	None	LOC, no abnormal movements	No drowsiness or confusion	Seconds (< 1 minute)
Postural hypotension	Seconds to 1 minute	LOC, no abnormal movements	No drowsiness or confusion	< 1 minute

suffers a secondary seizure that usually consists of a very brief tonic seizure lasting less than 20 seconds. In some patients syncope can occur with little or no warning, mimicking a Stokes–Adams attack (see below). Patients with shorter duration of warning symptoms may suffer traumatic injuries [3].

- **After ictus:** The patient rapidly regains consciousness (within 10–30 seconds) and, although they wonder what has happened, they are neither confused nor drowsy and can carry on a sensible conversation almost immediately after the episode, even when there has been a brief secondary seizure.

Unlike epilepsy, many patients who suffer from syncope can prevent LOC by lying or sitting down quickly when they experience the warning symptoms. This is an important diagnostic clue. Where there is uncertainty advise the patient to lie down immediately when the episode next occurs to see if LOC can be prevented by elevating the legs so that they are above the level of the head. There is a very rare condition in elderly patients where syncope can be related to carotid sinus sensitivity [4].

SOME NOTES OF CAUTION

1 Patients and eyewitnesses often have difficulty estimating time, and 'funny turns' always seem to last longer than they actually do.
2 Pallor by itself is not overly useful, as patients are invariably described as being pale or a dreadful colour with all types of funny turns of differing causes. Having said this, extreme pallor associated with sweating is very suggestive of a cardiovascular cause.
3 Feeling the pulse quickly is very difficult, even for people who are trained such as medical practitioners and nurses; the apparent absence of a pulse does not necessarily imply an arrhythmia.
4 Eyewitnesses and patients often interpret having no recollection of the event as post-ictal confusion.
5 Regarding confusion, it is very important to clarify what observers and patients mean when they say the patient was confused after the episode.

Tonic–clonic seizures

Only a few brief principles are discussed here, as Chapter 8, 'Seizures and epilepsy', deals with the subject of epilepsy in detail.

- **Immediately before ictus:** The pre-ictal phase or aura if present is very brief, lasting only a few seconds. In many patients with tonic–clonic seizures there is no warning before they lose consciousness.
- **During ictus:** The patient will fall to the ground and there is a brief stiffening of the limbs (tonic phase) lasting 10–20 seconds followed by jerking (clonic phase) of the limbs lasting on average 5–30 seconds. The duration of impaired consciousness is brief. Most tonic–clonic seizures last approximately 1 minute, although they can last as long as 10 minutes [5]. The eyes are usually open during the seizure and observers often say the eyes rolled up into the top of the head. The patient may bite their lip, cheek or tongue and they may suffer incontinence of urine and/or faeces during the seizure.
- **After ictus:** The post-ictal period is associated with drowsiness and confusion lasting from 30 seconds to several minutes [5]. The period of post-ictal drowsiness and confusion may be as long as 24 hours or even up to 1 week following prolonged seizures and in older patients [6].

Stokes–Adam's attack

This predominantly occurs in the elderly, although very rarely Stokes–Adam's attacks can occur in younger patients. These episodes are usually related to a bradyarrhythmia or complete heart block, although similar symptoms can occur with a tachyarrhythmia if it results in sudden hypotension [7].

- **Immediately before ictus:** There is no warning.
- **During ictus:** The patient suddenly finds themselves on the ground, wondering what has happened. They do NOT recall falling. The period of impaired consciousness (ictus) is very brief, usually only a matter of seconds, certainly less than 1 minute [8].
- **After ictus:** There is no post-ictal confusion.

Patients who lose consciousness due to a tachyarrhythmia may experience rapid palpitations, either just prior to the LOC or at other times, without losing consciousness. The presence of rapid palpitations at the time of the event provides a possible clue to an underlying cardiac cause for the transient LOC. The period of impaired consciousness may be longer if the patient suffers a head injury as a result of the fall.

Postural hypotension associated with loss of consciousness

This is the fourth most common cause of a fall associated with LOC. A VITAL clue is that, if the patient resumes a sitting or recumbent posture quickly, LOC may be prevented. Postural hypotension is suspected if episodes occur when the patient assumes an upright posture (e.g. stands up from sitting or lying).

- **Immediately before ictus:** The 'pre-ictal' symptoms are actually the initial symptoms of the event and are similar to those seen with syncope.
- **During ictus:** The LOC, if it occurs, is momentary. No abnormal movements.
- **After ictus:** There is no post-ictal confusion.

The diagnosis can be confirmed by measuring the blood pressure and pulse while lying and standing. The blood pressure falls and the pulse either increases or does not change at all depending on the aetiology of the postural hypotension. The commonest cause is drug-induced postural hypotension and in this case the blood pressure may not fall if it is measured several hours after the patient has taken the drug. The clue that the problem may be drug-induced is that the episodes occur at a similar time of the day, usually within 1 or 2 hours of the patient taking the medication.

The other causes of transient LOC listed in Table 7.1 are very rare and usually obvious because of the associated symptoms or circumstances when a very detailed history is obtained. Syncope due to aortic stenosis, idiopathic hypertrophic subaortic stenosis and pulmonary hypertension is precipitated by exertion. With these conditions, LOC can be avoided if the patient stops exercising with the very first symptom. There may also be associated dyspnoea with or without chest pain. Subarachnoid and intracerebral haemorrhage or a colloid cyst of the third ventricle will have associated severe explosive headache and vomiting. Pulmonary embolism causing a fall with LOC will be associated with severe chest pain, dyspnoea and hypotension. Gastrointestinal haemorrhage will be associated with haematemesis and/or melaena. The melaena may not be apparent when the patient is initially assessed.

FALLING WITHOUT LOSS OF CONSCIOUSNESS

Some patients will experience a fall but do not lose consciousness. There are three common causes as shown in Figure 7.4.

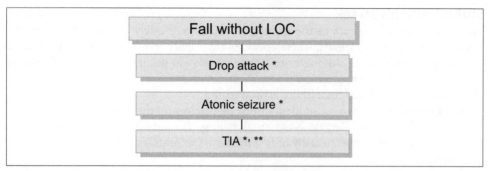

FIGURE 7.4   Causes of a fall without loss of consciousness

TIA = transient ischaemic attack

*Brief = seconds to less than 2 minutes

**Prolonged = many minutes to hours

Note: Patients with a TIA will fall only if the episode results in weakness of the leg(s) or the neurological symptoms are associated with severe vertigo. More commonly, patients with a TIA do not experience LOC nor do they fall. (See later in this chapter for more on TIA.)

Drop attacks

- **Immediately before ictus:** There is no warning.
- **During ictus:** The patient suddenly feels the legs go out from underneath them. The patient is able to say that they have fallen. The fall or ictus is very brief, lasting only a matter of seconds. The patient does not lose consciousness and may or may not feel themselves falling.
- **After ictus:** There are no post-ictal symptoms unless the patient has been injured in the fall, or is elderly with some physical disability. The patient is able to arise immediately and resume normal activities. In these episodes a patient may suffer serious injuries.

Drop attacks occur predominantly in middle-aged to elderly females. These falls may well relate to the same mechanisms that cause syncope in the elderly [9]. Drop attacks also occur in patients with advanced Ménière's disease [10], although if less severe the patient may simply experience an acute loss of balance without falling. Drop attacks are clinically identical to atonic seizures except that the latter are extremely rare in adults who have not had epilepsy (Lennox–Gastaut syndrome) in childhood.

Atonic seizures

As with patients with drop attacks, these patients suddenly fall or feel as if they are thrown to the ground.

- **Immediately before ictus:** There is no warning.
- **During ictus:** Very rarely there may be a momentary myoclonic jerk of the limbs preceding the sudden fall. The ictus is brief, usually lasting only seconds, or occasionally up to 1 minute. If an attack lasts for 1 minute there may be an associated LOC. No abnormal movements. Atonic seizures rarely, if ever, occur as an isolated phenomenon and are almost invariably associated with other types of seizures (see Chapter 8, 'Seizures and epilepsy').
- **After ictus:** There are no symptoms.

EPISODIC DISTURBANCES WITHOUT FALLING
Loss of awareness (consciousness) without falling

Most people interpret LOC as a dramatic event with profound impairment of consciousness and a collapse. In patients with impaired consciousness without falling perhaps a better term would be loss of awareness, where 'the lights are on but no one is at home' or, as a farmer once commented about his son, 'there are no sheep in the top paddock for 30 seconds'.[2] The patient remains sitting, standing or lying. They simply go off the air for a short period, unresponsive to external stimuli.

Figure 7.5 shows the more common intermittent disturbances of neurological function associated with a loss of awareness but no fall. The duration of the episodes is usually brief, seconds to less than 2–3 minutes.

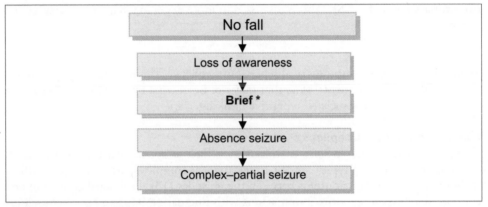

FIGURE 7.5   Intermittent disturbances without falling
*Brief = seconds to less than 2–3 minutes

BRIEF EPISODES
Absence seizure
Absence epilepsy is almost exclusively a problem in childhood. Very rarely it may present in adulthood, but in the form of recurrent absence seizures termed absence status (see Chapter 8, 'Seizures and epilepsy').
- **Immediately before ictus:** There is no warning.
- **During ictus:** The ictus is very brief, usually 4–9 (range 1–44) seconds [11]. During the seizure, the eyes are open and the patient stares into space without any abnormal movements apart from frequent blinking.
- **After ictus:** No symptoms, the patient behaves as if nothing had happened (unless driving, cycling or operating machinery where the seizure may result in an accident).

Complex–partial seizure
- **Immediately before ictus:** Most but not all patients with complex–partial seizures will experience brief pre-ictal symptoms (aura) lasting seconds. The nature of the symptoms during the aura reflects the site of origin of the seizure within the brain and is discussed in Chapter 8, 'Seizures and epilepsy'.

---

2 Two descriptions by relatives of patients with absence and complex–partial seizures.

- **During ictus:** During the ictus the patient remains in the same posture, stares into space and is unresponsive for approximately 1–3 minutes. Very rarely, complex–partial seizures can last up to 16 minutes [5]. Minor abnormal movements, especially of the mouth (lip-smacking), termed automatisms are not uncommon (see Chapter 8, 'Seizures and epilepsy').
- **After ictus:** There is a period of post-ictal confusion lasting several minutes, occasionally much longer.

PROLONGED EPISODES
Non-convulsive status epilepsy (NCSE) causes prolonged episodes lasting hours to days [12]. It presents more with confusion rather than unresponsiveness. Patients in NCSE may exhibit a wide range of clinical presentations including subtle memory deficits, bizarre behaviour, psychosis or coma. Absence status and complex partial status are the two primary types of NCSE. This is discussed in more detail in Chapter 8, 'Seizures and epilepsy'.

Absence status epilepsy
There are no pre-ictal symptoms of absence status epilepsy. This manifests as a prolonged period of depression in mental state that may not be noticed by eyewitnesses because it is mild. Often there is associated repetitive blinking.

Complex–partial status epilepsy
Complex–partial status epilepsy manifests as a fluctuating mental state with confusion related to repeated typical and at times atypical complex–partial seizures, with or without clearing of consciousness between the episodes [13]. Prolonged confusion and episodic stereotyped repetitive automatisms with fluctuating impairment of consciousness lasting days has also been described [12].

No fall and no loss of consciousness
Some intermittent disturbances are not associated with either LOC or falling. The diagnosis is based on the duration of the episode as well as the nature of the symptoms. In this setting there are some problems that produce symptoms lasting hours and occasionally days. Figure 7.6 shows the more common intermittent disturbances of neurological function that are not associated with a fall or loss of awareness (consciousness), distinguishing brief from prolonged episodes.

BRIEF EPISODES
Simple–partial seizure
- **Immediately before ictus:** There are no pre-ictal symptoms in a simple-partial seizure.
- **During ictus:** The ictus consists of brief stereotyped episodes lasting from 30 seconds to 3 minutes, and rarely up to 8 minutes [5]. There is no loss of awareness and in most instances the patient can continue normal activities during the episode but often chooses to halt them momentarily until the symptoms pass. The patient can describe all the symptoms; the nature of the symptoms reflects the site of origin within the cerebral hemisphere (see Chapter 8, 'Seizures and epilepsy').
- **After ictus:** There is no post-ictal confusion or drowsiness.

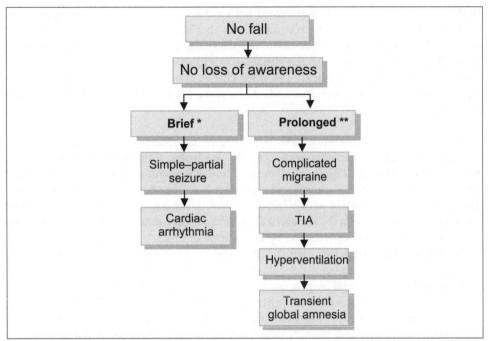

FIGURE 7.6 Causes of episodic disturbances without a fall or loss of consciousness

TIA = transient ischaemic attack

*Brief = seconds to less than 2 minutes

**Prolonged = many minutes to hours

Cardiac arrhythmia

- **Immediately before ictus:** There are no symptoms.
- **During ictus:** Although a patient presenting with palpitations with or without dyspnoea or chest pain presents little difficulty, many patients experience the symptoms related to hypotension secondary to the arrhythmia without being aware of the altered cardiac rhythm and in the absence of dyspnoea or chest pain. Here the diagnosis can present some difficulty, as the symptoms are non-specific and include light-headedness, nausea, sweating, blurred vision and a sensation of feeling unwell. The *one potential clue* is that these symptoms, which seem like hypotension, unlike postural hypotension or syncope may occur in the recumbent or sitting posture.
- **After ictus:** There are no symptoms.

PROLONGED EPISODES

Complicated migraine

This is discussed in more detail in Chapter 9, 'Headache and facial pain'. In essence, the symptoms come on gradually over minutes to less than 2 hours in 97% of patients [14] and persist on average for 24 hours but may persist for days [15]. The most important diagnostic feature, and the one that differentiates migraine from cerebral ischaemia, is the partial or complete resolution of the initial or early symptoms before the later symptoms have either appeared or fully evolved. In contrast, in cerebral ischaemia the symptoms are either of maximum intensity and distribution at onset or a cumulative neurological deficit develops with a stroke in evolution (see Chapter 10, 'Cerebrovascular disease'). The second clue is that the symptoms spread from their original site to other parts of the body, reflecting the spreading cortical depression of Leão. This is typically seen with the visual aura of migraine where the scotoma enlarges and moves across the visual field. The third clue is that the aura of migraine typically develops over 5 or more minutes and, when there is more than one symptom, they occur in succession [16].

Transient cerebral ischaemia attack including vertebrobasilar insufficiency

The great majority of patients with cerebral ischaemia, even those with widespread symptoms of VBI such as diplopia, dysarthria, visual loss and motor and sensory symptoms, can describe their symptoms and clearly have not lost consciousness or awareness. The exception is the patient with VBI where there is medial temporal lobe or thalamic involvement with amnesia for the event [17]. If the degree of weakness is severe patients with a TIA may fall if they are standing at the time of onset.

- **Immediately before ictus:** There are no clear-cut pre-ictal symptoms, although some patients describe being off-colour in the preceding few days.
- **During ictus:** The 'ictal' symptoms last from minutes to hours (by definition up to 24 hours, but usually 3–4 hours [18]). The nature of the symptoms depends on the vascular territory affected (carotid versus vertebrobasilar, large vessel versus small vessel). This is discussed in more detail in Chapter 10, 'Cerebrovascular disease'.
- **After ictus:** There are no obvious post-ictal symptoms.

Hyperventilation syndrome

Hyperventilation syndrome is a very common clinical problem that is often under-recognised.[3] Hyperventilation syndrome is characterised by a variety of somatic symptoms induced by physiologically inappropriate hyperventilation and usually reproduced in whole or in part by voluntary hyperventilation [19]. There is no pre-ictal or post-ictal phase.

- **Immediately before ictus:** There are no symptoms.
- **During ictus:** The symptoms gradually increase in intensity and then fluctuate in severity as the episode continues. The ictus consists of light-headedness that increases in severity over minutes and persists for hours, fluctuating in intensity during that period of time. There are often, but not invariably, associated symptoms with a sense of heaviness in the chest. Chest pain is rare; patients describe tightness in the chest. Occasionally, patients complain of shortness of breath; more often they complain of an inability to get enough air into the lungs, which is often associated with dryness of the mouth.
  When the symptoms become more severe, tingling that can at times be unilateral develops almost simultaneously around the mouth (peri-oral) and in the hands and/or feet. The tingling develops and increases in severity after the light-headedness has commenced and while it is still present. The tingling remains confined to the hands, feet and around the mouth. Unlike migraine, the paraesthesia does not migrate from one part of the body to another, although occasionally the tingling may commence in the foot or hands and spread to other parts of the body. If the patient has very severe hyperventilation the hands and wrists can develop an involuntary flexion termed 'carpopedal spasm'. Very rarely, subsequent LOC can occur. The patient may state that the limbs and body are shaking,

---

3 Personal observation.

suggesting epilepsy, but clarification of this symptom reveals that it is trembling rather than the involuntary jerking of epilepsy. The patient is fully alert during the time the limbs are shaking, which is not a feature of tonic–clonic epilepsy. In one study similar previous episodes were reported in 74% [20].

- **After ictus:** There are no symptoms.

Patients may have a background history of tension headache and neck discomfort, but in many cases hyperventilation appears as a recurrent symptom and is not necessarily associated with recent provocative stress [21]. A number of patients develop this problem after attending relaxation classes where they are instructed to take deep breaths in order to relax![4] The symptoms can be reproduced by asking the patient to take deep breaths (not panting) for 2–5 minutes. Alternatively, blood gases measured during an episode should reveal a low carbon dioxide (CO_2) level.

> Every single person will develop giddiness or dizziness when they hyperventilate and therefore it is imperative to confirm that the patient's symptoms have been reproduced exactly.

If the symptoms are not reproduced, the clinician should maintain a healthy scepticism about the diagnosis of hyperventilation syndrome. If the patient's symptoms are not reproduced exactly, and yet the symptoms strongly suggest hyperventilation, it is worthwhile sending the patient away with instructions to slow their breathing (see below). In many instances when it is hyperventilation syndrome the symptoms will resolve more rapidly with the patient slowing their breathing. The patient is instructed to return for further evaluation if the symptoms do not resolve. Treatment by breathing in and out of a paper bag, although effective, is embarrassing and impractical. A far more practical method is that the patient breathes in and then exhales and holds their breath for 15 or 20 seconds, repeating this procedure until the symptoms subside. This may take several minutes. It is easier to hold the breath after expiration than inspiration. The aim is to allow the CO_2 level to return to normal, having been lowered by the hyperventilation.

Transient global amnesia

Transient global amnesia (TGA) was first described in 1956 [22] and is a curious clinical syndrome characterised by the abrupt onset of severe anterograde amnesia [23]. It lasts several hours and is seen most often in the middle-aged or elderly. These patients are often not aware of any problems and are brought to medical attention by a concerned relative or an observer. During the attack the patient remains alert and communicative but keeps asking the same questions over and over again. Their personal identity is preserved and there are no focal neurological or epileptic features. Apart from short-term memory loss, the patient behaves as if nothing else is wrong; they can talk, walk etc. The ability to lay down new memories gradually recovers as the period of amnesia shrinks. There is a residual amnesia for events near the onset of the episode.

There are strict criteria for the diagnosis of TGA [24]:

1 The attack must be witnessed if it is to be diagnosed with a degree of certainty. Clear-cut anterograde amnesia must be present during the attack.
2 Clouding of consciousness and loss of personal identity must be absent.
3 The cognitive impairment must be limited to amnesia.
4 There should be no accompanying focal neurological symptoms.

---

4 Personal observation.

5 Epileptic seizures must be absent.
6 Attacks must resolve within 24 hours and patients with recent head injury or known active epilepsy are excluded.

Other causes of an acute amnestic syndrome include head injury, subarachnoid haemorrhage, Wernicke–Korsakoff syndrome and carbon monoxide poisoning. The associated symptoms of these other causes should enable easy differentiation from TGA.

Vertigo

Dizziness and giddiness are very non-specific terms that are commonly used by patients to describe their symptoms. Four types of dizziness have been defined: vertigo, presyncope, disequilibrium, and other [25]. Vertigo is a false sensation that the body or the environment is moving (head or room spinning). This is true vertigo and indicates a problem within the peripheral vestibular system (labyrinth or vestibular nerve) or the central vestibular connections in the brainstem or cerebellum. Table 7.3 lists the distinguishing features of central vertigo and peripheral vertigo as described by Swartz and Longwell [26]. Cerebellar infarction is discussed in greater detail in Chapter 10, 'Cerebrovascular disease'.

Vertigo essentially presents either as an acute severe episode or as recurrent attacks over months to years. Whatever the cause, vertigo is almost invariably associated with variable degrees of nausea and vomiting. Figure 7.7 shows the more common causes of vertigo. The two main causes of *acute severe vertigo* are 'acute vestibulopathy' (vestibular neuronitis, labyrinthitis) and cerebellar infarction [27].

Apart from cerebellar infarction, most conditions that cause vertigo do not have 'gold standard' tests to confirm the clinical diagnosis. Ménière's disease also lacks a diagnostic test but the syndrome is well defined in patients subsequently found to have the typical pathology in the ears, so the term has been retained.

TABLE 7.3 Central versus peripheral vertigo

Feature	Central vertigo	Peripheral vertigo
Deafness and tinnitus	Usually absent	May be present
Inability to stand	Yes	No
Dysarthria, diplopia	Yes	No
Findings on the Hallpike manoeuvre		
Delay in onset of vertigo	None	2–40 seconds
Severity of vertigo	Mild	Severe
Symptoms fatigue*	No	Yes
Symptoms habituate**	No	Yes
Duration of nystagmus	>1 minute	<1 minute

*Fatigue refers to the abatement of the vertigo and nystagmus after provocation while the head is still in the position that precipitated the symptoms.
**Habituation refers to a lessening of the severity of the symptoms with repeated Hallpike's testing.
Nystagmus is a rapid, involuntary, oscillatory motion of the eyeball.
Note: Vertigo is precipitated by the Hallpike manoeuvre in both central and peripheral lesions. The bottom 5 rows refer to the different findings on the Hallpike manoeuvre.

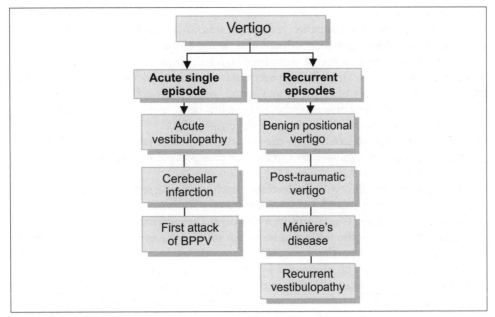

FIGURE 7.7 The more common causes of vertigo

BPPV = benign paroxysmal positional vertigo

As an isolated symptom, vertigo is most often peripheral in origin (inner ear or vestibular nerve including the root's entry zone in the brain stem) with benign positional vertigo, acute vestibular neuronitis and Ménière's disease accounting for 93% of patients with vertigo presenting to primary care physicians [28]. Very occasionally vertigo is central in origin, affecting the vestibular connections within the brainstem, but there are almost always other neurological symptoms and/or signs referable to the brainstem.

A sensation of imbalance (likened to being on a ship) may relate to the vestibular system and may represent a less severe form of vertigo. Patients use terms such as giddiness and dizziness to refer to this sense of imbalance. However, the more one deviates from the true definition of vertigo as a spinning sensation (either of the head or environment), the less one can be certain that the symptoms represent involvement of the vestibular pathway. In patients who complain that they are unsteady it is important to clarify whether there is an associated sensation of giddiness (suggesting either hypotension or a vestibular pathway cause for the instability) or a feeling of unsteadiness in the legs in the absence of giddiness, where the latter may be due to diseases affecting the central or peripheral nervous system and not involving the vestibular system. Rarely, vertigo can result from new spectacles or the sudden onset of diplopia due to an extraocular muscle paresis.

Acute single episode
Although the two conditions discussed in this section are monophasic illnesses, they are important causes of vertigo and it seems appropriate to include them in this chapter with the other causes of vertigo that result in episodic symptoms. In theory, patients with an initial attack of benign paroxysmal positional vertigo could present as an acute single episode; in reality these patients rarely if ever present after the first episode.

ACUTE VESTIBULOPATHY

The use of the term 'vestibulopathy' reflects the unknown aetiology of this clinical syndrome and, as already explained, is preferred to the terms 'labyrinthitis' or 'vestibular neuronitis' which imply a site of pathology and an infective or inflammatory process that is not proven [29]. By definition vestibular neuritis (or neuronitis) is confined to the vestibular system and hearing is unaffected, while labyrinthitis is a process that is thought to affect the inner ear as a whole or the 8th nerve as a whole and where hearing may be reduced or distorted in tandem with vertigo [30].

- **Immediately before ictus:** There may be an antecedent upper respiratory infection. In some patients a vague sense of imbalance may precede by some hours to days the more severe vertigo.
- **During ictus:** Vertigo typically develops slowly over a period of hours, is severe for a few days and then subsides over the course of a few weeks. Nausea and vomiting are marked but there is no tinnitus or deafness. The patients prefer to lie completely immobile on the side opposite to the affected ear as the slightest movement exacerbates the vertigo. There is unidirectional nystagmus with the fast phase to the unaffected ear. It can be suppressed by visual fixation (asking the patient to stare at an object). Examination of one retina with the ophthalmoscope while the other eye is covered can elicit the nystagmus as this removes visual fixation. Other than nystagmus there are no focal neurological symptoms or signs.

    Patients with an acute peripheral vestibular lesion as opposed to cerebellar infarction typically can stand, although they will veer toward the side of the lesion, especially if asked to walk on the spot with their eyes closed [31]. They may notice that their vision is disturbed or jumpy on looking to a particular side. This is termed oscillopsia, the symptom of nystagmus. Very rarely, anticlockwise rotary nystagmus with vertical (*not* horizontal) diplopia may occur (a skew deviation), related to dysconjugate larger deviation of the ipsilateral eye [32, 33]. This may give the impression that the vertigo is of central origin. Skew deviation can also occur with brainstem lesions and in these circumstances it can be difficult to differentiate between a central and a peripheral cause for the vertigo.
- **After ictus:** Some patients can have residual non-specific post-ictal giddiness and imbalance that lasts for months. Benign paroxysmal positional vertigo may develop as a sequela.

CEREBELLAR INFARCTION/HAEMORRHAGE

- **Immediately before ictus:** There are no 'pre-ictal' symptoms.
- **During ictus:** Onset is sudden if ischaemic or over many minutes if related to haemorrhage. 'Ictal' symptoms last for days. Although the patient may present with severe vertigo, cerebellar infarction or haemorrhage should be suspected in patients who present with:
    - severe nausea and vomiting
    - an inability to stand (see Chapter 10, 'Cerebrovascular disease').

    Unlike acute vestibulopathy, the patient is unable to stand. When there is associated dysarthria, diplopia and limb ataxia, the diagnosis of a central cause for the vertigo is apparent.
- **After ictus:** Residual symptoms will occur if recovery is incomplete.

In both cerebellar infarction and acute vestibulopathy the vomiting may be so severe and repeated that a Mallory–Weiss tear in the lower end of the oesophagus may occur and haematemesis may be the presenting symptom. It is not uncommon for these patients to be misdiagnosed with an acute gastrointestinal problem and admitted under the gastroenterology unit. The presence of severe vertigo or an inability to stand in these patients should alert the clinician to the correct diagnosis.

The head impulse test [34] detects severe unilateral loss of semicircular canal function clinically. It can distinguish between vestibular neuritis and cerebellar infarction as it is normal in a patient with cerebellar infarction but abnormal in a patient with vestibular neuritis or acute vestibulopathy. The head thrust test consists of holding the patient's face with both hands with the patient's head turned to one side slightly past the midline and then rapidly thrusting it to just past the midline on the opposite side. The patient is asked to fixate on a distant object. When the subject's head is turned to the side of the lesion, the vestibular ocular reflex is deficient and the eyes will move with the head so that they no longer fix on the point in the distance. A CT scan will detect haemorrhage but may be normal in the early hours after an infarct. An MRI scan will detect the infarction earlier.

Recurrent attacks of vertigo
POSITIONAL VERTIGO
Benign paroxysmal positional vertigo (BPPV) was first described in detail by Barany in 1921 [35]. This usually, but not invariably, occurs in the middle-aged to elderly where it is related to small deposits of calcium on the hair cells in the vestibule. Positional vertigo can also occur after a head injury or an acute vestibulopathy.

- **Pre-ictal:** There are no warning (pre-ictal) symptoms.
- **During ictus:** Patients describe paroxysms of true vertigo precipitated by head movement such as:
  - looking up to get something out of a cupboard or off the clothes line
  - bending over to tie shoe laces or to pick up an object
  - getting in and out of bed
  - lying down
  - rolling over in bed.
- **After ictus:** There are usually no symptoms.

Although the vertigo may be precipitated by all of these actions, in some patients only one or two of these head movements precipitate the vertigo. The symptoms are brief, lasting less than 2 minutes. Although nausea may occur, vomiting is rare. There are no other symptoms such as tinnitus (ringing in the ears), deafness, diplopia, dysarthria, slurred speech, blindness (termed amaurosis) weakness or sensory symptoms. Symptoms are present most days for weeks and occasionally months. Patients will notice good and bad days and on bad days there are repeated episodes in a day. The moment the patient gets out of bed they know if they are in for a good or bad day depending upon the appearance or not of symptoms. The crucial diagnostic clue is that the patient is free of vertigo when lying or sitting perfectly still.

The symptoms and the associated delayed onset of nystagmus that abates with maintenance of the fixed posture can be precipitated by the positioning test or Hallpike manoeuvre [36]:

1 The examiner should describe to the patient what the test involves and reassure them that it is safe and painless, but that it may reproduce their symptoms and make them very giddy. The patient should be reassured that they will not be allowed to fall off the examination couch.
2 Ask the patient to sit on an examination couch so that when they lie down the head is over and below the end of the couch. The movement has to be quick and the examiner needs to ensure that the patient does not suffer from back or neck problems before doing this procedure. Ensure that the back and neck are supported during the procedure.

3 When this test is performed the patient will want to close the eyes but must be encouraged to keep them open so that the nystagmus can be seen. Commence with the head looking to one side and then rapidly lie the patient down from the sitting position. If the problem is benign positional vertigo affecting the right ear, there is the delayed onset of a fast-phase clockwise (as the patient sees it, anti-clockwise from the examiner's perspective) torsional nystagmus with the affected right ear dependent or lower.

4 To complete the procedure the patient is returned to the seated position and the eyes are observed for reversal in the direction of the nystagmus, in this case a fast-phase anticlockwise nystagmus. The nystagmus settles within 30 seconds if the patient stays still in that position [36].

The rationale behind this is the observations of Schuknecht and Ruby who described small deposits of calcium (otoconia) on the hair cells, most often within the posterior semi-circular canals, as the cause of this problem [37]. These deposits are flushed out of the semi-circular canals using the Epley manoeuvre or a similar particle repositioning manoeuvre. The condition can be cured in 80% of patients, using the Canalith Repositioning Procedure or Epley manoeuvre [38]. This requires identification of whether it is the right or left ear in which the problem occurs and this is not always possible, particularly if the patient is having a good day and the Hallpike manoeuvre is negative. If one cannot provoke vertigo with the Hallpike manoeuvre, one cannot cure it with the Epley manoeuvre. In these circumstances the options are to bring the patient back on a bad day or alternatively recommend that they deliberately precipitate the symptoms many times in the morning and the evening until the problem resolves, using the Brandt–Daroff exercises [39]. This problem can recur on more than one occasion months or even years later.

MÉNIÈRE'S DISEASE

The term Ménière's disease is used to define the classic triad of:

1 vertigo of vestibular origin
2 tinnitus and hearing impairment (cochlear symptoms)
3 aural pressure.

Ménière's disease is manifested by episodic true vertigo associated with nausea and vomiting lasting longer than 1 hour and usually a few hours, together with a sense of fullness in the ear. Tinnitus may occur, and transient deafness during the attack that improves following the episode is a pathognomonic (this is a term that indicates that only one condition can cause the problem) symptom of Ménière's that can occur in two-thirds of patients [40]. The tinnitus and deafness may persist for days. The symptoms increase in intensity over several minutes and may continue to increase for up to half an hour. There may be a further period of up to half an hour of a sense of instability before the onset of the severe true vertigo with a sense of rotation. The patient prefers to lie still with the affected ear uppermost, but the vertigo persists even if the patient remains motionless. This condition recurs at variable intervals, as frequently as several attacks within a week or none for some years. *Two episodes of vertigo in 1 day are incompatible with the diagnosis of Ménière's.* Repeated attacks usually lead to progressive hearing loss over many years. In the early stages tinnitus, hearing impairment and/or fullness in the ear may appear prior to the onset of the first vertigo attack and vertigo can occur without tinnitus and deafness [41].

Three stages are identified in Ménière's disease:

• **Stage I**. In the early phase the predominant symptom is vertigo, characteristically rotatory or rocking, and it is associated with nausea or vomiting. The episode is often preceded by an aura of fullness or pressure in the ear or side of the head and usually lasts from 20 minutes to several hours. Between the attacks hearing reverts to normal and examination of the patient during this period of remission invariably shows normal results.

- **Stage II**. As the disease advances the hearing loss becomes established but continues to fluctuate. The deafness is sensorineural and initially affects the lower pitches. The paroxysms of vertigo reach their maximum severity and then tend to become less severe. The period of remission is highly variable, often lasting for several months.
- **Stage III**. In the last stage of the disorder the hearing loss stops fluctuating and progressively worsens; both ears tend to be affected so that the prime disability is deafness. The episodes of vertigo diminish and then disappear, although the patient may be unsteady, especially in the dark. [42].

RECURRENT VESTIBULOPATHY

Essentially, patients have recurrent *isolated vertigo* of unknown cause and without headache, neurological or auditory symptoms. Patients experience recurrent episodes of vertigo, with nausea and vomiting lasting hours or sometimes days [43]. These episodes occur at variable intervals and do not display the features of Ménière's syndrome, such as transient deafness and tinnitus during the attacks, and patients do not subsequently develop deafness. The precise aetiology of these episodes has not been established. At the time of writing there is a strong body of opinion that considers these episodes to be migrainous [44–50]. The increased incidence of migraine in patients with vertigo and vice versa and the response to 'migraine therapy' is cited as evidence for the link between migraine and vertigo. Diagnostic criteria have been proposed [47]. The evidence is circumstantial and, as there is no gold standard diagnostic test for migraine or migrainous vertigo, the episodes have been referred to as recurrent vestibulopathy.

Fleeting symptoms

Patients are occasionally encountered who describe fleeting symptoms lasting only 1 or 2 seconds. There may be a momentary sensation of impending LOC, particularly when a person is relaxed, referred to as the blip syndrome [51]. There may be transient symptoms of pain such as ice-pick headache (see Chapter 9, 'Headache and facial pain') or there may be transient sensory symptoms. These often defy explanation and are benign, and all investigations are normal[5].

REFERENCES

1 Official website of the Sir Arthur Conan Doyle Literary Estate, 2006. Available: http://www.sherlockholmes online.org/Biography/index.htm (14 Dec 2009).
2 Sheldon RS, Sheldon AG, Connolly SJ et al. Age of first faint in patients with vasovagal syncope. J Cardiovasc Electrophysiol 2006; 17:49–54.
3 Ammirati F, Colivicchi F, Velardi A et al. Prevalence and correlates of syncope-related traumatic injuries in tilt-induced vasovagal syncope. Ital Heart J 2001; 2:38–41.
4 Brignole M, Alboni P, Benditt D et al. Guidelines on management (diagnosis and treatment) of syncope. Eur Heart J 2001; 22:1256–1306.
5 Jenssen S, Gracely EJ, Sperling MR. How long do most seizures last? A systematic comparison of seizures recorded in the epilepsy monitoring unit. Epilepsia 2006; 47:1499–1503.
6 Godfrey JW, Roberts MA, Caird FI. Epileptic seizures in the elderly. II: Diagnostic problems. Age Ageing 1982; 11:29–34.
7 Johansson BW. Long-term ECG in ambulatory clinical practice. Analysis and 2-year follow-up of 100 patients studied with a portable ECG tape recorder. Eur J Cardiol 1977; 5:39–48.

5 Personal observation.

8   Harbison J, Newton JL, Seifer C et al. Stokes Adams attacks and cardiovascular syncope. Lancet 2002; 359:158–160.
9   Kenny RA, Traynor G. Carotid sinus syndrome – clinical characteristics in elderly patients. Age Ageing 1991; 20:449–454.
10 Kentala E, Havia M, Pyykko I. Short-lasting drop attacks in Ménière's disease. Otolaryngol Head Neck Surg 2001; 124:526–530.
11 Sadleir LG, Farrell K, Smith S et al. Electroclinical features of absence seizures in childhood absence epilepsy. Neurology 2006; 67:413–418.
12 Escueta AV, Boxley J, Stubbs N et al. Prolonged twilight state and automatisms: A case report. Neurology 1974; 24:331–339.
13 Ellis JM, Lee SI. Acute prolonged confusion in later life as an ictal state. Epilepsia 1978; 19:119–128.
14 Pryse-Phillips W, Aube M, Bailey P et al. A clinical study of migraine evolution. Headache 2006; 46:1480–1486.
15 Kelman L. Pain characteristics of the acute migraine attack. Headache 2006; 46:942–953.
16 Kirchmann M. Migraine with aura: New understanding from clinical epidemiologic studies. Curr Opin Neurol 2006; 19:286–293.
17 Akiguchi I, Ino T, Nabatame H et al. Acute-onset amnestic syndrome with localized infarct on the dominant side – comparison between anteromedial thalamic lesion and posterior cerebral artery territory lesion. Jpn J Med 1987; 26:15–20.
18 Crisostomo RA, Garcia MM, Tong DC. Detection of diffusion-weighted MRI abnormalities in patients with transient ischemic attack: Correlation with clinical characteristics. Stroke 2003; 34:932–937.
19 Lewis RA, Howell JB. Definition of the hyperventilation syndrome. Bull Eur Physiopathol Respir 1986; 22:201–205.
20 Saisch SG, Wessely S, Gardner WN. Patients with acute hyperventilation presenting to an inner-city emergency department. Chest 1996; 110:952–957.
21 Fejerman N. Nonepileptic disorders imitating generalized idiopathic epilepsies. Epilepsia 2005; 46(Suppl 9):S80–S83.
22 Courjon J, Guyotat J. [Amnesic strokes.] J Med Lyon 1956; 37:697–701.
23 Fisher CM, Adams RD. Transient global amnesia. Acta Neurol Scand 1964; 40(Suppl 9):S1–S83.
24 Hodges JR, Warlow CP. Syndromes of transient amnesia: Towards a classification. A study of 153 cases. J Neurol Neurosurg Psychiatry 1990; 53:834–843.
25 Drachman DA, Hart CW. An approach to the dizzy patient. Neurology 1972; 22:323–234.
26 Swartz R, Longwell P. Treatment of vertigo. Am Fam Physician 2005; 71:1115–1122.
27 Halmagyi GM. Diagnosis and management of vertigo. Clin Med 2005; 5:159–165.
28 Hanley K, O'Dowd T. Symptoms of vertigo in general practice: A prospective study of diagnosis. Br J Gen Pract 2002; 52:809–812.
29 Ryu JH. Vestibular neuritis: An overview using a classical case. Acta Otolaryngol Suppl 1993; 503:25–30.
30 Silvoniemi P. Vestibular neuronitis. An otoneurological evaluation. Acta Otolaryngol Suppl 1988; 453:1–72.
31 Fukuda T. The stepping test: Two phases of the labyrinthine reflex. Acta Otolaryngol 1959; 50:95–108.
32 Brandt TH, Dieterich M. Different types of skew deviation. J Neurol Neurosurg Psychiatry 1991; 54:549–550.
33 Safran AB, Vibert D, Issoua D et al. Skew deviation after vestibular neuritis. Am J Ophthalmol 1994; 118:238–245.
34 Halmagyi GM, Curthoys IS. A clinical sign of canal paresis. Arch Neurol 1988; 45:737–739.
35 Barany R. Diagnose von Krankheitserscheinungen im Bereiche des Otolithenapparates. Acta Otolaryng 1921; 2:434–437.
36 Dix MR, Hallpike CS. The pathology, symptomatology and diagnosis of certain common disorders of the vestibular system. Proc R Soc Med 1952; 45:341–354.
37 Schuknecht HF, Ruby RR. Cupulolithiasis. Adv Otorhinolaryngol 1973; 20:434–443.
38 Epley JM. The canalith repositioning procedure: For treatment of benign paroxysmal positional vertigo. Otolaryngol Head Neck Surg 1992; 107:399–404.
39 Brandt T, Daroff RB. Physical therapy for benign paroxysmal positional vertigo. Arch Otolaryngol 1980; 106:484–485.
40 Havia M, Kentala E, Pyykko I. Hearing loss and tinnitus in Ménière's disease. Auris Nasus Larynx 2002; 29:115–119.
41 Tokumasu K, Fujino A, Naganuma H et al. Initial symptoms and retrospective evaluation of prognosis in Ménière's disease. Acta Otolaryngol Suppl 1996; 524:43–49.
42 Saeed SR. Fortnightly review: Diagnosis and treatment of Ménière's disease. BMJ 1998; 316:368–372.
43 Lee H, Sohn SI, Jung DK et al. Migraine and isolated recurrent vertigo of unknown cause. Neurol Res 2002; 24:663–665.
44 Maione A. Migraine-related vertigo: Diagnostic criteria and prophylactic treatment. Laryngoscope 2006; 116:1782–1786.

45 Eggers SD. Migraine-related vertigo: Diagnosis and treatment. Curr Neurol Neurosci Rep 2006; 6:106–115.
46 Neuhauser HK, Lempert T. Diagnostic criteria for migrainous vertigo. Acta Otolaryngol 2005; 125: 1247–1248.
47 Neuhauser H, Leopold M, von Brevern M et al. The interrelations of migraine, vertigo, and migrainous vertigo. Neurology 2001; 56:436–441.
48 Gupta VK. Migraine-related vertigo: The challenge of the basic sciences. Clin Neurol Neurosurg 2005; 108:109–110:reply 111–112.
49 Lempert T, Neuhauser H. Migrainous vertigo. Neurol Clin 2005; 23:715–730, vi.
50 Brantberg K, Trees N, Baloh RW. Migraine-associated vertigo. Acta Otolaryngol 2005; 125:276–279.
51 Lance JW. Transient sensations of impending loss of consciousness: The "blip" syndrome. J Neurol Neurosurg Psychiatry 1996; 60:437–438.

chapter 8

Seizures and Epilepsy

This chapter is a brief discussion of the clinical aspects of **epilepsy**. It does not discuss pathophysiology. The numerous classification schemes [1–4] also are not discussed as it is inevitable that with advancing knowledge these will continue to evolve.

> In everyday clinical practice it is more practical to classify seizures on the basis of what happens to the patient and what can be witnessed.

The basic principles of clinical assessment and management of patients suffering from a suspected **seizure** or epilepsy (recurrent seizures) will be discussed. A comprehensive discussion of epilepsy can be found in numerous textbooks [5–7]. Treatment is documented in Appendix C but, as it will continue to evolve rapidly, any discussion in a textbook will quickly be out of date. Therefore, links to neurology- and epilepsy-related websites are included in Chapter 15, 'Further reading, keeping up-to-date and retrieving information'. It is anticipated that these websites will provide the reader with the up-to-date information that a textbook cannot provide.

CLINICAL FEATURES CHARACTERISTIC OF EPILEPSY

The clinical manifestations of epilepsy are extremely variable and depend on the site of origin of the seizures within the central nervous system. There are, however, certain characteristics of all forms of epilepsy that are independent of any classification scheme.

Epilepsy (apart from the very rare reflex epilepsies discussed below) is:
- an episodic disturbance
- that may or may not be preceded by a warning (**aura**)
- brief in duration
- unpredictable, with
  - stereotyped clinical manifestations
  - positive phenomena
  - impaired consciousness or awareness
  - often followed by a period of **post-ictal** (after the event) confusion.

Epilepsy is an *episodic disturbance* of function that occurs with variable frequency from a single seizure in a lifetime to many seizures per day. Apart from reflex epilepsy (see 'Reflex epilepsies' below), when seizures will occur is *unpredictable* and can be any time of the day or night and under any circumstances. Some patients may experience a brief warning (aura), lasting seconds only, leading up to the **ictus**. Unless a patient has more than one type of seizure each episode is identical or almost identical *(stereotyped)*, in terms of the clinical manifestations, to the previous one. If a patient suffers from multiple types of seizures each will be have their own stereotypical features. Seizures are *brief,* usually lasting less than 1–3 minutes (even tonic–clonic seizures) and rarely 5–10 minutes [8]. There are characteristic *positive phenomena,* i.e. abnormal movements or smell, taste, sensory, psychic or visual sensations. A loss of function, such as paralysis or sensory loss, is NOT a feature during a seizure but may follow a seizure; this is referred to as Todd's palsy (see 'Tonic–clonic seizures' below).

If the period of 'post-ictal' confusion and drowsiness is prolonged, this may reflect hypoxia during the seizure, or the seizure may be part of a disease process that in itself would cause prolonged confusion such as hypoglycaemic coma or infections such as meningitis and encephalitis.

THE PRINCIPLES OF MANAGEMENT OF PATIENTS WITH A SUSPECTED SEIZURE OR EPILEPSY

1 Confirm that the patient has suffered a seizure.
2 Characterise the type(s) of seizure(s).
3 Assess the frequency of seizures.
4 Identify any precipitating causes.
5 Establish the aetiology.
6 Decide whether to treat or not.
7 Choose the appropriate drug and dose and monitor the response to therapy.
8 Advise regarding lifestyle.
9 Consider surgery in patients who fail to respond to drug therapy.
10 Decide whether and when to withdraw therapy in 'seizure-free' patients.

CONFIRMING THAT THE PATIENT HAS HAD A SEIZURE OR SUFFERS FROM EPILEPSY

Epilepsy is an intermittent disturbance of neurological function. Unless the seizures are frequent, it is unlikely that the clinician, routine electroencephalography or even video-electroencephalography (EEG) telemetry will witness or capture an actual event. The diagnosis, therefore, is almost entirely dependent on the neurological history. If there is an eyewitness to the episode(s) they can be questioned; otherwise the history consists of what the patient is able to recall and, since many seizures are associated with loss of consciousness, this will be limited to what happened before and what the patient can recall after the ictus.

In patients with suspected seizure(s) the best history-taking technique is to obtain a blow-by-blow description of the episode or several of the episodes. Concentrate on the periods immediately before, during and after the event or ictus. These are referred to as the pre-ictal, ictal and post-ictal periods. The correct diagnosis depends on establishing the exact duration and nature of the symptoms that occur during each of these three phases. The alternative diagnoses that may be confused with epilepsy have been discussed in Chapter 7, 'Episodic disturbances of neurological function'.

> In patients with suspected seizure(s) the best history-taking technique is to obtain a blow-by-blow description of the episode or several of the episodes.

There are several useful questions that can be asked of the patient and any eyewitnesses and these are discussed next.

Useful questions to ask the patient

- *What were you doing just before the episode?* The circumstances under which the episode occurred may provide a vital clue in terms of aetiology or precipitating factors: flashing lights in a discotheque with photosensitive epilepsy or a seizure during venesection suggesting a seizure probably secondary to syncope.
- *Was there any warning? If so, what was the exact nature of this warning and how long did it last?* A brief warning or aura lasting only seconds is very typical of epilepsy; a more prolonged warning would point to a possible alternative diagnosis.
- *What was your next recollection? Can you establish how long this was after the episode commenced?* A short period of lost time, 10 minutes or at most 20 minutes, is more in keeping with epilepsy.
- *When you came to were you aware of anything the matter?* A period of post-ictal drowsiness or confusion in the absence of a head injury strongly suggests epilepsy.
- *Did you injure yourself?* This is non-specific, but a dislocated shoulder occasionally occurs with tonic–clonic seizures and an injury indicates a fall, thus reducing the number of diagnostic possibilities.
- *During the episode did you bite your tongue or cheek or lose control of your bladder or bowels?* These occur with tonic–clonic seizures.
- *Have you ever had any unexplained motor vehicle accidents?* An explanation may be a seizure without warning.
- *When you are watching a television program that you are interested in or having a conversation with a person, do you ever miss parts of the program or conversation?* An affirmative answer to this suggests the possibility of minor absence or complex–partial seizures that the patient may not have noticed. However, when patients are just sitting in front of the television it would be not uncommon through lack of concentration to miss parts of the program. On the other hand, if it interrupts a program that the patient is particularly interested in, it is more likely to be a minor seizure.
- *Do people accuse you of being a daydreamer?* It is not uncommon for children and adolescents to be thought of as daydreamers when they have been having unrecognised minor seizures. It is also not uncommon for children and teenagers to actually daydream, so interpret the answer to this question with caution. If the patient has suffered from repeated episodes, establish if each and every episode was identical or whether there may have been different types of seizures so that detailed questioning of several different events is necessary.
- *Have you ever been able to prevent one of these episodes and, if so, how?* Seizures secondary to syncope or hypotension may be prevented if the patient assumes a recumbent posture immediately after they experience the first warning.

Useful questions to ask an eyewitness or relative

Some patients can suffer unrecognised seizures for many years [9], particularly children and teenagers who are often thought to be daydreaming. Relatives may have witnessed a number of episodes and not recognised them as seizures.

A useful sequence of questions includes:

1 *Have you ever seen the patient suddenly interrupt what they were doing and stare into space, where their eyes were open but they did not respond to you?* If the answer is yes, this is in keeping with absence or complex–partial seizures.

2 *What was the patient doing at the time the episode commenced?*
3 *What was the first thing that you noticed and how long did it last?*
4 *What was the next thing that you noticed and how long did it last?*
5 *What was the next thing that you noticed and how long did it last?*

Keep asking this question until the whole episode has been described in detail. More specific questions include:

• *During the episode was the patient able to hear what you were saying or were they out to it?* If the answer is no, this indicates a loss of awareness suggesting a generalised seizure or complex–partial seizure.

• *Did you see any excessive blinking or abnormal chewing movements of the mouth?* These occur with absence and complex–partial seizures, respectively.

It is often useful to question more than one eyewitness or relative as one individual may not have observed all the details. When seeing a patient with suspected epilepsy or a seizure, more is to be gained by picking up the telephone and ringing a family member or an eyewitness than undertaking investigations.

> As a general rule, the more complex and varied the behaviour during an episode and the longer the duration of the abnormal behaviour, the less likely one is dealing with a seizure disorder.

Epilepsy in the elderly

It is a common misconception that epilepsy is a disease of childhood. While this is largely true of absence (petit-mal) seizures, which are very rare in adults and often present when they do occur with absence status epilepsy, seizures do occur in the elderly and the incidence increases with increasing age, as shown in Figure 8.1. Elderly patients with epilepsy most often present with tonic–clonic or complex–partial seizures that have a higher recurrence rate than in the younger population. The complex–partial seizures are often difficult to diagnose since they present with atypical symptoms, particularly prolonged post-ictal symptoms including memory lapses, confusion, altered mental status and inattention [10].

> Seizures can occur in any age group and either sex.

Although there is a continuing incidence of seizures throughout life, they are more common in the first 5 years. There is also a higher incidence in the 70- to 80-year-old age group [11].

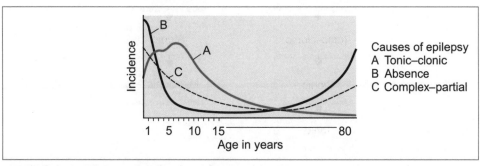

FIGURE 8.1   Incidence of epilepsy with age

Reproduced from 'Seizures and Epilepsy', by J Engel, Jr. In: *Contemporary Neurology Series,* edited by F Plum, Vol 31, 1989, FA Davis Company, Figure 5.3, p 115 [12]

CHARACTERISATION OF THE TYPE OF SEIZURE

The clinical manifestations of the more common types of seizures is discussed here; more detail can be found in textbooks [12–14]. The commonest seizures in clinical practice are:
* tonic–clonic
* absence
* complex–partial.

Less common are:
* simple–partial
* myoclonic
* clonic
* tonic
* atonic
* benign rolandic seizures.

Although the traditional approach is to classify seizures as focal versus generalised or primary (no obvious cause) versus secondary, an alternate way to characterise the various types of seizures is based on what can be witnessed:

1 seizures that cause the patient to fall with or without loss of consciousness (see Figure 8.2)
2 seizures that are not associated with a fall with or without loss of consciousness (awareness; see Figure 8.3).

Tonic–clonic seizures
* **Immediately before ictus:** The aura or warning if it occurs may indicate a focal onset such as **déjà vu**, **jamais vu** or unpleasant olfactory (smell) or gustatory (taste) phenomena that are suggestive of a temporal lobe origin. The aura may consist of a non-specific epigastric rising sensation, where an unpleasant feeling commences in the epigastrium and rises up towards the head very quickly over a few seconds, a non-specific light-headedness or an odd feeling in the head.

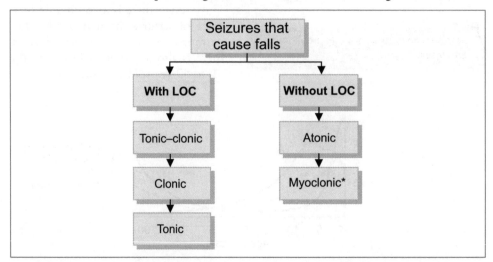

FIGURE 8.2   Seizures that cause a fall with or without loss of consciousness (LOC)

*A fall will result if the patient is standing and the myoclonus affects the legs. Patients with brief focal myoclonic seizures may not fall if they are seated.

Tonic–clonic seizures preceded by an aura are often referred to as focal seizures with secondary generalisation, as opposed to primary generalised epilepsy where the tonic–clonic seizure is not of focal origin. *The essential feature is that the aura is identical each time and more importantly is very brief,* usually lasting seconds only.

- **During ictus:** With or without warning (an aura) the patient will fall to the ground, rigid, with the teeth clenched, arms and legs extended and eyes open. At times the arms may be flexed instead of extended. Many eyewitnesses describe the eyes as rolling up into the top of the head, which means that the eyes are open. This tonic phase is brief, usually less than 30 seconds, and it is followed by repetitive jerking (clonic phase) of the arms and legs, which is also brief, usually less than 1 or 2 minutes, although it may be prolonged up to 10 minutes. Seizures may last longer if the patient develops status recurrent seizures without recovery of consciousness between seizures, referred to as status epilepsy. During a tonic–clonic seizure the patient may bite the tongue or cheek, froth at the mouth or be incontinent of urine and/or faeces. If urinary or faecal incontinence occurs, it is during the tonic phase.
- **After ictus:** Immediately following the seizure the patient is limp, drowsy and confused. This period of post-ictal confusion and drowsiness varies depending upon the duration of the seizure and the age of the patient. If seizures are brief the duration may be less than a few minutes; with more prolonged seizures, the period of confusion can last much longer, usually less than half an hour. In the elderly it may last for several days in the absence of any obvious metabolic or infective process to account for such confusion. Very rarely, paralysis of a limb(s) follows a seizure, an entity called Todd's palsy. Again, this tends to be more prolonged in the elderly.

Tonic seizures

Although these can occur at any age they are most commonly seen in childhood. When an adult has what seems like a tonic seizure it is often secondary to a hypotensive episode, e.g. vasovagal or neurocardiogenic syncope. Tonic contractions affect the face and limbs, resulting in flexion of the upper limbs and trunk and either flexion or extension of the lower limbs. Although consciousness is impaired, these seizures are very brief often lasting only seconds. It is rare for these to occur in isolation and usually patients have other types of seizures.

Atonic seizures

Atonic seizures, also referred to as drop attacks, are rare and consist of a sudden loss of postural tone: if brief only the head may drop, but if more severe the person will fall to the floor, often sustaining injury. There may be a brief period (seconds) of impaired consciousness but no post-ictal confusion. Patients usually have other seizure types, including a few brief myoclonic jerks, prior to the atonic seizure but most often tonic–clonic epilepsy.

Drop attacks due to epilepsy mainly occur in childhood; drop attacks that occur in elderly adults are thought not to be epileptic in origin and are discussed in Chapter 7, 'Episodic disturbances of function'. The Lennox–Gastaut syndrome is seen in childhood and consists of multiple seizure types including atypical absence seizures, myoclonic, tonic–clonic and atonic seizures with often a degree of intellectual disability [5].

Myoclonic seizures

Myoclonus is a shock-like contraction of a muscle or a group of muscles. Myoclonus occurs in people without epilepsy, often when they are just falling asleep but also occasionally any time of the day. The frequency would usually be less than once a month. There is also an entity called segmental myoclonus that is not a seizure disorder, where a particular muscle or group of muscles supplied by a particular nerve or nerve root will have myoclonic jerks.

In patients with myoclonic epilepsy, these myoclonic jerks are more frequent, often occur during sleep but characteristically occur first thing in the morning on awakening. They affect the whole body or a single limb and may be single or repetitive jerks. In myoclonic seizures the patient is fully aware of what is happening. There is no aura, loss of awareness or post-ictal confusion, i.e. the patient is normal immediately before and after the event. Myoclonus induced by movement is a feature of post-hypoxic myoclonus [15].

JUVENILE MYOCLONIC EPILEPSY

Juvenile myoclonic epilepsy (JME) is myoclonus, absence seizures and occasional tonic–clonic seizures. This usually presents between ages 6 and 22, but there is a lifelong predisposition to recurrent seizures without treatment [16, 17].

Complex–partial seizures

Complex–partial seizures most commonly arise from the temporal lobe in association with mesial temporal sclerosis. Complex–partial epilepsy (CPE) was originally referred to as temporal lobe epilepsy. However, the recognition that minor seizures that impair consciousness without causing the patient to fall may arise from the occipital, frontal or parietal lobes has led to the use of the term CPE.

- **Immediately before ictus:** The duration of the aura is usually measured in seconds; the symptoms of aura have been described above.
- **During ictus:** The ictus usually lasts seconds to a few minutes. The patient is not aware of what is happening, nor are they able to respond to any verbal or painful stimuli. In the words of two relatives witnessing minor seizures: 'the lights were on

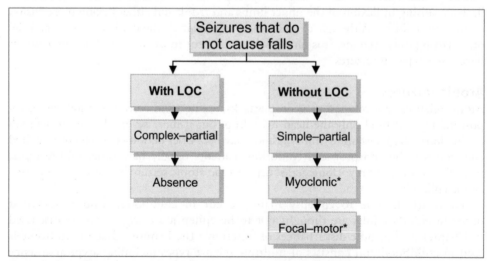

FIGURE 8.3 Seizures that do not cause a fall with or without loss of consciousness (LOC)

*Patients with myoclonic or focal–motor seizures may fall if they are standing but there is no LOC.

but no one was at home' or 'there were no sheep in the top paddock'. There may be involuntary movements of the mouth or limbs, depending on which area of the brain is the focus for the seizure.

- **After ictus:** There is a period of post-ictal confusion lasting several minutes during which the patient can usually respond to outside stimuli but is clearly disoriented and confused [18]. The patient is unable to relate what happened during the event.

Absence (petit-mal) seizures

Absence epilepsy generally occurs in childhood and is very rare as a primary presentation in adults. In retrospect, however, when one takes a careful history from a patient with their first tonic–clonic seizure, many patients have had unrecognised absence seizures [9] in childhood and have simply been regarded as either dull or a daydreamer.

- **Immediately before ictus:** The absence seizure is characterised by no warning unless it is an atypical absence.
- **During ictus:** The period of impaired consciousness is brief. In one study the average seizure duration was 9.4 seconds (range 1–44 seconds, SD 7 seconds), 26% of seizures were shorter than 4 seconds and 8% were longer than 20 seconds [19]. The patient simply stares into space and may blink, but they are clearly unresponsive to either verbal or painful stimuli. They have no recollection of what happened or was said to them during the episode.
- **After ictus:** Immediately following the ictus, the patient is able to resume a conversation and the activity that they were undertaking without any post-ictal confusion.

It is surprising how many absence seizures patients can experience without people actually noticing them because they are so brief. Absence seizures can readily be induced by hyperventilation (HV). In one study of 47 children with childhood absence seizures, HV induced seizures in 83% (39/47) of children. Of the eight children who did not have seizures induced by HV, four were too young to perform HV. In the other four children, HV was performed but may not have been performed well [19].

The important clue that helps differentiate absence seizures from daydreaming is that with absence seizures the patient will interrupt their behaviour. For example, they will momentarily pause unexpectedly during a conversation or a game they have been playing, and then appear to resume it as if nothing has happened. Many children daydream or are concentrating on television or some other activity and, although it can be difficult to attract their attention, they are not unresponsive. One common presentation of absence epilepsy is the child who has previously done well at school and who begins to fail. Unfortunately, many children in the past were assumed to be daydreamers who were not working hard enough when in fact they were missing large parts of the lesson because of minor absence seizures. In the author's experience, many teachers fail to detect children with minor epilepsy. It is when these children who fail have further teaching that the seizures are actually discovered by the tutor who spends more time with them on a one-to-one basis.

The EEG in absence seizures shows a characteristic 3 per second spike and wave (see Figure 8.4).

Simple partial seizures

The essential characteristic of simple partial seizures is that they can occur at any age in either sex and consist of a brief stereotyped sensation without loss of awareness, i.e. the patient is fully conscious of what is happening and is able to describe the whole episode

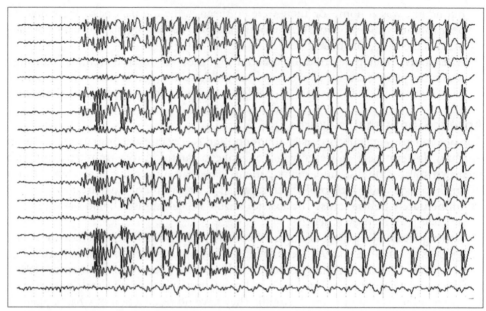

FIGURE 8.4   EEG in absence epilepsy showing 3 per second spike and wave

from start to finish. There is no warning or aura, nor is there any post-ictal drowsiness or confusion. Examples of this type of epilepsy are patients who experience a tingling sensation that may commence in their feet and rise up to the top of the head and sometimes go back down again to their feet, over a matter of seconds.

Focal motor seizures

These episodes are very brief, usually lasting less than a minute or two, although they can go on repetitively in patients, in which case the term focal motor status epilepsy is used. The patient is fully aware of what is going on around them, there is usually no warning and certainly there is no post-ictal drowsiness or confusion. The seizures consist of repetitive contractions down one side of the body.

Benign focal seizure of childhood

There are a number of benign focal seizures of childhood [20, 21]. There are currently three identifiable electroclinical syndromes recognised by the International League against Epilepsy (ILAE) [22]: rolandic epilepsy, Panayiotopoulos syndrome (PS) or common autonomic epilepsy and the idiopathic childhood occipital epilepsy of Gastaut (ICOE-G). They produce terrifying manifestations. Details are given in Appendix B, 'Benign focal seizures of childhood', because they are rare and atypical with the duration of symptoms being longer than for most other seizure types.

Febrile convulsions

Febrile convulsions affect 2% to 5% of all children and usually appear between 3 months and 5 years of age. Febrile convulsions may be provoked by any febrile bacterial or viral illness and no specific level of fever is required to diagnose febrile seizures. It is essential to exclude underlying meningitis either clinically or, if any doubt remains, by lumbar puncture. The risk of epilepsy following a febrile seizure is 1% to 6% [23].

Reflex epilepsies

Reflex epilepsies are very rare, but are discussed briefly so that the reader is familiar with this entity. The clue to the clinical diagnosis is repeated precipitation of a brief stereotyped episode by a particular stimulus. One of the commonest is the tonic–clonic seizure that is precipitated by the stroboscope at a dance.

The reflex epilepsies are syndromes in which all epileptic seizures are precipitated by sensory stimuli. Generalised reflex seizures are precipitated by visual light stimulation, thinking and decision making. Numerous triggers can induce focal reflex seizures, including reading, writing, other language functions, startle, somatosensory stimulation, proprioception, auditory stimuli, immersion in hot water, eating and vestibular stimulation [24].

Consider possible multiple types of seizures

Having established that the patient has suffered a seizure, the next step is to determine whether they suffer from any other seizure types and whether they have suffered from undiagnosed seizures in the past. Although most patients who present with their first tonic–clonic seizure have not had other manifestations of epilepsy, with detailed questioning it is not uncommon for patients to have had unrecognised myoclonic seizures and/or minor absence or complex–partial seizures in the past [9].

Most seizures conform to the common seizure types listed above and the diagnosis rarely presents any difficulty. On the other hand, there are rare cases where the events during the ictus are atypical and can lead to an erroneous diagnosis of a non-organic event. Consider the following actual case history (Case 8.1) where the principles discussed earlier in this chapter are highlighted.

CASE 8.1

Dear Doctor,

Thank you for seeing this young man with very strange behaviour. He has had recurrent episodes lasting less than a minute or two. He is witnessed to walk across the room and shakes whoever is in the room a few times. After this he is confused for a few more minutes and states that he does not recall what happened.

Yours sincerely,

This patient did exhibit very strange behaviour. However, the episodes were stereotyped and brief, lasting less than 90 seconds, and during the episode there were positive phenomena in that he walked, grabbed people and shook them. He lost awareness and was amnestic during the episode and it was followed by a short period of post-ictal confusion. Subsequent video-EEG monitoring confirmed that these episodes were complex–partial seizures.

Pseudoseizures

Pseudoseizures are paroxysmal changes in behaviour that resemble epileptic seizures, but which are without organic cause and the expected EEG changes. Longer ictal duration and less stereotypy (variation of the manifestations from one episode to the next) are characteristic. Other characteristic features include asynchronous extremity movements, atypical vocalisation, alternating head movements, talking or screaming, opisthotonic posturing (arching of the back) and pelvic thrusting [25].

An increasing frequency of 'seizures' with escalating doses of anticonvulsants should alert the clinician to the possible diagnosis [26]. The diagnosis can be very difficult as up to 30% of patients with pseudoseizures have epileptic seizures as well and pelvic thrusting can be a very rare manifestation of temporal lobe or frontal lobe epilepsy [27]. The diagnosis of psychogenic pseudoseizures has improved with the availability of video-EEG monitoring [28]. If pseudoseizures are suspected, one way to confirm the diagnosis is to instruct family members, nursing staff on the ward or anyone who may witness an episode to try and interrupt what is happening either by talking to the patient or by employing a painful stimulus, e.g. pinching the skin over the medial aspect of the elbow. Organic seizures, as opposed to pseudoseizures, cannot be interrupted.

ASSESSING THE FREQUENCY OF SEIZURES

The patient with their 'first seizure'

As already stated it is not uncommon to see patients with their first apparent tonic–clonic seizure who have had a previous seizure or a long history of unrecognised minor seizures or myoclonus [9]. Ask the patient whether they have frequent involuntary brief jerking of one limb or all of the body, similar to the sensation that they experience when they are just falling asleep. These involuntary jerks (termed myoclonus) can occur infrequently, perhaps a few times per year in normal individuals, whereas in patients with epilepsy they occur more frequently and often first thing in the morning upon wakening, particularly in patients with juvenile myoclonic epilepsy syndrome. Although the patient is very aware of these myoclonic jerks, they interfere so little with their life that often they do not seek medical attention. Similarly, minor seizures may go undetected or undiagnosed for many, many years. Often detailed questioning of relatives or friends using the questions described above will elicit a prior history of previously unrecognised minor seizures. Ascertain how frequently the various types of seizures occur (i.e. many times per day, daily, weekly etc).

Status epilepsy

Status epilepsy is a seizure that 'persists for a sufficient length of time or is repeated frequently enough that recovery between attacks does not occur'. Both convulsive and non-convulsive status epilepsy are recognised.

CONVULSIVE STATUS EPILEPSY

Status tonic–clonic (convulsive) epilepsy consists of continuous or rapidly repeating seizures and is a medical emergency. **The treating doctor should not leave the bedside until seizures cease.** There are published guidelines for the management of status epilepsy [29–31]. Guidelines are often updated and every institution should have access to them. Patients who do not respond to initial therapy should be treated in an intensive care unit, as artificial ventilation and haemodynamic support are required.

NON-CONVULSIVE STATUS EPILEPSY

Non-convulsive status epilepsy is an epileptic state in which there is some impairment of consciousness associated with ongoing seizure activity on the EEG [32]. It is often a sequel to convulsive status epilepsy [32]. Patients may present in a coma without any overt signs of seizure activity [33].

IDENTIFYING ANY PRECIPITATING CAUSES

Identifying a reversible precipitating cause is important as avoidance in the future can reduce the risk of subsequent seizures. Most seizures are due to an abnormal electrical discharge within the brain, often referred to as primary epilepsy. Seizures can also be secondary to the hypotension that occurs for example with syncope, a Stokes–Adams attack, alcohol abuse or withdrawal of sedative or hypnotic drugs.

- In patients with primary epilepsy, sleep deprivation, photic stimulation, alcohol abuse [34], menstruation and an intercurrent infective illness may potentially predispose to recurrence [35].
- Vomiting and/or diarrhoea alter drug levels, predisposing to recurrent seizures, and many drugs, including psychotropics, local and general anaesthetics, narcotics, antiarrhythmics and antibiotics, are recognised precipitating factors for seizures [36].
- Poor compliance is one, if not the commonest, cause of recurrent seizures in patients on anticonvulsants [34].

ESTABLISHING AN AETIOLOGY

Most patients with epilepsy do not have any identifiable underlying pathology. It is possible that with future advancements in the understanding of epilepsy more causes will be identified. Focal-motor seizures, complex–partial seizures and, particularly, seizures associated with a focal neurological deficit are more likely to have identifiable pathology on imaging [37].

Seizures may occur with alcohol or drug withdrawal, infective processes within the central nervous system, drugs, benign and malignant tumours, just to mention a few possible aetiologies. Seizures can be the presenting symptom of disturbances of cardiac rhythm [38] or, rarely, secondary to severe pain, for example in patients with trigeminal neuralgia [39]. Detailed lists can be found in textbooks on epilepsy [5–7, 14, 40, 41]. This means that it is not possible to be dogmatic about what investigation(s) should be performed in an individual patient; suffice to say that every effort should be made to find a cause.

> A word of warning: the presence of a family history of epilepsy or a past history of a head injury *only suggests* that the seizure may be familial or post-traumatic, and other pathological processes need to be considered.

Investigations

- Some would argue that it is justifiable to perform medical imaging of all adult patients who present with tonic–clonic, complex–partial and focal motor seizures [42, 43]. Others would argue that there is currently insufficient data to support or refute recommending any of these tests for the routine evaluation of adults presenting with an apparent first unprovoked seizure [43]. The yield of currently available imaging techniques is about 10%. Current recommendations advocate an EEG, CT or MRI brain scan in all patients presenting with a first unprovoked seizure [43]. In reality most, if not all, patients will demand imaging for reassurance that they do not have a brain tumour.
- Laboratory tests, such as blood counts, blood glucose and electrolytes, particularly sodium, lumbar puncture and toxicology screening may be helpful as determined by the specific clinical circumstances based on the history, physical and neurological examination, but there are insufficient data to support or refute recommending any of these tests for the routine evaluation of adults presenting with an apparent first unprovoked seizure [43].
- On the other hand, although metabolic disturbances causing seizures are rare they are readily correctable, particularly hypoglycaemia. When a patient presents with a

seizure, probably the single most important test to perform immediately is a serum glucose to exclude hypoglycaemia. Other metabolic disturbances, such as hyponatraemia, hypocalcaemia and an elevated urea, may cause seizures and, as a general principle, these investigations are without risk and the subsequent management is easy. It would seem reasonable to exclude metabolic causes in all patients.

DECIDING WHETHER TO TREAT OR NOT

In many patients with simple partial seizures, reassurance that nothing sinister is the matter suffices and they do not wish to take medication to stop such trivial symptoms. In patients with an isolated idiopathic (no particular cause) tonic–clonic seizure the subsequent risk of further seizures varies from study to study. In one study of children it was 54% [44], while in another study of adults there was a 27% risk of recurrence at 36 months [45]. A first seizure provoked by an acute brain disturbance is unlikely to recur (3–10%), whereas a first unprovoked seizure has a recurrence risk of 30–50% over the next 2 years [46].

The number of seizures of all types at presentation, the presence of a neurological disorder and an abnormal EEG are significant risk factors for recurrent seizures. An abnormal EEG is defined as specific focal or generalised epileptiform or slow wave abnormalities. Individuals with two or three seizures plus a neurological disorder and/or an abnormal EEG have been identified as a high-risk group with a 73% incidence of recurrent seizures at 5 years [47]. In the same study the recurrence rate at 5 years in patients with a single seizure, a normal EEG and no neurological abnormality was 39% [47].

In a study of immediate versus delayed treatment with currently available anticonvulsants, immediate treatment did not reduce the long-term recurrence rate. At 5-year follow-up, 76% of patients in the immediate treatment group and 77% of those in the deferred treatment group were seizure free (difference –0.2%, 95% CI –5.8% to 5.5%) [48]. When confronted with such a low risk of recurrence many patients elect not to take antiepileptic drug (AED) treatment after a first seizure [46]. It would therefore seem reasonable not to recommend therapy in patients with an isolated tonic–clonic seizure in the absence of a positive family history, an abnormal EEG and pre-existing cerebral pathology, particularly if there was an easily reversible precipitating cause such as sleep deprivation. The patient in this situation often decides. The question to put to the patient is: 'What effect would another seizure have on your life?' The commonest reason patients give for wanting to go onto medication is that a further seizure would terrify them, although more often it is the unacceptable social implications and the effect on their ability to drive, and thus on their employment, that influences their decision whether to take medication or not. Being employed is a major reason why patients continue to drive against medical advice [49].

Occasional patients can have two seizures many years apart. If the patient had been placed on medication after the first seizure, the clinician would have regarded the treatment as excellent when in fact the natural history was such that the patient was not going to experience a second seizure for many years. In general, AEDs should be offered after a first tonic–clonic seizure if:
- the patient has had previous myoclonic, absence or partial seizures
- the EEG shows unequivocal epileptic discharges
- the patient has a congenital neurological deficit
- the patient considers the risk of recurrence unacceptable.

CHOOSING THE APPROPRIATE DRUG, DOSE AND ONGOING MONITORING OF THE RESPONSE TO THERAPY

Choosing a drug

Treatment is targeted primarily to:

- assist the patient in adjusting psychologically to the diagnosis and in maintaining as normal a lifestyle as possible
- reduce or eliminate seizure occurrence
- avoid or minimise the side effects of long-term drug treatment.

Most patients with more than one seizure require prophylactic AED therapy. Some seizure types or epilepsy syndromes may respond to certain drugs while other drugs may exacerbate the seizures [50, 51].

The general principle is to choose a drug with the greatest efficacy in terms of preventing seizures, provided there is no contraindication to its use. If there are several possible drugs, the 'correct drug' is the drug the patient deems to have the fewest undesirable potential side effects from their perspective, e.g. the risks of weight gain or interference with oral contraceptives are common reasons why young females refuse a particular drug. Patients can only make such a decision when they receive detailed information regarding the proposed treatment options.

Side effects are a significant reason for discontinuing an AED, particularly in the elderly [52].

When monotherapy does not control seizures, review the diagnosis of epilepsy and check for compliance with medication. Failure of the first AED due to lack of efficacy (and not due to incorrect choice of drug, wrong dose, incorrect dosing schedule or poor compliance) implies refractoriness and trying multiple AEDs one after another is unlikely to be successful [53]. Combination therapy should be considered when treatment with two first-line AEDs has failed or when the first well-tolerated drug substantially improves seizure control but fails to produce freedom from seizure at maximal dosage. In this instance, an AED with different and perhaps multiple mechanisms of action should be added. Strategies for combining drugs should involve individual assessment of the patient's seizure type, together with an understanding of the pharmacology, side effects and interaction profiles of the AEDs [54]. The choice of drugs to use in combination should be limited to two or at most three AEDs.

An important principle when altering therapeutic regimens is to *avoid changing two things at a time*. In that situation it is difficult to know what has done the good or harm.

Current treatment recommendations and the potential side effects of specific drugs are given in Appendix C, 'Currently recommended drugs for epilepsy', and links to websites that should provide more up-to-date information are given in Chapter 15, 'Further reading, keeping up-to-date and retrieving information'.

Choosing the dose

Other than with status epilepsy, there is no need to reach a therapeutic dose rapidly. Therefore, treatment should commence with the lowest possible dose and increase very slowly over weeks as this *may* reduce the incidence of side effects [55, 56]. The number of doses per day is dependent on the half-life of the drug, but medications prescribed more than twice a day are associated with an increasing incidence of poor compliance [57].

Monitoring the response

In many patients complete freedom from seizures is not possible and sensible decisions regarding the efficacy of medication can be made only with careful assessment of seizure frequency. Seizure frequency has a significant impact on quality of life [58]. Although it is recommended that patients keep a diary to record the frequency of their seizures, very few do. It is important for the treating doctor to keep detailed notes on behalf of the patient and refer to these notes when deciding if a particular AED has been effective in reducing the number of seizures. Monitoring the response to treatment at times can be extraordinarily difficult, particularly in young patients who through embarrassment will often deny forgetting their medication, drinking too much alcohol or staying out all night.

Intractable epilepsy

One of the major difficulties in patients with intractable epilepsy is that many do not know what drugs have been used, what the doses were and whether they were stopped due to an apparent lack of efficacy or because of side effects. The lack of efficacy may relate to an incorrect choice of drug or drug dosage and scheduling. It is sometimes useful to show patients pictures of the specific drugs or, better still, have all the common AEDs stuck onto cardboard so that patients can identify the drug they have taken. Unfortunately, even when they can identify the drug, they are usually unaware of the dose tried, the frequency of dosing and the reason for stopping the drug. It is useful to advise patients to keep a diary of the date and time of any seizures that occur for two reasons:

1 To see whether there is a decrease in the frequency of seizures when therapy is modified.
2 Perhaps more importantly, to determine what time of the day the seizures occur in relation to the timing of medication.

In patients on a twice daily dosage regimen, a number will experience seizures in the hour or two before or within the first half hour after the dose. Simply increasing the individual dose in this setting results in symptoms of toxicity as the peak serum level increases but then falls below the threshold for the patient's seizures just prior to the next dose. The appropriate course of action is to increase the frequency of the medication if the drug has a half-life of 8–12 hours (although compliance is better when drugs are prescribed less frequently) or, alternatively, change the patient to a drug that has a longer half-life.

Unfortunately, with many drugs, there is a 'honeymoon period' during the first 6 months of treatment when the number of seizures decreases, but subsequently seizures may become just as frequent.

Measuring serum levels

Serum AED measurements are useful when the level directly reflects efficacy; this is not the case for all drugs. Other clinical situations where AED monitoring is useful include checking for compliance or toxicity, as a guide to adjusting the dose when another drug is added or during pregnancy [59].

ADVICE REGARDING LIFESTYLE

Driving and epilepsy

Each country has different regulations with regard to driving and epilepsy, and it is important for all clinicians who care for patients with epilepsy to have a copy of their respective country's (or state's) guidelines. In recent years restrictions have been less stringent, reflecting the low contribution of seizures to the overall road toll [60]. In some countries the restriction on driving is very severe, whereas in others a more lenient approach is taken.

Essentially, a sufficient period of time needs to elapse to be certain that a recurrent seizure is unlikely to occur. In one study patients who had seizure-free intervals of 12 months or longer had 93% reduced odds of motor vehicle accidents compared to patients with shorter seizure-free intervals. The majority (54%) of patients who crashed were driving illegally, with seizure-free intervals shorter than legally permitted [61], and 20% had missed an AED dose just prior to the crash. Patients should be informed that, although the risk of a seizure is small, the potential consequences could be disastrous. It is also a useful tactic to show patients the guidelines, explaining that the medical practitioner does not make the rules and that these rules are not there to punish patients with epilepsy but to protect the patient from hurting themselves or innocent people.

The risk of a seizure occurring while driving is also a reflection of the time spent driving. If the patient drives for only half an hour per day the risk of a seizure while driving is much lower than if they drive for 12 hours per day. For this reason in many countries the requirements are more stringent for commercial and heavy goods vehicle licenses than for private motor vehicle licenses [62].

Pregnancy and epilepsy

Although the increased risk of major congenital malformations in patients with epilepsy taking AED(s) during pregnancy is possibly 2–3 times that of the normal population [63], most pregnancies will result in a normal child. There is some debate about the exact role of AED exposure in pregnancy and any increased risk [64]. Some AEDs and the use of multiple AEDs (polypharmacy) may be associated with a greater risk [65–67]. Long-term cognitive problems in the child may also occur [65].

In clinical practice many patients attend their doctor to discuss withdrawal of medication when they are 2–3 months pregnant. Any teratogenic effects will have already occurred, and it is probably unwise and essentially too late to withdraw medication at this stage of the pregnancy. The risk of uncontrolled seizures during pregnancy needs to be weighed against the risk of AED exposure. An increased risk to the mother and infant is often quoted but it is difficult to find good evidence to justify this statement. In the European Registry of Antiepileptic Drugs and Pregnancy (EURAP) study, of 1956 pregnancies 58.3% were seizure-free throughout pregnancy. Seizures occurred during delivery in 60 pregnancies (3.5%), more commonly in women with seizures during pregnancy (odds ratio (OR): 4.8; 2.3–10.0). There were 36 cases of status epilepsy (12 convulsive), which resulted in stillbirth in only 1 case, but no cases of miscarriage or maternal mortality [68]. A Cochrane review has concluded that, based on the best current available evidence, it would seem advisable for women to continue medication during pregnancy using monotherapy at the lowest dose required to achieve seizure control [65].

Some patients seek advice about ceasing their AEDs prior to pregnancy and here the decision is more difficult. Even if the epilepsy is easily controlled, the patient has to be willing to run the risk of a recurrent seizure and the subsequent consequences regarding the alteration in their lifestyle, in particular driving. In general, if the epilepsy has been difficult to control, an argument can be made for the patient to remain on medication throughout the pregnancy. Accumulating evidence from drug registries suggests that the lowest possible dose and avoidance of certain drugs may be appropriate

[68–70]. Patients willing to consider a mid-trimester termination can have testing for major malformations.

Some patients may experience an increased seizure frequency while others have fewer seizures [68]. Occasionally, patients not known to suffer from epilepsy have a tonic–clonic seizure during labour and, although other serious disorders need to be considered, often a detailed history will elicit a long history of infrequent minor and previously unrecognised seizures.[1] Most patients with epilepsy will maintain control during pregnancy [68].

Potentially hazardous activities
Patients should be warned that it may be dangerous to go swimming or fishing, have a bath or walk near water if they are alone as a seizure could result in drowning [71]. Patients should also be advised not to scale heights, walk near the edge of cliffs, sky dive or scuba dive.

CONSIDERATION OF SURGERY IN PATIENTS WHO FAIL TO RESPOND TO DRUG THERAPY

Approximately one-third of patients with epilepsy are refractory to AED therapy and many of these patients are candidates for surgical treatment [72]. Among patients who do not respond to the first drug, the percentage who subsequently become seizure-free with additional AEDs is smaller (11%) [53]. Patients with refractory epilepsy should be referred to an appropriate centre earlier rather than later for potential surgery.

Investigation and treatment
The use of magnetic resonance imaging (MRI) has been pivotal in the evaluation of patients with partial seizures [73]. Patients with MRI-negative partial epilepsy may be candidates for additional neuroimaging techniques including positron emission tomography, MR spectroscopy and single photon emission tomography. Peri-ictal imaging may allow identification of the epileptogenic zone in patients with normal MRI scans.

In patients with refractory epilepsy, vagal nerve [74], hippocampal [75] and bilateral cerebellar [76] electrical stimulation have been advocated. These techniques have resulted in a modest reduction in seizure frequency but none has eliminated seizures altogether. On the other hand surgery, in particular temporal lobectomy for mesial temporal sclerosis, has been shown to be highly effective in a randomised controlled trial, with more than 50% of patients seizure-free as opposed to 8% in the non-surgical group [77].

Macroscopic and radiological evidence of total lesional excision with isolated structural lesions such as dysembryoplastic tumours, low-grade astrocytomas or focal vascular abnormalities is associated with excellent seizure-free outcome [78].

Corpus callosotomy is recommended for patients with atonic seizures or drop attacks [79, 80].

Hemispherectomy is now a widely accepted procedure for medically refractory, catastrophic hemispheric epilepsy. The classic anatomical hemispherectomy procedure has been abandoned in favour of functional or modified hemispherectomy [81].

---

1 Personal observation.

WHETHER AND WHEN TO WITHDRAW THERAPY IN 'SEIZURE-FREE' PATIENTS

A patient who has been free of seizures for some time often asks whether AEDs can be stopped. The juvenile myoclonic epilepsy syndrome consisting of absence and myoclonic seizures and infrequent tonic–clonic seizures is associated with a lifelong predisposition to seizures and AEDs should not be ceased.

In other forms of epilepsy where remission can occur and a trial off AEDs is not unreasonable, the initial question to the patient must be: 'What effect would a recurrent seizure have on your life?' For example, the patient would be unable to drive for a prescribed period after the seizure and this could impact on their life and work. A recurrent seizure may occur in a situation where it would cause significant embarrassment or, worse still, possible injury. A minimum of 2 years free of seizures is recommended before considering withdrawal of medication [82]. Even when the risk of recurrence is low, it must be stated that *there is no guarantee that there will not be a recurrent seizure*. Recurrent seizures may occur after as many as 8 years off medication.[2]

In a review of 28 studies accounting for 4571 patients (2758 children, 1020 adults and a combined group of 793), most with at least 2 years of seizure remission, the proportion of patients with relapses during or after AED withdrawal ranged from 12% to 66% [83].

A higher-than-average risk of seizure relapse included:
- adolescent-onset epilepsy
- partial seizures
- the presence of an underlying neurological condition
- abnormal EEG findings at the time of AED withdrawal in children [83].

Most relapses occur during or within the first 6 months after withdrawal [84]. At the time of writing there was no evidence to determine the rate of withdrawal [85], but it seems reasonable to reduce the dose slowly over several weeks to months.

COMMON TREATMENT ERRORS

In 1999 Feely [86] elegantly summarised many common treatment errors and most of his observations apply today. They include:
1 Incorrect or incomplete identification of seizure type(s), resulting in inappropriate choice of treatment: for example confusion between brief complex–partial seizures and absences or failure to recognise juvenile myoclonic epilepsy.
2 A drug appropriate for the patient's seizure type(s) is chosen, but it is not appropriate for that patient: for example, phenytoin for an adolescent female (coarsening of facial features), valproic acid for a woman likely to become pregnant (increased risk of congenital malformations) or carbamazepine for a woman on the oral contraceptive pill (reduced contraceptive efficacy).
3 The diagnosis and choice of drug are correct, but the patient is given too low a dose (for example, only the 'starting' dose is tried) or the patient is given too high a dose too quickly.
4 The epilepsy is controlled, but the patient has problems with side effects and no change in the treatment (drug or dosage) is made.

2 Personal observation.

5 The patient is seen by a specialist and referred back to the general practitioner with an appropriate recommendation regarding treatment, but when this proves ineffective further advice is not sought.

6 This author would add that, although a detailed explanation regarding treatment, lifestyle etc is provided at the time of the consultation, this information is often forgotten. It is for this reason that this author provides a copy of his letter to the referring doctor to all patients.

THE ELECTROENCEPHALOGRAM

No chapter on epilepsy would be complete without a discussion of the electro-encephalogram (EEG).

Perhaps the single most important point to make is that a NORMAL EEG does not exclude epilepsy and an ABNORMAL EEG can very occasionally be seen in patients without epilepsy.

Points to consider are:
- A single inter-ictal (between seizures) EEG has a sensitivity of approximately 50% [87, 88] and a specificity of 97–98% [89, 90]. The sensitivity can be increased to 92% if a further three EEGs are performed [88].
- Sleep deprivation increases the number of abnormal EEGs [9, 91].
- Epileptiform abnormalities are more likely to be detected if the EEG is performed within the first 24 hours after a seizure [9].
- In adults the EEG is more likely to be abnormal in patients with generalised seizures than partial seizures [9].
- Prolonged monitoring with or without video monitoring is useful for patients with refractory epilepsy [92] or frequent seizures, particularly in childhood [93].
- Video-EEG monitoring is useful for patients with suspected pseudoseizures [94].
- EEG abnormalities have been found in 3.5% of 3726 children without epilepsy [90].

REFERENCES

1 Fisher RS et al. Epileptic seizures and epilepsy: Definitions proposed by the International League Against Epilepsy (ILAE) and the International Bureau for Epilepsy (IBE). Epilepsia 2005; 46(4):470–472.

2 Engel J, Jr. A proposed diagnostic scheme for people with epileptic seizures and with epilepsy: Report of the ILAE task force on classification and terminology. 2006. Available: http://www.ilae-epilepsy.org/Visitors/Centre/ctf/overview.cfm (14 Dec 2009).

3 Engel J, Jr. Classifications of the International League Against Epilepsy: Time for reappraisal. Epilepsia 1998; 39(9):1014–1017.

4 Everitt AD, Sander JW. Classification of the epilepsies: Time for a change? A critical review of the International Classification of the Epilepsies and Epileptic Syndromes (ICEES) and its usefulness in clinical practice and epidemiological studies of epilepsy. Eur Neurol 1999; 42(1):1–10.

5 Engel J, Jr. Seizures and epilepsy. In: Plum F (ed). Contemporary neurology series, vol 31. Philadelphia: FA Davis Company; 1989:165, 203–207.

6 Shorvon SD. Handbook of epilepsy treatment: Forms, causes and therapy in children and adults. Oxford: Blackwell Publishing; 2005:304.

7 Engel J, Pedley TA (eds). Epilepsy: A comprehensive textbook. Philadelphia: Lippincott Williams & Wilkins; 2007:3056.

8 Jenssen S, Gracely EJ, Sperling MR. How long do most seizures last? A systematic comparison of seizures recorded in the epilepsy monitoring unit. Epilepsia 2006; 47(9):1499–1503.

9 King MA et al. Epileptology of the first-seizure presentation: A clinical, electroencephalographic, and magnetic resonance imaging study of 300 consecutive patients. Lancet 1998; 352(9133):1007–1011.

10 Jetter GM, Cavazos JE. Epilepsy in the elderly. Semin Neurol 2008; 28(3):336–341.

11 Anderson VE. Family studies of epilepsy. In: Anderson VE et al (ed). Genetic basis of the epilepsies. New York: Raven; 1982:103–112.

12 Engel J, Jr. Seizures and epilepsy. In: Plum F (ed). Contemporary neurology series, vol 31. Philadelphia: FA Davis Company; 1989:536.

13 Lüders H. Textbook of Epileptology. Boca Raton, Florida: Taylor & Francis CRC Press; 2001:400.

14 Shorvon S. Handbook of epilepsy treatment. Massachusetts: Blackwell Publishing; 2000:248.

15 Fahn S. Posthypoxic action myoclonus: Literature review update. Adv Neurol 1986; 43:157–169.

16 Alfradique I, Vasconcelos MM. Juvenile myoclonic epilepsy. Arq Neuropsiquiatr 2007; 65(4B):1266–1271.

17 Auvin S. Treatment of juvenile myoclonic epilepsy. CNS Neurosci Ther 2008; 14(3):227–233.

18 Caicoya AG, Serratosa JM. Postictal behaviour in temporal lobe epilepsy. Epileptic Disord 2006; 8(3): 228–231.

19 Sadleir LG et al. Electroclinical features of absence seizures in childhood absence epilepsy. Neurology 2006; 67(3):413–418.

20 Panayiotopoulos CP et al. Benign childhood focal epilepsies: Assessment of established and newly recognized syndromes. Brain 2008; 131(Pt 9):2264–2286.

21 Doose H, Baier WK. Benign partial epilepsy and related conditions: Multifactorial pathogenesis with hereditary impairment of brain maturation. Eur J Pediatr 1989; 149(3):152–158.

22 Engel JJ. Report of the ILAE classification core group. Epilepsia 2006; 47:1558–1568.

23 Fetveit A. Assessment of febrile seizures in children. Eur J Pediatr 2008; 167(1):17–27.

24 Xue LY, Ritaccio AL. Reflex seizures and reflex epilepsy. Am J Electroneurodiagnostic Technol 2006; 46(1):39–48.

25 King DW et al. Pseudoseizures: Diagnostic evaluation. Neurology 1982; 32(1):18–23.

26 Boon PA, Williamson PD. The diagnosis of pseudoseizures. Clin Neurol Neurosurg 1993; 95(1):1–8.

27 Geyer JD, Payne TA, Drury I. The value of pelvic thrusting in the diagnosis of seizures and pseudoseizures. Neurology 2000; 54(1):227–229.

28 Harden CL, Burgut FT, Kanner AM. The diagnostic significance of video-EEG monitoring findings on pseudoseizure patients differs between neurologists and psychiatrists. Epilepsia 2003; 44(3):453–456.

29 Eriksson K, Kalviainen R. Pharmacologic management of convulsive status epilepticus in childhood. Expert Rev Neurother 2005; 5(6):777–783.

30 Meierkord H et al. EFNS guideline on the management of status epilepticus. Eur J Neurol 2006; 13(5):445–450.

31 Riviello JJ, Jr et al. Practice parameter: Diagnostic assessment of the child with status epilepticus (an evidence-based review): Report of the Quality Standards Subcommittee of the American Academy of Neurology and the Practice Committee of the Child Neurology Society. Neurology 2006; 67(9):1542–1550.

32 DeLorenzo RJ et al. Persistent nonconvulsive status epilepticus after the control of convulsive status epilepticus. Epilepsia 1998; 39(8):833–840.

33 Towne AR et al. Prevalence of nonconvulsive status epilepticus in comatose patients. Neurology 2000; 54(2):340–345.

34 Bauer J et al. Precipitating factors and therapeutic outcome in epilepsy with generalized tonic–clonic seizures. Acta Neurol Scand 2000; 102(4):205–208.

35 Goulden KJ et al. Changes in serum anticonvulsant levels with febrile illness in children with epilepsy. Can J Neurol Sci 1988; 15(3):281–285.

36 Zaccara G, Muscas GC, Messori A. Clinical features, pathogenesis and management of drug-induced seizures. Drug Saf 1990; 5(2):109–151.

37 Ramirez-Lassepas M et al. Value of computed tomographic scan in the evaluation of adult patients after their first seizure. Ann Neurol 1984; 15(6):536–543.

38 Phizackerley PJ, Poole EW, Whitty CW. Sino-auricular heart block as an epileptic manifestation; a case report. Epilepsia 1954; 3:89–91.

39 Garretson HD, Elvidge AR. Glossopharyngeal neuralgia with asystole and seizures. Arch Neurol 1963; 8:26–31.

40 Rowland LP (ed). Merritt's textbook of neurology, vol 11e. Philadelphia: Lippincott Williams & Wilkins; 2005.

41 Walton JN. Brain's diseases of the nervous system, 8th edn. New York: Oxford Medical Publications; 1977:1277.

42 Quality Standards Subcommittee of the American Academy of Neurology in cooperation with American College of Emergency Physicians, American Association of Neurological Surgeons, and American Society of Neuroradiology. Practice parameter: neuroimaging in the emergency patient presenting with seizure – summary statement. Neurology 1996; 47(1):288–291.

43 Krumholz A et al. Practice parameter: Evaluating an apparent unprovoked first seizure in adults (an evidence-based review): Report of the Quality Standards Subcommittee of the American Academy of Neurology and the American Epilepsy Society. Neurology 2007; 69(21):1996–2007.

44 Stroink H et al. The first unprovoked, untreated seizure in childhood: A hospital based study of the accuracy of the diagnosis, rate of recurrence, and long term outcome after recurrence. Dutch study of epilepsy in childhood. J Neurol Neurosurg Psychiatry 1998; 64(5):595–600.

45 Hauser WA et al. Seizure recurrence after a first unprovoked seizure. N Engl J Med 1982; 307(9):522–528.

46 Pohlmann-Eden B et al. The first seizure and its management in adults and children. BMJ 2006; 332(7537):339–342.

47 Kim LG et al. Prediction of risk of seizure recurrence after a single seizure and early epilepsy: Further results from the MESS trial. Lancet Neurol 2006; 5(4):317–322.

48 Marson A et al. Immediate versus deferred antiepileptic drug treatment for early epilepsy and single seizures: A randomised controlled trial. Lancet 2005; 365(9476):2007–2013.

49 Bautista RE, Wludyka P. Driving prevalence and factors associated with driving among patients with epilepsy. Epilepsy Behav 2006; 9(4):625–631.

50 Verrotti A et al. Levetiracetam in absence epilepsy. Dev Med Child Neurol 2008; 50(11):850–853.

51 Posner EB, Panayiotopoulos CP. The significance of specific diagnosis in the treatment of epilepsies. Dev Med Child Neurol 2008; 50(11):807.

52 Rowan AJ et al. New onset geriatric epilepsy: A randomized study of gabapentin, lamotrigine, and carbamazepine. Neurology 2005; 64(11):1868–1873.

53 Kwan P, Brodie MJ. Early identification of refractory epilepsy. N Engl J Med 2000; 342(5):314–319.

54 Brodie MJ. Medical therapy of epilepsy: When to initiate treatment and when to combine? J Neurol 2005; 252(2):125–130.

55 Stephen LJ. Drug treatment of epilepsy in elderly people: Focus on valproic acid. Drugs Aging 2003; 20(2):141–152.

56 Hirsch LJ et al. Predictors of lamotrigine-associated rash. Epilepsia 2006; 47(2):318–322.

57 Claxton AJ, Cramer J, Pierce C. A systematic review of the associations between dose regimens and medication compliance. Clin Ther 2001; 23(8):1296–1310.

58 Leidy NK et al. Seizure frequency and the health-related quality of life of adults with epilepsy. Neurology 1999; 53(1):162–166.

59 Patsalos PN et al. Antiepileptic drugs – best practice guidelines for therapeutic drug monitoring: A position paper by the subcommission on therapeutic drug monitoring, ILAE Commission on Therapeutic Strategies. Epilepsia 2008; 49(7):1239–1276.

60 Sheth SG et al. Mortality in epilepsy: Driving fatalities vs other causes of death in patients with epilepsy. Neurology 2004; 63(6):1002–1007.

61 Krauss GL et al. Risk factors for seizure-related motor vehicle crashes in patients with epilepsy. Neurology 1999; 52(7):1324–1329.

62 Austroads. Assessing fitness to drive. Sydney: Austroads Incorporated; 2003.

63 Perucca E. Birth defects after prenatal exposure to antiepileptic drugs. Lancet Neurol 2005; 4(11):781–786.

64 Tomson T, Perucca E, Battino D. Navigating toward fetal and maternal health: The challenge of treating epilepsy in pregnancy. Epilepsia 2004; 45(10):1171–1175.

65 Adab N et al. Common antiepileptic drugs in pregnancy in women with epilepsy. Cochrane Database Syst Rev 2004(3):CD004848.

66 Holmes LB, Wyszynski DF, Lieberman E. The AED (antiepileptic drug) pregnancy registry: A 6-year experience. Arch Neurol 2004; 61(5):673–678.

67 Wyszynski DF et al. Increased rate of major malformations in offspring exposed to valproate during pregnancy. Neurology 2005; 64(6):961–965.

68 The EURAP Study Group. Seizure control and treatment in pregnancy: Observations from the EURAP epilepsy pregnancy registry. Neurology 2006; 66(3):354–360.

69 Morrow J et al. Malformation risks of antiepileptic drugs in pregnancy: A prospective study from the UK Epilepsy and Pregnancy Register. J Neurol Neurosurg Psychiatry 2006; 77(2):193–198.

70 Vajda FJ et al. Foetal malformations and seizure control: 52 months data of the Australian Pregnancy Registry. Eur J Neurol 2006; 13(6):645–654.

71 Ryan CA, Dowling G. Drowning deaths in people with epilepsy. CMAJ 1993; 148(5):781–784.

72 Arango MF, Steven DA, Herrick IA. Neurosurgery for the treatment of epilepsy. Curr Opin Anaesthesiol 2004; 17(5):383–387.

73 Cascino GD. Neuroimaging in epilepsy: Diagnostic strategies in partial epilepsy. Semin Neurol 2008; 28(4):523–532.

74 The Vagus Nerve Stimulation Study Group. A randomized controlled trial of chronic vagus nerve stimulation for treatment of medically intractable seizures. Neurology 1995; 45(2):224–230.

75 Tellez-Zenteno JF et al. Hippocampal electrical stimulation in mesial temporal lobe epilepsy. Neurology 2006; 66(10):1490–1494.

76 Velasco F et al. Double-blind, randomized controlled pilot study of bilateral cerebellar stimulation for treatment of intractable motor seizures. Epilepsia 2005; 46(7):1071–1081.

77 Wiebe S et al. A randomized, controlled trial of surgery for temporal-lobe epilepsy. N Engl J Med 2001; 345(5):311–318.

78 Shaefi S, Harkness W. Current status of surgery in the management of epilepsy. Epilepsia 2003; 44(Suppl 1): 43–47.

79 Rathore C et al. Outcome after corpus callosotomy in children with injurious drop attacks and severe mental retardation. Brain Dev 2007; 29(9):577–585.
80 Jea A et al. Corpus callosotomy in children with intractable epilepsy using frameless stereotactic neuronavigation: 12-year experience at The Hospital for Sick Children in Toronto. Neurosurg Focus 2008; 25(3):E7.
81 Spencer S, Huh L. Outcomes of epilepsy surgery in adults and children. Lancet Neurol 2008; 7(6):525–537.
82 Sirven JI, Sperling M, Wingerchuk DM. Early versus late antiepileptic drug withdrawal for people with epilepsy in remission. Cochrane Database Syst Rev 2001(3):CD001902.
83 Specchio LM, Beghi E. Should antiepileptic drugs be withdrawn in seizure-free patients? CNS Drugs 2004; 18(4):201–212.
84 Aktekin B et al. Withdrawal of antiepileptic drugs in adult patients free of seizures for 4 years: A prospective study. Epilepsy Behav 2006; 8(3):616–619.
85 Ranganathan LN, Ramaratnam S. Rapid versus slow withdrawal of antiepileptic drugs. Cochrane Database Syst Rev 2006(2):CD005003.
86 Feely M. Clinical review: Fortnightly review drug treatment of epilepsy. BMJ 1999; 318:106–109.
87 Marsan CA, Zivin LS. Factors related to the occurrence of typical paroxysmal abnormalities in the EEG records of epileptic patients. Epilepsia 1970; 11(4):361–381.
88 Salinsky M, Kanter R, Dasheiff RM. Effectiveness of multiple EEGs in supporting the diagnosis of epilepsy: An operational curve. Epilepsia 1987; 28(4):331–334.
89 Zivin L, Marsan CA. Incidence and prognostic significance of "epileptiform" activity in the eeg of non-epileptic subjects. Brain 1968; 91(4):751–778.
90 Cavazzuti GB, Cappella L, Nalin A. Longitudinal study of epileptiform EEG patterns in normal children. Epilepsia 1980; 21(1):43–55.
91 Degen R. A study of the diagnostic value of waking and sleep EEGs after sleep deprivation in epileptic patients on anticonvulsive therapy. Electroencephalogr Clin Neurophysiol 1980; 49(5-6):577–584.
92 Boon P et al. Interictal and ictal video-EEG monitoring. Acta Neurol Belg 1999; 99(4):247–255.
93 Watemberg N et al. Adding video recording increases the diagnostic yield of routine electroencephalograms in children with frequent paroxysmal events. Epilepsia 2005; 46(5):716–719.
94 Jedrzejczak J, Owczarek K, Majkowski J. Psychogenic pseudoepileptic seizures: Clinical and electroencephalogram (EEG) video-tape recordings. Eur J Neurol 1999; 6(4):473–479.

chapter 9

Headache and Facial Pain

Headache is one of the commonest problems encountered in neurology. This chapter is not intended to be a comprehensive review of headache. The approach to the more common headache and facial pain syndromes encountered in clinical practice will be discussed. There are many excellent textbooks that contain more detailed information [1–5].

The various labels given to different types of headache have arisen from clinicians observing recurring patterns of similar symptoms in large number of patients in the *absence of any gold standard for the diagnosis*. Thus, the diagnosis of the cause of most headaches or facial pain is almost entirely dependent on a detailed and accurate history because, at this point in time, there are no diagnostic tests to confirm most of the common causes of headache such as migraine, cluster and tension-type headache. Imaging techniques such as computerised tomography (CT) and magnetic resonance imaging (MRI) detect abnormalities that can explain the clinical presentation in only 2% of cases [6].

> - The single most important question to ask a patient presenting with headache is: 'From the moment you first noticed the headache how long did it take to reach maximum severity?' This is the vital clue to the likely pathology.
> - 'If you only have 30 minutes with a patient presenting with headache, spend 29 on the history and 1 on the examination' (quote attributed to Alfred Sahs).

Consider the following case history:

CASE 9.1

A 26-year-old man presents with headache, nausea, vomiting, **photophobia** and **phonophobia**.

Write down your diagnosis or diagnoses for Case 9.1 below before reading on.

Most students will say **subarachnoid haemorrhage** (SAH), some will say meningitis or migraine but in fact this young man had a hangover! All four diagnoses will result in headache, nausea, vomiting and **photophobia**. Although fever should differentiate SAH from meningitis, migraine and hangovers and neck stiffness should raise the suspicion of SAH or meningitis, occasionally patients with migraine complain of neck stiffness and rarely fever [7]. Similarly, if a young man had been out drinking heavily the night before, it would be wrong to assume he had a hangover if he experienced the *thunderclap onset* of severe generalised headache with nausea and vomiting as this is more in keeping with a SAH. *This case reiterates the point made in Chapter 2, 'The neurological history', which is that the nature and distribution of symptoms DO NOT define the aetiology.* The time course (mode of onset and subsequent progression of symptoms) will differentiate between these various entities, with the headache of SAH being of sudden onset and maximum severity at onset, whereas the headache of migraine, meningitis and that of a hangover will usually evolve over a variable period of time from minutes to hours.

The International Headache Society [8] classifies headaches as:

*   primary – migraine, tension-type headache, cluster headache and other trigeminal autonomic cephalalgias, other primary headaches
*   secondary – headache due to another disorder that resolves within 3 months of treatment of that disorder.

> In any patient suffering from headache, establish the exact mode of onset and progression of the headache and other associated symptoms that may be present.

Most patients with headache fear they may have a brain tumour. Although headache is a common symptom of a brain tumour, brain tumour as a cause of headache is extremely rare [9].

The commonest causes are the primary headache syndromes such as episodic tension-type headache and migraine and the commonest secondary causes are a hangover and fever [10] (see Table 9.1).

TABLE 9.1 The lifetime prevalence (the number of people in a given group or population who are reported to have a disease) of various types of primary and secondary headaches

Headache type	%	95% CI
Primary (non-symptomatic)		
Episodic tension-type headache	66	62–69
Chronic tension-type headache	3	2–5
Migraine with **aura**	6	5–8
Migraine without aura	9	7–11
Idiopathic stabbing headache	4	1–4
External compression headache	15	12–17
Cold stimulus headache	1	0–2
Benign cough headache	1	0–2
Headache associated with sexual activity	1	0–2
Secondary (symptomatic)		
Hangover	72	68–75
Fever	63	59–66
Head injury	4	2–5
Disorder of the nose or sinuses	15	12–17
Intracranial neoplasm	0	
Metabolic disorders	22	19–25

Note: The International Headache Society criteria current at the time of the study were used.
Note: Figures are derived from a random sample of 925 individuals from the community in Denmark [10]. External compression headache relates to compression by helmets or swimming goggles. The prevalences are likely to be similar in other countries.

WHAT QUESTIONS TO ASK

There are three scenarios (see Figure 9.1):

1 It is the first headache that the patient has ever experienced.
2 It is an identical headache in a patient who suffers from recurrent headaches.
3 It could be a completely different headache in a patient who has suffered from recurrent headaches.

If you know the patient and the diagnosis and the patient says the headache is identical, it is not unreasonable to treat the patient's headache accordingly. On the other hand, if you do not know the patient, or if the headache is different from those which the patient has had in the past, it is imperative that you treat this headache as if it were the first headache that the patient has ever experienced. When seeing a patient for the first time with a prior diagnosis of headache, **do not assume that the previous diagnosis is correct**. The lack of diagnostic tests to confirm most diagnoses means there is always a degree of uncertainty.

Use the technique below to obtain a blow-by-blow description, similar to that outlined in Chapter 2, 'The neurological history'. Enquire what the patient was doing at the precise moment the headache commenced; what they had been doing just prior to this; what was the time from the onset of the headache until the headache reached its maximum severity; what were the exact nature, distribution and time taken to reach

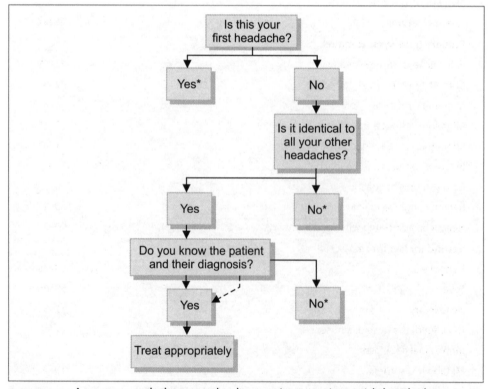

FIGURE 9.1 A recommended approach when seeing a patient with headache

Note: The asterisk (*) indicates that it is important to obtain a very detailed history using the technique outlined below.

maximum intensity or extent of involvement of the body; what was the duration of all associated symptoms and the time they took to resolve, both individually and in relation to each other. Ascertaining the time taken to reach maximum intensity is the vital clue as to the likely pathological process.

Classical teaching has suggested students ask: whether the headache is unilateral or bilateral; constant or throbbing; frontal, temporal, parietal or occipital; made worse by straining, moving or coughing; whether it awakens the patient from sleep; and whether there is associated photophobia or phonophobia. *In most instances the answers to these questions are unhelpful.* As anyone who has suffered from migraine, tension-type headaches or hangovers will know, most of these features are non-specific (as highlighted in Case 9.1 above). Although migraine (see below) is typically a unilateral, throbbing headache associated with visual, gastrointestinal or neurological symptoms, it can be bilateral, constant and is not always accompanied by associated symptoms. Although trigeminal neuralgia is almost exclusively unilateral pain, cases of bilateral pain have been described and are more likely to represent symptomatic (underlying pathology other than compression of the nerve by a vascular loop) trigeminal neuralgia [11]. Similarly, cluster headache is unilateral but even here atypical cases with bilateral headache occur [12–14].

Virtually all headaches are exacerbated by exercise, coughing, sneezing and straining. The exception is cluster headache where the patient often paces the floor or even hits their head on the wall in order to reduce the severity.

In everyday clinical practice if patients are simply asked to describe their headache(s), they often omit vital information.

Obtaining a detailed history

A recommended approach when taking a history is:

1 *What were you doing at the time (circumstances) the headache first commenced?*
2 *What had you been doing beforehand?*
3 *What was the first thing you noticed and how long did it take from when you first noticed this symptom until it reached its maximum severity?*
4 *What was the next thing you noticed and how long did it take from when you first noticed this symptom until it reached its maximum severity?*
5 *And then what happened?*
6 *And then what happened? and so on, until the entire episode is described from start to finish.*

The phrase 'and then what happened' is one of the most useful questions to ask patients with episodic disturbances of neurological function; it ensures the patient does not omit any details. This approach often elucidates pieces of information that are the clues to the likely underlying pathological process, as discussed below.

Case 9.2 demonstrates the value of this history-taking technique.

The value of this method of obtaining histories can also be highlighted by re-examining the Case 9.1 which was described at the beginning of this chapter.

This is a typical history of someone with either migraine or suffering from

> A word of warning: a patient with a past history of recurrent headaches, e.g. related to migraine or tension-type headache, is not precluded from developing another cause such as a SAH. If the headache is not identical to those of the past, take the history as if it is the patient's first headache.

a hangover. The presence of **photopsia** and neurological symptoms would indicate a likely diagnosis of migraine.

An alternative diagnosis becomes apparent in Case 9.3 who on the surface initially appears to present with identical symptoms.

CASE 9.1 *cont'd*

A 26-year-old man presents with headache, nausea, vomiting, photophobia and phonophobia.
What were you doing at the time the headache first commenced?
'I woke up with a headache.'
What had you been doing before?
'I was out with the lads celebrating our victory in the football match. I had drunk more than my fair share of alcohol and felt a bit under the weather when I went to bed.'
What was the first thing you noticed?
'I awoke with a headache all over my head, I felt nauseated and every time I moved I would feel very dizzy.'
How long did it take from when you first noticed the headache until it reached its maximum severity?
'About half an hour.'
Then what happened?
'I got out of bed to go to the toilet and I felt worse; the bright light coming in through the bathroom window hurt my eyes, the nausea and dizziness increased and I vomited.'

CASE 9.2

A 50-year-old man presents with the sudden onset of excruciatingly severe headache. The initial suspicion is that he may have suffered a SAH. However, the history was obtained using the above approach:
What were you doing at the time the headache first commenced?
'Having a shower.'
What was the first thing you noticed?
'A headache at the back of my head.'
How long did it take from when you first noticed this symptom until it reached its maximum severity?
'About 30 seconds to 1 minute.'
Then what happened?
'The headache became very severe and was all over my head.'
This is not the history of a SAH and, after further questioning, the patient admitted that he had been masturbating and the correct diagnosis was benign orgasmic headache.

CASE 9.3

A 26-year-old man presents with headache, nausea, vomiting, photophobia and phonophobia.
What were you doing at the time the headache first commenced?
'I was sitting watching television.'
What had you been doing before?
'Nothing, I was perfectly well until that time.'

CASE 9.3 *cont'd*

What was the first thing you noticed and how long did it take from when you first noticed this symptom until it reached its maximum severity and then what happened?
'I noticed flashing lights in my vision.'
Where in your vision?
'They started on the left side.'
Then what happened?
'They gradually enlarged and spread to the right side.'
How long did they take to spread to the right side?
'Approximately 10–15 minutes.'
Then what happened?
'Just as I thought I was getting better because the trouble with my vision was resolving, I developed a very severe headache all over my head.'
How long did it take from when you first noticed the headache until the headache reached its maximum severity?
'Approximately 30 minutes. When the headache reached its maximum severity I began to feel nauseated and the light was hurting my eyes.'
Then what happened?
'The nausea increased over the next 15 minutes.'
Then what happened?
'Then I started to vomit and I vomited several times; every time I vomited my head felt worse.'
Then what happened?
'I decided to come to the hospital for treatment.'
Have you ever had this headache before?
'No.'
Is there a family history of migraine?
'No.'

In this patient, symptoms evolved gradually with the initial symptoms disappearing before subsequent symptoms either developed or reached their maximum intensity, typical of a migraine. The last two questions would strengthen the diagnosis had the answer been yes, but remember that a past or a family history of migraine is circumstantial evidence (see Chapter 2, 'The neurological history').

In the next example, once again the initial presenting symptoms appear identical.

CASE 9.4

A 26-year-old man presents with headache, nausea, vomiting, photophobia and phonophobia.
What were you doing at the time the headache first commenced?
'I was sitting watching television.'
What had you been doing before?
'I was perfectly well until that time.'
What was the first thing you noticed?
'It felt as if someone had hit me over the head with an axe. I developed this very severe headache at the back and over the top of my head.'
How long did it take from when you first noticed the headache until it reached its maximum severity?
'It was at its most severe when it first started.'

CASE 9.4 *cont'd*

And then what happened?
'At the same time I felt very nauseated and began to vomit. As I walked to the bathroom I noticed that the light coming in through the window hurt my eyes.'
Then what happened?
'I decided to come to the hospital for treatment.'

The diagnosis of SAH is inescapable when the exact mode of onset and progression of the headache and associated symptoms are established.

The above discussion would suggest that taking a history from patients with headache is easy. Unfortunately this is not always the case. The CT scan in Figure 9.2 is from a patient who was incapable of giving a detailed history because of the cognitive impairment resulting from the hydrocephalus. The patient complained of vague headache, non-descript blurring of vision and a change in her personality (her sister's psychiatrist had diagnosed schizophrenia when her sister told him about her symptoms). The two clues to the underlying diagnosis were the fact that her legs gave way when her brother hugged her (this would have increased intrathoracic and intracranial pressure) and the presence of papilloedema when examined.

> Do not diagnose a psychiatric problem because of your inability to obtain a history that makes sense. This could reflect cognitive impairment as a result of the underlying disease process.

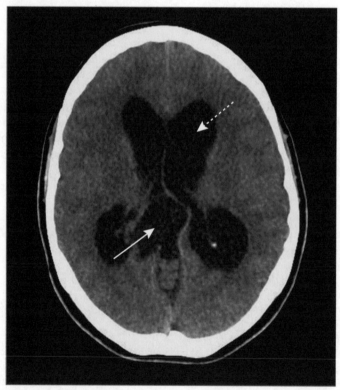

FIGURE 9.2 A CT scan of the brain demonstrating a large dermoid cyst (straight arrow) with secondary hydrocephalus (dotted arrow)

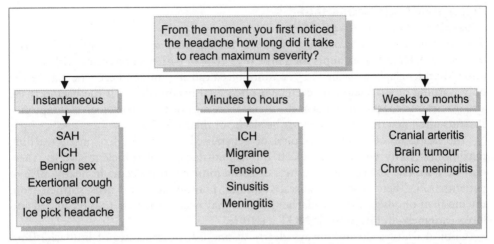

FIGURE 9.3 The three broad categories of headache. ICH = intracerebral haemorrhage

There are many different ways to approach patients with headache. The International Headache Society classification is into primary and secondary headache. In clinical practice when evaluating patients with headache there are three broad categories based on the rapidity of onset of the headache (see Figure 9.3).

The remainder of this chapter will initially discuss the approach to patients presenting with a single headache, followed by the approach to patients with recurrent headaches.

A SINGLE (OR THE FIRST) EPISODE OF HEADACHE

Sudden onset 'thunderclap headache'
- Intracranial haemorrhage
  - Subarachnoid haemorrhage
  - Intracerebral haemorrhage
  - Intraventricular haemorrhage
- Cough headache
- Exertional headache
- Benign sex headache
- Ice-cream headache
- Ice-pick headache

All these conditions have one thing in common and that is the sudden onset of severe headache. (The slight exception is the headache related to exertion or orgasm; see below.) What differentiates one from the other are the associated symptoms, the duration of the headache and, to a lesser extent, the circumstances under which the headache occurs. **It is important to remember that the most lethal condition NOT to miss is a subarachnoid haemorrhage (SAH)** and that it can occur under any circumstances including when patients exert themselves, cough, sneeze or during sexual intercourse. There are extremely rare causes of sudden severe headache such as hydrocephalic attack with or without the presence of a third ventricular colloid cyst acting as a ball valve, and very rarely sudden onset headache may be the presenting symptom of aseptic or viral meningitis [15].

INTRACRANIAL HAEMORRHAGE
Subarachnoid haemorrhage (SAH)

The single most important, although probably not the commonest, cause of sudden severe headache is SAH. SAH accounts for a little over 10% of patients presenting with sudden onset 'thunder clap' headache [15]. A minor bleed causing sudden headache may be the only warning of a subsequent severe and often fatal haemorrhage. If the haemorrhage also occurs into the parenchyma of the brain, there may be focal neurological symptoms. Patients often describe it as the worst headache of their life [16].

The headache of SAH is occipital or generalised and of sudden onset, reaching maximum severity within seconds. If the haemorrhage is of sufficient severity, there may be transient loss of consciousness or coma induced; this occurs in nearly 50% of patients [17]. There is severe nausea, vomiting, photophobia and neck stiffness from the moment of onset of the headache. Seizures may occur. The patient is obtunded and looks extremely ill. Photopsia is NOT a feature.

Clinical features do not always clearly distinguish other causes of headache from SAH [15, 18]. The presence or lack of accompanying symptoms like nausea, vomiting, photophobia and collapse at onset does not seem a reliable means of distinguishing between SAH and benign causes of acute headache [15].

> The moment the possibility of SAH is entertained, all patients should be thoroughly investigated with imaging and, if negative, a lumbar puncture (LP).

In almost 20–40% of patients with SAH a warning leak (minor haemorrhage) may occur 1–8 weeks prior to a major SAH. The associated headache (referred to as a sentinel headache) is often short-lived and the patient may not seek immediate medical attention [19]. Even if the patient consults a physician the headache seems so trivial that often the diagnosis is missed [20]. Some of these patients are seen some days to weeks later [21] with the story of a sudden, explosive severe headache, usually in the absence of any other symptoms. The briefer the headache, the less likely it was related to a warning bleed. Here the question arises as to whether they have suffered a SAH and how extensively they should be investigated, and there is no easy answer to this question.

The probability of detecting an aneurysmal haemorrhage on CT scans performed at various intervals after the ictus is [9]:
- day 0, 95%
- day 3, 74%
- 1 week, 50%
- 2 weeks, 30%
- 3 weeks, almost nil.

The probability of detecting xanthochromia with spectrophotometry of the CSF at various times after a SAH is [9]:
- 12 hours, 100%
- 1 week, 100%
- 2 weeks, 100%
- 3 weeks, > 70%
- 4 weeks, > 40%.

Magnetic resonance angiography will detect aneurysms of > 3 mm in diameter and is recommended in patients with thunderclap headache with a low index of suspicion for SAH (normal CT scan and CSF) [9], as the risk of subsequent SAH is negligible [21, 22]. If the index of suspicion for SAH is high standard angiography should be performed.

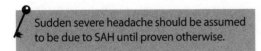

Sudden severe headache should be assumed to be due to SAH until proven otherwise.

A 3rd nerve palsy with a dilated pupil is a classic sign of a sentinel bleed.

Intracerebral haemorrhage
The headache of intracerebral haemorrhage is associated with nausea and vomiting due to raised intracranial pressure. It is often sudden in onset and of maximum severity at onset; however, it can increase in severity more slowly over a period of minutes to hours. In this situation the patient will usually have depression of the conscious state and often focal neurological signs.

Intraventricular haemorrhage
Primary intraventricular haemorrhage is rare and usually results from parenchymal (intracerebral) haemorrhage rupturing into the ventricle. The headache is of sudden onset and maximum intensity within seconds; it is usually associated with nausea, vomiting, photophobia and neck rigidity. If the haemorrhage is more severe or if it leads to secondary hydrocephalus, depression of the conscious state will occur. There are no focal neurological symptoms unless the intraventricular haemorrhage is secondary to a parenchymal haemorrhage.

COUGH, BENIGN EXERTIONAL, BENIGN SEX, ICE-CREAM AND ICE-PICK HEADACHES
Although these headaches have a tendency to recur, they have one thing in common and that is the headache is of sudden onset and therefore they are discussed in this section.

Anybody who has suffered from a headache knows that coughing, sneezing or straining momentarily exacerbates the headache. *Headache precipitated by coughing* is referred to as cough headache. A similar headache can also be precipitated by anything that increases intrathoracic pressure such as sneezing, straining, laughing or stooping [24]. In the majority of patients with this headache, no structural pathology is present, although in as many as 25% it may be symptomatic (indicating the presence of an underlying pathology) with a significant proportion related to a Chiari malformation [25].

Cough headache
Benign cough headache is a headache precipitated by coughing in the absence of any intracranial disorder. The headache is of maximum severity at onset, coming on within seconds of coughing, sneezing or straining. It is very brief, lasting only a few seconds to less than a minute. There are no associated symptoms. The headache is generalised, frontal or occipital. The headaches usually resolve within 1 or 2 years although cases have been described lasting up to 12 years [26].

TREATMENT of BENIGN COUGH HEADACHE

In general reassurance only is required. Occasionally symptomatic relief can be provided with indomethacin or other non-steroidal anti-inflammatory drugs [26, 27].

Exertional headache
Benign exertional headache is a bilateral, throbbing headache, lasting from 5 minutes to 24 hours specifically provoked by physical exercise and not associated with any systemic or intracranial disorder [28]. A small percentage of patients with exertional headache

may have structural pathology [28]. This headache is of sudden onset (but not usually described as explosive in nature), generalised frontal or occipital and precipitated by activities such as weight lifting or any other activity that causes the patient to Valsalva. Similar to coital headache, there may be an antecedent dull occipital pain that builds up in severity over seconds to minutes as the intensity of the exercise increases and, if the person stops exerting themselves, this warning headache will resolve and they will not experience the sudden severe headache. The aetiology of this headache is unknown. Recurrent episodes may occur for weeks, occasionally months.

Benign sex (orgasmic or coital) headache

'Headache associated with sexual activity' describes bilateral headaches precipitated by masturbation or coitus in the absence of any intracranial disorder [29, 30]. The headache is sudden in onset and excruciatingly severe, occurring at the moment of orgasm. It is predominantly occipital, but may be frontal or generalised. It is brief, lasting minutes, rarely hours. There are no associated symptoms. *There is often a valuable clue that is not seen with SAH*: the patient may experience a dull pain in the occipital or suboccipital region that increases in severity as excitement increases, subsides if they interrupt sexual activity and recurs if they become aroused again. If the patient interrupts sexual activity and avoids orgasm, this dull headache subsides without the subsequent severe explosive headache. If you can obtain a history of this headache preceding the sudden explosive headache, then the diagnosis is quite straightforward. On the other hand, if the history of this warning headache is not elicited, the major differential diagnosis, particularly if the headache lasts hours, is SAH. The aetiology of this headache is unclear but it is almost invariably seen in patients who are experiencing considerable stress in their lives and, once the stress resolves, so do the headaches.

Rarely, patients may experience their first SAH when coughing, sneezing, straining, exerting themselves or during sexual intercourse [25]. Here, although the headache will be explosive in onset, there will not be an antecedent warning headache in the seconds before the explosive headache, and the headache will persist for hours to days and is usually associated with nausea, vomiting, neck stiffness and possibly a focal neurological deficit and/or depression of the conscious state.

TREATMENT of COUGH, EXERTIONAL AND BENIGN SEX HEADACHE

The most important aspect of the management of cough, exertional and benign sex headaches is to reassure the patient of their benign nature and to advise them that they will resolve with the passage of time. Cough, exertional and benign sex headaches may be helped by the introduction of indomethacin 25–100 mg per day, other non-steroidal anti-inflammatory drugs or a beta-blocker.

Ice-cream or cold-induced headache

Cold-induced headache occurs when the patient is eating or drinking something very cold such as ice cream that touches the palate or posterior pharyngeal wall. The patient experiences the onset over seconds of an excruciating, unilateral frontal headache that can be so severe that it may induce a profound bradycardia and syncope. This is a common cause of headache in adolescents [31] and is not influenced by eating ice cream more slowly [32].

Ice-pick headache
Ice-pick headache is also termed 'jabs and jolts' and refers to a curious entity in which the patient experiences recurrent, brief stabbing pains, often localised to one part of the head, rarely in other parts of the body. The patient describes the pain as lancinating like a needle, a nail or an ice pick being stabbed into their scalp. The pain lasts seconds only, may occur as a single jab of pain or there may be many stabs of pain within seconds to a minute. The commonest site is the temples. The same site on the opposite side (mirror image) of the head may be similarly affected. Ice-pick headaches occur more commonly in patients with migraine, where they can occur during or before the migraine [33]. They are benign and do not represent any sinister underlying pathology; reassurance is all that is required.

Aseptic or viral meningitis
Very rarely, aseptic or viral meningitis may present with the very abrupt onset of severe headache [15]. The associated fever and sweats and the presence of an antecedent upper respiratory tract infection provide clues to the possible diagnosis, but a lumbar puncture may be required to differentiate aseptic meningitis from SAH.

Posture-induced headache
Severe headache on standing that resolves with lying flat is characteristic of a reduced cerebrospinal fluid (CSF) pressure. This most often occurs after a lumbar puncture but may develop with a CSF leak, the so-called spontaneous low-pressure headache.

POST-LUMBAR PUNCTURE HEADACHE
The characteristic and **pathognomonic** feature is a headache that worsens within 15 minutes of standing and *resolves within 30 minutes if the patient lies completely flat* [8], particularly if the foot of the bed or the legs are elevated. If the patient lies down on several pillows the headache will be less severe but will not be abolished. It is important that the headache resolves as all headaches are usually less severe when a patient lies down. The headache can be dull or throbbing, frontal, occipital or generalised, worsened by coughing, sneezing and straining, i.e. non-specific features.

There is often neck discomfort; other associated symptoms include a change in hearing (hyperacusis), nausea, blurred vision, photophobia, horizontal diplopia, occasionally facial numbness, cognitive abnormalities and even coma. All these symptoms resolve when the patient lies completely flat.

The headache usually develops within 1 or 2 days of the lumbar puncture (LP) or epidural, although rare cases occurring 12 days later have been reported [34]. CSF pressures, by definition, are quite low and can be measured to confirm the diagnosis [35]. Although it usually resolves spontaneously, there are reports of it persisting for up to 19 months [36].

Post-LP headache occurs in as many as 30% of patients [37]. The incidence is reduced to as low as 5% when a smaller gauge needle is used, inserting the bevel parallel rather than at right angles to the fibres of the dura, the stylet is re-inserted before removing the needle or non-cutting (pencil-point) needles are used [38, 39]. There is *no evidence that bedrest following an LP reduces the incidence* of headache. The incidence is also not influenced by whether the LP is performed in the sitting or lying position or whether increased oral or IV fluids are administered. The volume of CSF removed does not increase the incidence of post-LP headache, thus *there should be no hesitation in removing copious amounts of CSF for diagnostic purposes.*

LOW-PRESSURE HEADACHE OR SPONTANEOUS INTRACRANIAL HYPOTENSION
The clinical features are identical to the headache seen after an LP. This headache relates to a leak of CSF either from the nose following a head injury (rarely a spontaneous leak) or, in the majority of patients, the leak is at the level of the spine, particularly the thoracic spine and cervicothoracic junction [35].

INVESTIGATION AND TREATMENT of LOW-PRESSURE AND POST-LP HEADACHE

Typical imaging findings consist of subdural fluid collections, pachymeningeal enhancement, pituitary hyperaemia and brain sagging on CT scans. MRI may be normal. Myelography or CSF isotope studies can often identify the CSF leak [35, 40] but are not necessary to make the diagnosis. Radioisotope cisternography typically shows absence of activity over the cerebral convexities, even at 24 or 48 hours, and early appearance of activity in the kidneys and urinary bladder.

Initial treatment is effective in as many as 85% of patients [41] and consists of lying the patient completely flat with the foot of the bed elevated, copious fluids (unproven benefit) and, if this fails, an epidural blood patch is often effective [42]. Occasionally more than one epidural blood patch may be required [43], up to as long as 19 months after the onset [36].

Headaches of gradual onset
Migraine, cluster and tension-type are the commonest headaches that develop gradually and these are discussed in the next section.

Cranial arteritis, bacterial meningitis and ethmoid sinusitis are three causes of headache of gradual onset that must not be missed.

> There is one overarching principle in clinical medicine and that is: DO NOT MISS the treatable or the diagnosis that if missed could lead to disastrous consequences.

CRANIAL ARTERITIS
Cranial arteritis (also known as giant cell or temporal arteritis as most often the temporal arteries are affected) is a vasculitis that distinctly targets large- and medium-sized arteries, preferentially the aorta and its extracranial branches, and in particular the temporal and occipital arteries [44]. This is a disorder of the older patient (the mean age is almost 75 [45]) and is rarely seen below the age of 50 [46]. It is more common in women and age-specific incidence rates increase with age [47]. Cranial arteritis should be treated as an emergency as a delay in diagnosis may lead to irreversible blindness due to ophthalmic artery occlusion.

The patient presents with the insidious onset of severe headache increasing in severity over days or even weeks and often but not invariably associated with one or more of the following:
- scalp tenderness (pain on brushing or washing the hair)
- jaw claudication (pain in the jaw with chewing)
- polymyalgia rheumatica (aches and pains in the shoulder region and often in the proximal legs, occurring in up to 50% of patients).

Occasionally the patient has prominent, tender thrombosed extracranial arteries (see Figure 9.4). Headache is not the only presentation of cranial arteritis: it can present with or be associated with anorexia, weight loss, joint pains, a fever of unknown origin, transient visual obscurations (lasting minutes or up to 2 hours), central retinal artery occlusion or anterior ischaemic optic neuropathy [AION] resulting in unilateral or even

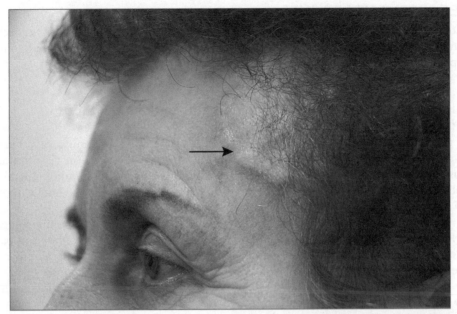

FIGURE 9.4 Prominent temporal arteries that are tender and non-pulsatile indicating thrombosis of the vessel

bilateral blindness [48–50]. Diplopia (double vision) that relates to ischaemia of the ocular muscles or nerves innervating those muscles has been described [48].

Investigation of suspected cranial arteritis

The erythrocyte sedimentation rate (ESR) is invariably elevated as is the C-reactive protein (CRP), *although early on both these tests may be normal.* If cranial arteritis is suspected, repeated testing over the ensuing days and weeks is necessary. Biopsy of the temporal or occipital artery can be diagnostic, but it is important to remember that the disease process is not contiguous along the vessel and, unless a long segment of artery is obtained, the biopsy may be normal [51]. The diagnostic yield is higher with a minimum length of 1 cm [52].

ACUTE BACTERIAL OR VIRAL MENINGITIS

Isolated headache, particularly in the absence of fever, is unlikely to be due to meningitis.

In general, patients present with increasingly severe generalised headache developing over several hours or rarely days, either constant or throbbing in nature. Headache, fever and neck stiffness occur in more than 90% of patients [53]. Photophobia, nausea and vomiting, a change in mental status, seizures and focal neurological deficits may also occur. *Worsening of headache with eye movement is a characteristic feature.*

The clinical features of meningitis in its early stages can, however, often be non-specific and yet patients with fulminant meningitis, particularly meningococcal meningitis, may deteriorate rapidly over hours, so that it is important to have a high index of suspicion. Meningococcal meningitis and septicaemia are often associated with a petechial or purpuric rash [54].

Viral meningitis can be mild such that patients may not present in the early stages and, by the time they seek advice, the headache is already resolving.

RECURRENT HEADACHES

Most patients with recurrent headaches will suffer from one of the primary headache syndromes such as migraine, tension-type headache or one of the trigeminal autonomic cephalalgias.

Migraine with aura, migraine without aura and aura without migraine headache

In the original International Headache Society classification [55], migraine was referred to as classical, common or migraine equivalents. In the revised criteria the classification was changed such that migraine with **aura** replaced classic migraine, common migraine became migraine without aura and migraine equivalents are referred to as aura without migraine headache [8].

When the subacute onset of headache is accompanied by photopsia (flashing lights), scotomata (patches of visual loss), nausea, vomiting, photophobia, phonophobia or paraesthesia, the most likely diagnosis is migraine with aura. However, migraine is not the only cause of such a constellation of symptoms. The simultaneous onset of headache, photopsia, nausea and vomiting can occur with vertebrobasilar ischaemia (see Chapter 10, 'Cerebrovascular disease').

> It is the progressive evolution of the headache and associated symptoms, with the initial symptoms showing signs of either improvement or resolution before the later symptoms appear or reach their full intensity in terms of severity or distribution, which is characteristic of migraine.

It was long thought, based on the work of Wolff [56], that the aura was related to vasoconstriction of the intracranial vessels and the headache was due to dilatation of the extracranial vessels. Although unique changes in brain blood flow seen in patients during attacks of migraine with aura [57] have been replicated in animal experiments [58], a recent controversial [59] MRI study has failed to confirm any changes in cerebral blood flow during nitroglycerin-induced migraine [60]. Cortical spreading depression (CSD) of Leäo [61] is a short-lasting depolarisation wave heralded by a brief phase of excitation, which is immediately followed by prolonged nerve cell depression synchronous with a dramatic failure of brain ion homeostasis, efflux of excitatory amino acids from nerve cells and enhanced energy metabolism [58]. CSD is now widely recognised as the neurophysiological substrate of classical migraine aura and may be involved in migraines without a perceived aura as well [62]. CSD moves across the cortex at a rate of 3–5 mm/min. This slow spread of cortical depolarisation is reflected in the gradual evolution of the associated visual and other focal neurological symptoms that occur with migraine.

The more common varieties of migraine as classified by the International Headache Society are listed below [8].

- Classical or migraine with aura
- Migraine without aura
- Aura without headache (migraine without headache or migraine equivalents)
- Basilar artery migraine
- Hemiplegic migraine
- Status migrainosus
- Menstrual migraine

MIGRAINE WITH AURA

This is headache associated with visual, gastrointestinal and neurological symptoms with or without photophobia and phonophobia. A number of patients may experience non-specific symptoms such as changes in appetite, drowsiness, yawning and alterations of mood (irritability or depression) up to 24 hours before the onset of headache.

An aura occurs in a little over one-third of patients and lasts on average 27 minutes, and the headache follows within approximately 10 minutes [63]. The characteristic feature is that there is a separation in time between each aspect of the aura; the visual, sensory and other focal neurological symptoms *do not develop simultaneously.* The visual and neurological symptoms evolve gradually with the initial symptoms disappearing or lessening in intensity or area affected as the later ones either commence or increase in severity.

The aura

VISUAL SYMPTOMS

A variety of visual symptoms may occur during the aura. Photopsia (flashing lights) consists of zigzag or jagged lines, bright spots or stars referred to as fortification spectra that may leave an area of impaired vision in the centre, 'the scintillating scotoma'. Scotomata may occur in the absence of any fortification spectra, resulting in patchy areas of loss of vision replaced by greyness or blackness, and at times a contralateral hemianopia or even total blindness may occur.

> Photopsia are not specific to migraine and may occur with posterior vitreous detachment, retinal detachment or occipital lobe infarction.

SENSORY SYMPTOMS

The sensory symptoms, usually described as a tingling or numbness, commence in one part of the body (e.g. the hand) and gradually spread over 10–20 minutes to involve a greater area of the body, including the face. Usually by the time the sensory symptoms have reached the foot they are no longer present at the site where they originated. The sensory symptoms persist for seconds up to 20 minutes. They may be ipsilateral or contralateral to the headache [64].

OTHER SYMPTOMS

Alterations in speech (dysphasia) and weakness may occur but are much less common.

The headache

The headache of migraine is more commonly unilateral and frontal but may be bilateral, occipital or generalised. In some patients the headache begins in the neck and radiates up to the head. Very rarely, migraine can affect predominantly the face, an entity referred to as lower-half headache. Ice-pick pains are common in patients with migraine [33]. The headache increases in severity over minutes to an hour or two (more rapidly than tension-type headache). A common misconception is that migraine headache is throbbing in character but this occurs in only 50% of patients; constant non-throbbing headache is equally as common. The headache of migraine is severe, lasting less than 4 hours in 27%, 4–24 hours in 40%, 1–2 days in 11% and more than 2 days in 22% of patients [65].

MIGRAINE WITHOUT AURA

This consists of recurrent moderate to severe unilateral, pulsating headaches lasting 4–72 hours, aggravated by routine physical activity and associated with mild nausea and/or photophobia and phonophobia. If one takes patients with classic migraine (migraine with aura) and carefully analyses the headache, there are three characteristic features that seem to occur in most patients.[1] Patients with migraine typically retire to bed without headache and either:

- awake in the middle of the night or
- awake at their normal time the following morning with severe headache.
- The other characteristic is that the headache increases in severity over a short period, usually minutes up to 2 hours.

These features may help differentiate migraine without aura from tension-type headache. Patients with tension-type headache or chronic daily headache typically retire to bed with a headache and awake the next morning with the same headache, which fluctuates in severity and increases in severity slowly over hours.

It is uncertain whether migraine with aura and migraine without aura are the same disorder as far as treatment is concerned [66].

AURA WITHOUT HEADACHE (MIGRAINE WITHOUT HEADACHE OR MIGRAINE EQUIVALENTS)

These are episodes of completely reversible visual and/or sensory symptoms with or without speech disturbance that develop gradually, lasting less than 60 minutes and without subsequent headache [67, 68]. In essence these patients experience the symptoms typical of the aura of migraine without subsequently developing a headache. When the symptoms have occurred in the past as the typical aura of a migraine headache, the diagnosis is not difficult. If this has not occurred it can be difficult to differentiate such symptoms from transient ischaemic attacks. As already stated, the clue to the diagnosis is that the first symptoms are showing signs of resolving before subsequent symptoms either appear or fully develop. If the neurological symptoms develop simultaneously or if the initial symptoms are not showing signs of resolving as the later symptoms are developing then, although this can very rarely occur in migraine, a diagnosis of cerebral ischaemia should be considered.

BASILAR ARTERY MIGRAINE

Basilar artery migraine is migraine headache with aura symptoms clearly originating from the brainstem and/or from both hemispheres simultaneously but *without motor weakness*. To the uninitiated these patients can be terrifying, presenting with altered conscious state, total blindness, visual hallucinations, photopsia, fortification spectra, vertigo, ataxia and perioral and peripheral tingling or numbness. The symptoms last from 2 to 45 minutes and are followed by a severe throbbing headache and vomiting lasting several hours [69]. Basilar artery migraine is more common in young females but fortunately the attacks are infrequent.

HEMIPLEGIC MIGRAINE

Migraine with aura associated with weakness is referred to as familial hemiplegic migraine if a first- or second-degree relative is also affected [70]. Hemiplegic migraine is extremely rare and this diagnosis should be made with caution and, in the first instance, probably by a neurologist. The unilateral motor symptoms of hemiplegic migraine differ from the more common forms of aura. There is no apparent spread of symptoms over the course of an hour and the duration of motor weakness is much greater than in the other aura types. Patients with hemiplegic migraine often have unilateral weakness for hours to days [71].

---

1 Personal unpublished and unproven observations.

MENSTRUAL MIGRAINE

This is defined as attacks of migraine without aura in menstruating women occurring exclusively on day 1 (± 2 days) of menstruation in at least two out of three menstrual cycles and at no other times of the cycle. Menstrual migraine occurs during or after the time at which oestradiol and progesterone levels fall to their lowest [72, 73]. In some patients migraine occurs only at the time of menstruation; other patients experience migraines both at the time of menstruation and at other times during the cycle. In the latter patients the migraine related to menstruation may not necessarily have a hormonal basis.

PRINCIPLES OF TREATMENT OF MIGRAINE

The most appropriate treatment is to identify any precipitating factor and eliminate that element. Some patients are adamant that their migraine is precipitated by certain foods, and this is particularly observed in children [74, 75]. The commonest foods include cow's milk, egg, chocolate, oranges and orange juice, wheat, cheese, artificial colourings and preservatives such as benzoic acid and tartrazine found in tinned, packet and junk food, while in others alcohol seems to be the offending agent. Elimination of the offending substance in theory should reduce the frequency of migraine. However, a careful study by McQueen et al [76] could not demonstrate any benefit from an elimination diet. Despite this, one encounters patients who are adamant that they have experienced fewer migraine headaches when they eliminated a particular substance from their diet.[2] Treatment begins with a headache and diet diary and the selective avoidance of foods presumed to trigger attacks [74].

Non-pharmacological treatments are often advocated. Although psychological factors are important triggers of migraine, there are no controlled trials confirming psychological therapy is effective. Biofeedback/relaxation therapy is effective in some patients [77]. A meta-analysis of acupuncture as therapy concluded that there is weak evidence for efficacy [78]. Hypnotherapy is difficult to subject to randomised controlled trials, but one unblinded study claimed efficacy [79]. Some patients have claimed that their migraine is helped by a chiropractor or a naturopath performing neck manipulation but there is no objective evidence of benefit.

The pharmacological treatment of migraine is influenced by:

1 the frequency and the severity of the attacks
2 the patient's willingness to accept the potential risk of side effects from drugs
3 whether vomiting occurs early during the migraine, thus preventing the use of oral therapy. In this latter circumstance subcutaneous, intravenous, sublingual, intranasal or rectal therapy will need to be employed.

If the migraine attacks are frequent, prophylaxis is indicated. If the migraine attacks are infrequent, but are very severe and difficult to treat when they occur, many patients will prefer to take prophylactic medication. If the migraines are infrequent many patients will opt not to expose themselves to the potential risk of side effects of drugs taken on a daily basis.

Ultimately it is the patient's decision whether to choose therapy at the time of the migraine or prophylactic therapy.

There are a large number of drugs that may be used to treat the acute migraine or as prophylactic therapy [80]. These are likely to change over the ensuing years. As migraine is an unpredictable illness, only the results of randomised controlled trials should be used to decide what therapies are useful. Currently recommended therapies for both the individual migraine and for prophylaxis are detailed in Appendix D.

---

2 Personal observation.

Unfortunately, there is no way of predicting which patient will respond or not respond to a particular therapy. In clinical practice it is often a matter of trial and error. The principle is to use the drugs with the fewest potential side effects initially and then move to perhaps more potent therapies that may be associated with a greater risk of side effects.

TREATMENT of MIGRAINE IN ADULTS

The principles of treatment have been discussed. Appendix D contains two tables listing the currently recommended drugs for the treatment of acute attacks (Table D.1) and those recommended for prophylaxis (Table D.2) of migraine. Only drugs for which there is level 1 evidence (randomised controlled trials) have been included.

Krymchantowski has recommended for acute treatment combination therapy to suit the individual patient profile, with the use of analgesics or a non-steroidal anti-inflammatory drug together with a triptan or a gastro kinetic drug [81]. A multicentre randomised, double-blind, single-dose, placebo-controlled study found that administering two tablets of the fixed combination of 250 mg acetylsalicylic acid (ASA) + 200 mg paracetamol + 50 mg caffeine (thomapyrin) was statistically more effective than giving two tablets of 250 mg ASA + 200 mg paracetamol, two tablets of 500 mg ASA, two tablets of 500 mg paracetamol, two tablets of 50 mg caffeine or placebo in patients who were used to treating their episodic tension-type headache or migraine attacks with non-prescription analgesics [82].

Botulinum toxin type A (BoNTA) is safe, effective and well tolerated for reducing the frequency of headache episodes in patients with chronic daily headache [83, 84] but not migraine [85, 86]. Recently, a placebo-controlled (sham surgery) study demonstrated that surgical deactivation of peripheral migraine headache trigger sites is an effective alternative treatment for patients who suffer from frequent moderate to severe migraine headaches that are difficult to manage with standard protocols [87].

TREATMENT of MENSTRUAL-RELATED MIGRAINE

Menstrual-related migraine does not respond very well to the usual prophylactic measures but oestradiol implants or oestradiol gel can render some patients headache-free [88]. Some patients who experience migraine at the time of menstruation also experience migraine at other times. These patients do not respond as well to oestradiol implants.

A number of drugs, such as non-steroidal anti-inflammatory drugs and the triptans, started 2 days prior to the expected onset of menses and continuing for 7 days, reduce the severity and duration of the headache but, unlike the oestradiol implants, do not abolish the headaches altogether. Naproxen 550 mg twice daily [89] and zolmitriptan 2.5 mg oral tablet 2 or 3 times per day has been proven to be efficacious, with 3 doses per day more effective than 2 per day [90]. Sumatriptan 85 mg combined with naproxen sodium 500 mg in a single fixed dose taken within 1 hour of onset of menstruation has also been shown to be effective but only in a little less than one-third of patients [91].

Trigeminal autonomic cephalalgias

Cluster headaches together with short-lasting, unilateral, neuralgiform headache attacks with conjunctival injection and tearing (SUNCT) syndrome and paroxysmal hemicranias belong to a group of disorders that the International Headache Society classifies as trigeminal autonomic cephalalgias [8].

CLUSTER HEADACHE

The pain of cluster headache must be *strictly unilateral*. It is almost invariably in or around the eye, although it may involve the temple, frontal or maxillary regions (see Figure 9.5). The pain increases in severity over minutes to an hour or so and is excruciatingly severe. The headaches last 15–180 minutes and occur every second day or up to eight times per day. There is often reddening and watering of the ipsilateral eye and blockage of the ipsilateral nostril. A *transient* Horner's syndrome (see Figure 4.9) during the headache is virtually pathognomonic.

It is most often seen in men, and is also referred to as suicide headache because of the severity of the pain. When it does occur in women it is very similar, except that women experience more vomiting and other 'migrainous symptoms' [92].

The attacks occur in bouts or clusters, thus the name. These may be hours or days apart and there is a curious periodicity with headaches often occurring at the same time of the day or night with each subsequent headache until the cluster resolves. The patient can almost set a clock to the headaches. Alcohol can exacerbate the problem and patients voluntarily refrain during the bouts.

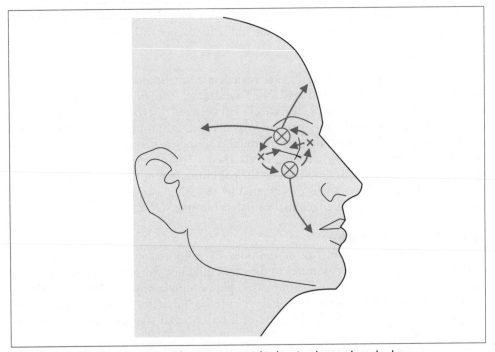

FIGURE 9.5   The distribution of pain seen with classic cluster headache
Reproduced from *Headache*, 2nd edn, by NH Raskin, 1988, Churchill Livingstone, Figure 6.1, p 230 [3]

TREATMENT of CLUSTER HEADACHE, PAROXYSMAL HEMICRANIA AND SUNCT SYNDROME

• For the acute treatment of cluster headache attacks, oxygen (100%) with a flow rate of at least 7 L/min over 15 min or 6 mg subcutaneous sumatriptan are the treatments of first choice for acute cluster headache. Prophylaxis of cluster headache should initially be with verapamil 240 mg/day (maximum dose depends on efficacy or tolerability). Although no class I or II trial results are available, steroids are clearly effective in cluster headache.[3] Therefore, the use of at least 100 mg methylprednisolone (or equivalent corticosteroid) given orally or at up to 500 mg intravenously per day over 5 days (then tapering down) is recommended. Methysergide, lithium and topiramate are recommended as alternative treatments [93].

• For paroxysmal hemicranias, indomethacin at a daily dose of up to 225 mg is the drug of choice.

• For treatment of SUNCT syndrome, a large series suggest that lamotrigine is the most effective preventive agent, with topiramate and gabapentin also being useful. Intravenous lidocaine may also be helpful as an acute therapy when patients are extremely distressed and disabled by frequent attacks.

PAROXYSMAL HEMICRANIA

Paroxysmal hemicrania may either be episodic or chronic. It consists of paroxysmal headache attacks where the character and localisation of the pain and the autonomic symptoms (although less severe) are very similar to those observed in cluster headache. However, the attacks are more frequent (by definition more than five per day for half of the time), of shorter duration and lack the circadian rhythm seen with cluster headache. One of the diagnostic criteria is the complete abolition of the headaches with indomethacin.

SUNCT SYNDROME

There are other short-lasting unilateral neuralgia form headaches with conjunctival injection and tearing, referred to as SUNCT syndrome. As opposed to cluster headache this is more common in females. The attacks last between 5 seconds and 4 minutes and occur from as few as three times per day to as many as 200 times per day. These headaches are also strictly unilateral and periorbital, and they are triggered by touching the periorbital region, talking or chewing food. There is mild conjunctival injection and watering of the eye and this differentiates the pain from trigeminal neuralgia. The other clue is that triggered pain (pain precipitated by touching a trigger point on the face) shows a refractory period in trigeminal neuralgia but not SUNCT syndrome.

Tension-type headache

Tension-type headache consists of episodes of mild to moderately severe non-throbbing headache lasting minutes to days that does not worsen with routine physical activity and is not associated with nausea, phonophobia or photophobia. Probably the most characteristic feature is that the headache fluctuates in severity from hour to hour, day to day. It is the main cause of headache that lasts all day every day for months on end.

The headache is typically bilateral, although it can be unilateral, and is often described as a tight sensation around the head or a pressure sensation in the head. Some authorities consider tension-type headache and migraine headache without associated features (common migraine) virtually indistinguishable, except that with migraine the headaches are relatively brief and episodic in nature [94]. Episodic tension-type headache is more likely to be seen in primary care practice [95] whereas chronic daily headache is more likely seen in the specialist clinic [96].

---

3 Personal observation. Steroids are often very effective during the first bout but seem to be less so for subsequent bouts.

Many patients with the clinical features of tension-type headache take issue with the term 'tension-type', denying that there is tension or stress in their life. Some have commented that they could understand it if the headache had developed some time ago when there was considerable stress in their life, others deny any stress at all. The absence of stress should not preclude a diagnosis of tension-type headache if all other criteria are fulfilled. Similarly, the presence of stress in someone with headaches is only circumstantial evidence that the headaches are tension-type; it is important to use the diagnostic criteria for tension-type headache and look for the tension in a patient's life to explain why they have tension-type headache. 'Lifestyle headache' is a term that patients are comfortable with and refers to the fact that they are experiencing a headache because of a lack of balance between the personal, professional and family aspects of their life.[4]

TREATMENT of TENSION-TYPE HEADACHE

Textbooks advise a multifaceted approach to the treatment of tension-type headache, employing psychological, physiological and pharmacological therapies [97]. Most young patients shun pharmacological therapy. Some patients may be persuaded to use short-term pharmacological therapy if presented with the analogy of the ability to save oneself from drowning if the head is above water as opposed to having no chance to do so if the head is below the water. It is suggested to the patient that they take medication for a short time while they are altering their lifestyle.[5]

Hypnotherapy, relaxation, biofeedback and acupuncture have all been advocated in the treatment of tension-type headache. Acupuncture has not been confirmed in randomised controlled trials [78]; hypnotherapy resulted in less frequent, less prolonged and less intense headaches in a single blind study [98]. A recent Internet-delivered behavioural regimen composed of progressive relaxation, limited biofeedback with autogenic training and stress management claimed significant benefit compared to symptom monitoring waitlist control [99].

Sinusitis

Sinusitis is a very rare but commonly over-diagnosed cause of headache and facial pain. Of patients with either a self-diagnosis or physician diagnosis of sinusitis, 80% fulfil the International Headache Society migraine criteria [100, 101]. The problem is compounded by the fact that many patients' sinuses have thickened mucosa and this is incorrectly interpreted as sinusitis. The presence of a fluid level in the sinus is required for the diagnosis of acute sinusitis.

Frontal or maxillary sinusitis usually presents with facial pain and both are discussed below. Ethmoid or sphenoid sinusitis presents with malaise, severe headache in the midline behind the nose and low-grade fever. The problem can be very difficult to diagnose if the ostium to the sinus is occluded as there will be no nasal discharge. The ethmoid and sphenoid sinuses are deep within the skull and therefore tenderness is not present. As the sinusitis progresses, pain usually increases over the ethmoidal area; however, the pain can be referred to the medial orbit, eye and brow. More severe cases of acute ethmoid sinusitis, especially in immune-compromised patients, can rapidly progress and

---

4 Personal observations. These patients have not found a balance between time for themselves, time for their work and time for their families. Many of these patients' headaches have resolved once they resume the physical or social activity that they have given up because they had become too busy.
5 Personal observation.

present with facial cellulitis, orbital cellulitis and meningitis. Although it can have a bacterial, viral, fungal or allergic aetiology, it is most often bacterial.

Chronic headaches
CHRONIC DAILY HEADACHE

If tension-type headaches have been present for 6 months or more, they are referred to as *chronic daily headache*.

Chronic daily headache is defined as headache on more than 15 days per month or 180 days per year. Approximately 35–40% of patients who seek treatment at head-ache centres suffer from daily or near-daily headache [102]. Some 80% of patients with chronic daily headache have evolved from episodic headache, predominantly migraine, and this is referred to as 'transformed migraine'. In 20% of patients the headache is daily from onset [103].

Chronic daily headache may be constant or throbbing; mild, moderate or severe; and often is associated with mild photophobia, photophobia and nausea. Consistently uni-lateral headache is seen in only 2% of patients [104]. The headache fluctuates in severity from hour to hour and day to day. Patients retire with a headache and awaken with the headache the following morning.

Excess analgesics or ergotamine overuse (termed *medication or analgesic overuse head-ache*) and stress are the two leading factors that appear to increase the risk of developing chronic daily headache. In many patients, however, no obvious reason for the chronic daily headaches can be identified. Episodic migraine can transform into chronic daily headache and often continues once chronic daily headache has developed.

Medication overuse syndrome is also referred to as rebound headache and is defined as the perpetuation of head pain in chronic headache sufferers, caused by frequent and excessive use of immediate relief medication. The International Headache Society [105] defines medication overuse headache as:

A headache that is present on ≥ 15 days/month fulfilling criteria C and D
B regular overuse for > 3 months of one or more drugs that can be taken for acute and/ or symptomatic treatment of headache
C headache that has developed or markedly worsened during medication overuse
D headache that resolves or reverts to its previous pattern within 2 months after discon-tinuation of overused medication.

Medications that can cause medication overuse headache include: ergotamine prepa-rations, opiates, triptans and simple analgesics such as aspirin or paracetamol.

TREATMENT of CHRONIC DAILY HEADACHE

Spontaneous improvement can occur on discontinuation of the medications causing the problem. The combination of a tricyclic antidepressant and cessation of analgesia reduces headache frequency more than cessation of analgesia alone [106]. Kudrow, in his landmark study [106], demonstrated that only 18% resolved if nothing was changed, but resolu-tion was seen in 30% with addition of a tricyclic antidepressant, 43% when analgesia was ceased and 70% with a combination of an antidepressant and ceasing analgesia.

HEADACHE IN CHRONIC MENINGITIS

Chronic meningitis is defined as irritation and inflammation of the meninges persist-ing for more than 4 weeks and associated with pleocytosis (increased white cell count) in the CSF [107]. In reality, the average duration of symptoms varies from 17 to

43 months [108]. Chronic meningitis can be infective (cryptococcus, tuberculosis, listeria), non-infective (sarcoidosis, mollaret, drugs) or related to malignancy [109].

Low-grade fever, headache and mild neck stiffness may be extremely subtle and variable and any one feature may be absent. Mental status changes, seizures or focal deficits may evolve over time [110]. The headache can slowly worsen, fluctuate or remain static. The headache is bilateral, frontal and retro-orbital, and may be associated with photophobia, nausea and vomiting and generalised malaise. The presence of a fever suggests an infective aetiology and, although significant weight loss can occur with all causes, it is more common with malignancy. Night sweats, neck stiffness, papilloedema and possibly cranial nerve abnormalities have been described [111, 112].

HEADACHE AND IDIOPATHIC INTRACRANIAL HYPERTENSION

The headache is constant or throbbing, worse with coughing or straining (like most headaches) and may mimic chronic tension-type headache. The headache is generalised and of low to moderate severity. At times it can be pulsatile and awaken the patient from sleep. Retro-ocular pain worse with eye movement can occur [113]. The presence of visual obscurations (transient blindness lasting seconds) may occur, especially when straining. Bilateral papilloedema is the only sign unless the patient develops cranial nerve palsies (most commonly a 6th) secondary to the raised intracranial pressure.

WHEN TO WORRY

The great majority of patients encountered with headache will have one of the primary headache syndromes and not a serious underlying pathology. It is often taught that a change in the character or nature of headaches suggests a possible sinister underlying cause but this scenario is very common in patients with transformed migraine. Any of the following features should alert the clinician to a possible underlying serious disorder:
- headache awakening patients from sleep
- thunderclap onset of headache
- headaches associated with focal neurological symptoms that accompany or outlast the headache [114]
- long-lasting headaches (weeks or months) [114]
- headache with systemic symptoms such as anorexia, weight loss or fever, scalp tenderness or jaw claudication
- new onset headache in the elderly.

Headache and brain tumours

Many patients with headache fear they have a brain tumour (see Figure 9.6). Fortunately these are very rare. Although headache is a common symptom of brain tumours, occurring in up to 70% of adults [115] and 60% of children [116], it is the sole manifestation in only 2% of patients [117]. *In primary care, the risk of brain tumour with a headache presentation is less than 0.1%* [10, 118]. This implies a primary care physician will have to do 1000 imaging procedures on patients with headache to detect one tumour!

Many of the features of the brain tumour-associated headache are non-specific. It is mild to moderately severe lasting for hours (not all day every day like chronic daily or tension-type headache) and develops over weeks or months [119]. Headache that awakens the patient from sleep and the presence of unsteadiness are the two main clinical

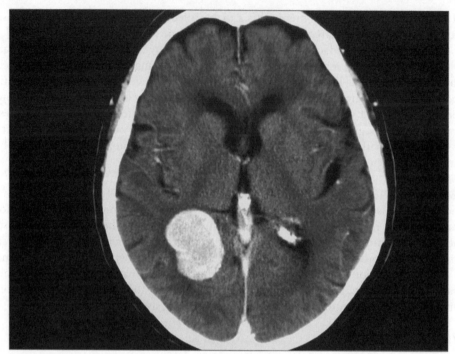

FIGURE 9.6 CT scan of the brain demonstrating a large intraventricular meningioma

features that should alert the clinician to the possibility of a brain tumour [115, 119]. Increasingly severe headache and the development of headache for the first time in elderly patients is also an indication of a possible brain tumour [120].

INVESTIGATING HEADACHE

The American Academy of Neurology practice guidelines [120] recommend imaging if the headache:
* is worsened by Valsalva manoeuvre
* causes the patient to awaken from sleep
* is a new headache in an older patient
* is a progressively worsening headache
* is accompanied by the presence of abnormal neurological findings.

Neuroimaging is not usually warranted for patients with migraine and a normal neurological examination. For patients with atypical headache features or patients who do not fulfill the strict definition of migraine (or have some additional risk factor), a lower threshold for neuroimaging may be applied.

The American Academy of Neurology guidelines state that there is insufficient evidence for choosing between a CT scan and an MRI scan, nor is there sufficient evidence to indicate whether an enhanced CT scan is better than an unenhanced CT scan when evaluating patients with migraine or other non-acute headaches [120]. Unfortunately most patients with headache are terrified that they have a brain tumour and virtually demand some form of imaging of the brain, and most have had a CT scan well before referral to the neurologist.

FACIAL PAIN

There are many causes of facial pain. The more common ones include:
- trigeminal neuralgia
- pain of dental origin
- sinusitis
- glossopharyngeal neuralgia
- atypical facial pain
- herpes zoster ophthalmicus and post-herpetic neuralgia
- Tolosa–Hunt syndrome.

Trigeminal neuralgia

Trigeminal neuralgia consists of brief lancinating pain abrupt in onset and termination that *MUST be within the distribution of the trigeminal nerve* (see Figure 1.7), most often the 2nd and 3rd divisions and occasionally the 1st division. Although the paroxysms of pain may occur spontaneously, they are frequently precipitated by trivial stimuli such as washing, shaving, talking, brushing teeth, applying make-up or the wind blowing on the face.

Dental pain, which is discussed below, will also be in the distribution of the 2nd or 3rd divisions of the trigeminal nerve but never the 1st division. The two entities are very commonly confused [121]. Both dental pain and trigeminal neuralgia may be precipitated by eating or chewing but *the vital clue that the problem is trigeminal neuralgia is the presence of a trigger point on the face*, an area that if touched or sometimes even if the wind blows onto it will trigger a severe paroxysm of pain. The pain is so severe it makes the patient wince and hence the term 'tic douloureux', which is derived from the French meaning literally a painful tick.

In general, this is a condition of older patients and the aetiology is most often compression of the trigeminal nerve in the posterior fossa by an aberrant loop of a vessel [122]. Less commonly, it is symptomatic of another disorder, for example a tumour or multiple sclerosis. Younger age, bilateral trigeminal neuralgia and abnormal trigeminal sensation and corneal reflexes indicate a possible secondary cause [11].

TREATMENT of TRIGEMINAL NEURALGIA

- Carbamazepine or oxcarbazepine are the drugs of choice for trigeminal and glossopharyngeal neuralgia. Baclofen and lamotrigine are alternatives [11].
- If medical therapy fails, posterior fossa microvascular decompression is the treatment of choice [122].
- In patients unable to undergo intracranial surgery a percutaneous rhizotomy of the trigeminal ganglion is useful [11].

Pain of dental origin

Pain of dental origin is at times very difficult to diagnose, particularly when it is related to a deep root abscess where often the dentist cannot see anything wrong with the tooth. The pain is a constant aching sensation, often fluctuating in severity and at times very distressing. *The vital clue is that pain of dental origin is precipitated or exacerbated by contact of hot (and to a lesser extent cold) fluids on the affected tooth* [123].

A useful bedside test is to put ice blocks in a glass of water and ask the patient to swirl the cold water around on the suspected side of the mouth. WARN the patient that this may cause a very severe attack of pain but it is a very effective way to sort out the problem. Start with the lower jaw and then the upper jaw. This may help localise the offending tooth as on occasion the pain is referred to the cheek when the problem is in the lower jaw.

Facial pain confined to the distribution of the 2nd or 3rd divisions of the trigeminal nerve is either trigeminal neuralgia or dental pain. The vital clue is the presence of trigger spots on the face in trigeminal neuralgia that are absent with dental pain, where the pain will be precipitated by drinking predominantly hot or occasionally cold fluids.

Sinusitis

Acute sinusitis frequently follows upper respiratory tract infections. Although patients may complain of ipsilateral headache, ipsilateral facial pain over the region of the infected sinus is more common and usually associated with fever and purulent rhinorrhoea [124]. Clinical signs and symptoms most helpful in the diagnosis of maxillary and frontal sinusitis are the presence of a purulent nasal discharge, cough, purulent secretions observed on nasal examination and tenderness over the sinus [125].

Glossopharyngeal neuralgia

The pain of glossopharyngeal neuralgia is severe transient (seconds only) stabbing pain experienced in the ear, tonsillar fossa, base of the tongue or beneath the angle of the jaw. It is commonly provoked by coughing, swallowing or talking. In between paroxysms of pain there may be a dull discomfort. In some patients the pain is predominantly in the ear, in others it is in the pharynx. Unlike trigeminal neuralgia, the pain is beyond the distribution of the glossopharyngeal nerve also affecting the auricular and pharyngeal branches of the vagus nerve [126]. Occasionally, the pain is so severe that it results in transient asystole (no cardiac electrical activity) [127].

TREATMENT of GLOSSOPHARYNGEAL NEURAGIA

Carbarnazepine is the drug of choice.

Persistent idiopathic facial pain

Persistent idiopathic facial pain was previously referred to as atypical facial pain. This consists of persistent facial pain that does not have the features of the cranial neuralgias and is not attributable to any other cause, i.e. does not fit a recognised pattern. The pain is deep, poorly localised, although most commonly it is in the region of the nasolabial fold or chin, and present most of the day almost every day. Occasionally, the condition follows surgery or trauma in the distribution of the trigeminal nerve [128]. There are no abnormal neurological signs and no cause is found despite detailed investigation, although occasional patients presenting with facial pain will have a nasopharyngeal carcinoma. The aetiology of this condition is unclear; some authorities suggest depression plays a significant role although this is controversial.

TREATMENT of PERSISTENT IDIOPATHIC FACIAL PAIN

Tricyclic antidepressants, such as amitryptiline, imipramine or nortryptiline, are the treatment of choice for persistent idiopathic facial pain [96, 129, 130].

Herpes zoster ophthalmicus and post-herpetic neuralgia

Facial pain, usually burning in nature and in the distribution of the 1st division of the trigeminal nerve, may precede the onset of the characteristic rash of herpes zoster by several days. Once the rash, consisting of blisters, appears the diagnosis is straightforward (see Figure 9.7). Post-herpetic neuralgia may develop in as many as 50% of patients (more commonly in the elderly) and pain may persist for months or even years after the rash has resolved. The pain is stabbing or burning in nature and the skin is very sensitive to touch (hyperaesthesia).

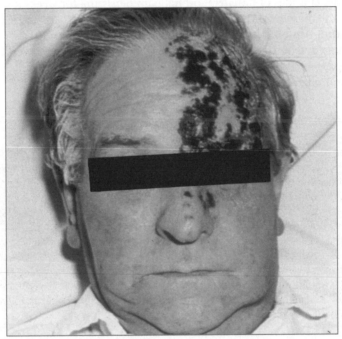

FIGURE 9.7   Severe herpes zoster ophthalmicus

TREATMENT of HERPES ZOSTER AND POST-HERPETIC NEURALGIA

* Herpes zoster vaccine has been shown to reduce the incidence of herpes zoster and post-herpetic neuralgia [131] and is recommended for all persons aged ≥ 60 years who have no contraindications, including persons who report a previous episode of zoster or who have a chronic medical condition [132].
* Treatment with antiviral therapy [133] and a small dose of a tricyclic antidepressant, such as amitryptiline 25 mg [134], once herpes zoster develops will lead to a more rapid improvement in the pain and reduce the incidence of post-herpetic neuralgia.
* Corticosteroids have been claimed to reduce the incidence of post-herpetic neuralgia in small unblinded, controlled trials [135, 136], but a Cochrane review has concluded that there is insufficient evidence to justify their use [137].
* Tricyclic antidepressants, such as amitryptiline, imipramine or nortriptyline are the treatment of choice for post-herpetic neuralgia [96, 129, 130].

Tolosa–Hunt syndrome

Tolosa–Hunt syndrome is a rare disorder due to a granulomatous inflammatory process and is characterised by episodic orbital and periorbital pain, with paralysis of the 3rd, 4th or 6th cranial nerves developing within 2 weeks of the onset of pain. Occasionally, the 1st division of the 5th cranial nerve may be affected. It can remit spontaneously over days to weeks but may relapse and remit. There are many conditions that can produce a painful ophthalmoplegia, such as Graves' disease, Wegener's granulomatosis, sarcoidosis, diabetes and cavernous sinus thrombosis; aneurysm and lymphoma need to be excluded. An excellent discussion can be found in the review by Lutt et al [138].

The International Headache Society diagnostic criteria are:
* one or more episodes of unilateral orbital pain persisting for weeks if untreated
* paresis of the muscles of the eye, of one or more of the 3rd, 4th and/or 6th cranial nerves and/or demonstration of granulomas by MRI or biopsy
* paresis coinciding with the onset of pain or following it within 2 weeks
* pain and paresis resolving within 72 hours when treated adequately with corticosteroids
* exclusion of other causes by appropriate investigations.

INVESTIGATION AND TREATMENT of TOLOSA–HUNT SYNDROME

An MRI scan is abnormal in more than 90% of patients and reveals a convex enlargement of the symptomatic cavernous sinus by an abnormal tissue isointense with gray matter on short repetition time/echo time (TR/TE) spin echo images and isohypointense on long TR/TE images. This abnormal tissue markedly increases in signal intensity after contrast injection [139]. The MRI scan may remain abnormal following resolution of symptoms. The mass may extend into the superior orbital fissure [140].

High-dose corticosteroids are the treatment of choice and are more likely to induce resolution and avoid recurrence than lower dose regimens. Pain, but not the neurological signs, usually subsides rapidly, often within 72 hours, and this is used as a diagnostic criterion. It is important to remember that a response to treatment DOES NOT confirm the diagnosis and many of the other conditions causing a painful ophthalmoplegia also respond to corticosteroids, probably not as promptly.

REFERENCES

1 Selby G. Migraine and its variants. NSW: ADIS Health Science Press; 1983:153.
2 Vinken PJ, Bruyn GW, Klawans HL (eds). Headache. Handbook of clinical neurology. Amsterdam: Elsevier; 1986:556.
3 Raskin NH. Headache, 2nd edn. London: Churchill Livingstone; 1988:396.
4 Lance JW, Goadsby PJ. Mechanism and management of headache, 7th edn. New York: Elsevier; 2005.
5 Olesen J et al. The headaches, 3rd edn. London: Lippincott Williams & Wilkins; 2005.
6 You JJ et al. Indications for and results of outpatient computed tomography and magnetic resonance imaging in Ontario. Can Assoc Radiol J 2008; 59(3):135–143.
7 Jacob J. Mechanisms of fever occurring in migraine. Adv Neurol 1982; 33:127–133.
8 Olsen J et al. The international classification of headache disorders: 2nd edition. Cephalalgia 2004; 24(Suppl 1):1–160.
9 Evans RW. Diagnostic testing for the evaluation of headaches. Neurol Clin 1996; 14(1):1–26.
10 Rasmussen BK, Olesen J. Symptomatic and nonsymptomatic headaches in a general population. Neurology 1992; 42(6):1225–1231.
11 Gronseth G et al. Practice parameter: The diagnostic evaluation and treatment of trigeminal neuralgia (an evidence-based review): Report of the Quality Standards Subcommittee of the American Academy of Neurology and the European Federation of Neurological Societies. Neurology 2008; 71(15):1183–1190.
12 Young WB, Rozen TD. Bilateral cluster headache: Case report and a theory of (failed) contralateral suppression. Cephalalgia 1999; 19(3):188–190.

13 Leone M, Rigamonti A, Bussone G. Cluster headache sine headache: Two new cases in one family. Cephalalgia 2002; 22(1):12–14.
14 Rozen TD. Atypical presentations of cluster headache. Cephalalgia 2002; 22(9):725–729.
15 Landtblom AM et al. Sudden onset headache: A prospective study of features, incidence and causes. Cephalalgia 2002; 22(5):354–360.
16 Morgenstern LB et al. Worst headache and subarachnoid hemorrhage: Prospective, modern computed tomography and spinal fluid analysis. Ann Emerg Med 1998; 32(3 Pt 1):297–304.
17 Bo SH et al. Acute headache: A prospective diagnostic work-up of patients admitted to a general hospital. Eur J Neurol 2008; 15(12):1293–1299.
18 Seet CM. Clinical presentation of patients with subarachnoid haemorrhage at a local emergency department. Singapore Med J 1999; 40(6):383–385.
19 Verweij RD, Wijdicks EF, van Gijn J. Warning headache in aneurysmal subarachnoid hemorrhage. A case-control study. Arch Neurol 1988; 45(9):1019–1020.
20 Jakobsson KE et al. Warning leak and management outcome in aneurysmal subarachnoid hemorrhage. J Neurosurg 1996; 85(6):995–999.
21 Markus HS. A prospective follow-up of thunderclap headache mimicking subarachnoid haemorrhage. J Neurol Neurosurg Psychiatry 1991; 54(12):1117–1118.
22 Wijdicks EF, Kerkhoff H, van Gijn J. Long-term follow-up of 71 patients with thunderclap headache mimicking subarachnoid haemorrhage. Lancet 1988; 2(8602):68–70.
23 Qureshi AI et al. Spontaneous intracerebral hemorrhage. N Engl J Med 2001; 344(19):1450–1460.
24 Symonds C. Cough headache. Brain 1956; 79(4):557–568.
25 Pascual J et al. Cough, exertional, and sexual headaches: An analysis of 72 benign and symptomatic cases. Neurology 1996; 46(6):1520–1524.
26 Diamond S, Medina JL. Prolonged benign exertional headache: Clinical characteristics and response to indomethacin. Adv Neurol 1982; 33:145–149.
27 Mathew NT. Indomethacin responsive headache syndromes. Headache 1981; 21(4):147–150.
28 Rooke ED. Benign exertional headache. Med Clin North Am 1968; 52(4):801–808.
29 Kriz K. [Coitus as a factor in the pathogenesis of neurologic complications.] Cesk Neurol 1970; 33(3):162–167.
30 Lance JW. Headaches occurring during sexual intercourse. Proc Aust Assoc Neurol 1974; 11:57–60.
31 Fuh JL et al. Ice-cream headache – a large survey of 8359 adolescents. Cephalalgia 2003; 23(10):977–981.
32 Kaczorowski M, Kaczorowski J. Ice cream evoked headaches (ICE-H) study: Randomised trial of accelerated versus cautious ice cream eating regimen. BMJ 2002; 325(7378):1445–1446.
33 Raskin NH, Schwartz RK. Icepick-like pain. Neurology 1980; 30(2):203–205.
34 Reamy BV. Post-epidural headache: How late can it occur? J Am Board Fam Med 2009; 22(2):202–205.
35 Mokri B. Spontaneous intracranial hypotension. Curr Neurol Neurosci Rep 2001; 1(2):109–117.
36 Wilton NC, Globerson JH, de Rosayro AM. Epidural blood patch for postdural puncture headache: It's never too late. Anesth Analg 1986; 65(8):895–896.
37 Thoennissen J et al. Does bed rest after cervical or lumbar puncture prevent headache? A systematic review and meta-analysis. CMAJ 2001; 165(10):1311–1316.
38 Evans RW et al. Assessment: Prevention of post-lumbar puncture headaches: Report of the Therapeutics and Technology Assessment Subcommittee of the American Academy of Neurology. Neurology 2000; 55(7):909–914.
39 Armon C, Evans RW. Addendum to assessment: Prevention of post-lumbar puncture headaches. Report of the Therapeutics and Technology Assessment Subcommittee of the American Academy of Neurology. Neurology 2005; 65(4):510–512.
40 Moriyama E et al. Quantitative analysis of radioisotope cisternography in the diagnosis of intracranial hypotension. J Neurosurg 2004; 101(3):421–426.
41 Turnbull DK, Shepherd DB. Post-dural puncture headache: Pathogenesis, prevention and treatment. Br J Anaesth 2003; 91(5):718–729.
42 van Kooten F et al. Epidural blood patch in post dural puncture headache: A randomised, observer-blind, controlled clinical trial. J Neurol Neurosurg Psychiatry 2008; 79(5):553–558.
43 Ho KY, Gan TJ. Management of persistent post-dural puncture headache after repeated epidural blood patch. Acta Anaesthesiol Scand 2007; 51(5):633–636.
44 Schwedt TJ, Dodick DW, Caselli RJ. Giant cell arteritis. Curr Pain Headache Rep 2006; 10(6):415–420.
45 Salvarani C et al. Reappraisal of the epidemiology of giant cell arteritis in Olmsted County, Minnesota, over a fifty-year period. Arthritis Rheum 2004; 51(2):264–268.
46 Pipinos II et al. Giant-cell temporal arteritis in a 17-year-old male. J Vasc Surg 2006; 43(5):1053–1055.
47 Salvarani C et al. The incidence of giant cell arteritis in Olmsted County, Minnesota: apparent fluctuations in a cyclic pattern. Ann Intern Med 1995; 123(3):192–194.
48 Danesh-Meyer HV, Savino PJ. Giant cell arteritis. Curr Opin Ophthalmol 2007; 18(6):443–449.

49 Tal S, Guller V, Gurevich A. Fever of unknown origin in older adults. Clin Geriatr Med 2007; 23(3):649–668, viii.

50 Schmidt D. Ocular ichemia syndrome – a malignant course of giant cell arteritis. Eur J Med Res 2005; 10(6):233–242.

51 Tehrani R et al. Giant cell arteritis. Semin Ophthalmol 2008; 23(2):99–110.

52 Taylor-Gjevre R et al. Temporal artery biopsy for giant cell arteritis. J Rheumatol 2005; 32(7):1279–1282.

53 Roos KL. Acute bacterial meningitis. Semin Neurol 2000; 20(3):293–306.

54 Rosenstein NE et al. Meningococcal disease. N Engl J Med 2001; 344(18):1378–1388.

55 Headache Classification Committee of the International Headache Society. Classification and diagnostic criteria for headache disorders, cranial neuralgias and facial pain. Cephalalgia 1988; 8(Suppl 7):1–96.

56 Wolff H. Headache and other head pain, 2nd edn. New York: Oxford University Press; 1963.

57 Olesen J, Larsen B, Lauritzen M. Focal hyperemia followed by spreading oligemia and impaired activation of rCBF in classic migraine. Ann Neurol 1981; 9(4):344–352.

58 Lauritzen M. Pathophysiology of the migraine aura: The spreading depression theory. Brain 1994; 117(Pt 1):199–210.

59 VanDenBrink AM, Duncker DJ, Saxena PR. Migraine headache is not associated with cerebral or meningeal vasodilatation – a 3T magnetic resonance angiography study. Brain 2009; 132(Pt 6):e112:author reply e113.

60 Schoonman GG et al. Migraine headache is not associated with cerebral or meningeal vasodilatation – a 3T magnetic resonance angiography study. Brain 2008; 131(Pt 8):2192–2200.

61 Leao AAP. Spreading depression of activity in cerebral cortex. J Neurophysiol 1944; 7:359–390.

62 Ayata C. Spreading depression: From serendipity to targeted therapy in migraine prophylaxis. Cephalalgia 2009; 29(10):1095–1114.

63 Kelman L. The aura: A tertiary care study of 952 migraine patients. Cephalalgia 2004; 24(9):728–734.

64 Jensen K et al. Classic migraine: A prospective reporting of symptoms. Acta Neurol Scand 1986; 73:359–362.

65 Selby G, Lance JW. Observations on 500 cases of migraine and allied vascular headache. J Neurol Neurosurg Psychiatry 1960; 23:23–32.

66 Welch KM. Drug therapy of migraine. N Engl J Med 1993; 329(20):1476–1483.

67 Fisher CM. Late-life migraine accompaniments as a cause of unexplained transient ischemic attacks. Can J Neurol Sci 1980; 7(1):9–17.

68 Kunkel RS. Acephalgic migraine. Headache 1986; 26(4):198–201.

69 Bickerstaff ER. The basilar artery and the migraine epilepsy syndrome. Proc R Soc Med 1962; 55:167–169.

70 Glista GG, Mellinger JF, Rooke ED. Familial hemiplegic migraine. Mayo Clin Proc 1975; 50(6):307–311.

71 Foroozan R, Cutrer FM. Transient neurologic dysfunction in migraine. Neurol Clin 2009; 27(2):361–378.

72 Somerville BW. The role of progesterone in menstrual migraine. Neurology 1971; 21(8):853–859.

73 Somerville BW. The role of estradiol withdrawal in the etiology of menstrual migraine. Neurology 1972; 22(4):355–365.

74 Millichap JG, Yee MM. The diet factor in pediatric and adolescent migraine. Pediatr Neurol 2003; 28(1):9–15.

75 Egger J et al. Is migraine food allergy? A double-blind controlled trial of oligoantigenic diet treatment. Lancet 1983; 2(8355):865–869.

76 McQueen J et al. A controlled trial of dietary modification in migraine. In: New advances in headache research. Rose FC (ed). London: Smith-Gordon; 1989:235–242.

77 Holroyd KA, Penzien DB. Pharmacological versus non-pharmacological prophylaxis of recurrent migraine headache: A meta-analytic review of clinical trials. Pain 1990; 42(1):1–13.

78 Melchart D et al. Acupuncture for recurrent headaches: A systematic review of randomized controlled trials. Cephalalgia 1999; 19(9):779–786:discussion 765.

79 Anderson JA, Basker MA, Dalton R. Migraine and hypnotherapy. Int J Clin Exp Hypn 1975; 23(1):48–58.

80 Goadsby PJ. Advances in the pharmacotherapy of migraine: How knowledge of pathophysiology is guiding drug development. Drugs R D 1999; 2(6):361–374.

81 Krymchantowski AV. Acute treatment of migraine: Breaking the paradigm of monotherapy. BMC Neurol 2004; 4:4.

82 Diener HC. Medication overuse is more than just taking too much. Cephalalgia 2005; 25(7):481.

83 Silberstein SD et al. Botulinum toxin type A for the prophylactic treatment of chronic daily headache: A randomized, double-blind, placebo-controlled trial. Mayo Clin Proc 2005; 80(9):1126–1137.

84 Mathew NT et al. Botulinum toxin type A (BOTOX) for the prophylactic treatment of chronic daily headache: A randomized, double-blind, placebo-controlled trial. Headache 2005; 45(4):293–307.

85 Aurora SK et al. Botulinum toxin type A prophylactic treatment of episodic migraine: a randomized, double-blind, placebo-controlled exploratory study. Headache 2007; 47(4):486–499.

86 Relja M et al. A multicentre, double-blind, randomized, placebo-controlled, parallel group study of multiple treatments of botulinum toxin type A (BoNTA) for the prophylaxis of episodic migraine headaches. Cephalalgia 2007; 27(6):492–503.

87 Guyuron B et al. A placebo-controlled surgical trial of the treatment of migraine headaches. Plast Reconstr Surg 2009; 124(2):461–468.

88 Magos AL, Zilkha KJ, Studd JW. Treatment of menstrual migraine by oestradiol implants. J Neurol Neurosurg Psychiatry 1983; 46(11):1044–1046.

89 Sances G et al. Naproxen sodium in menstrual migraine prophylaxis: A double-blind placebo controlled study. Headache 1990; 30(11):705–709.

90 Tuchman MM et al. Oral zolmitriptan in the short-term prevention of menstrual migraine: a randomized, placebo-controlled study. CNS Drugs 2008; 22(10):877–886.

91 Mannix LK et al. Combination treatment for menstrual migraine and dysmenorrhea using sumatriptan-naproxen: Two randomized controlled trials. Obstet Gynecol 2009; 114(1):106–113.

92 Rozen TD et al. Cluster headache in women: clinical characteristics and comparison with cluster headache in men. J Neurol Neurosurg Psychiatry 2001; 70(5):613–617.

93 May A et al. EFNS guidelines on the treatment of cluster headache and other trigeminal-autonomic cephalalgias. Eur J Neurol 2006; 13(10):1066–1077.

94 Zeigler AK, Hassanein RT. Migraine muscle contraction headache dichotomy studied by statistical analysis of headache symptoms. In: Advances in migraine research and therapy. Rose FC (ed). New York: Raven Press; 1995:7–11.

95 Rasmussen BK et al. Epidemiology of headache in a general population – a prevalence study. J Clin Epidemiol 1991; 44(11):1147–1157.

96 Lance JW, Curran DA. Treatment of chronic tension headache. Lancet 1964; 1(7345):1236–1239.

97 Lance JW, Goadsby PJ. Mechanisms and Management of Headache, 7th edn. : Elsevier, Butterworth, Heinemann; 2005.

98 Melis PM et al. Treatment of chronic tension-type headache with hypnotherapy: a single-blind time controlled study. Headache 1991; 31(10):686–689.

99 Devineni T, Blanchard EB. A randomized controlled trial of an internet-based treatment for chronic headache. Behav Res Ther 2005; 43(3):277–292.

100 Blau JN. A note on migraine and the nose. Headache 1988; 28(7):495.

101 Schreiber CP et al. Prevalence of migraine in patients with a history of self-reported or physician-diagnosed "sinus" headache. Arch Intern Med 2004; 164(16):1769–1772.

102 Mathew NT, Reuveni U, Perez F. Transformed or evolutive migraine. Headache 1987; 27(2):102–106.

103 Mathew NT. Transformed migraine, analgesic rebound, and other chronic daily headaches. Neurol Clin 1997; 15(1):167–186.

104 Solomon S, Lipton RB, Newman LC. Clinical features of chronic daily headache. Headache 1992; 32(7):325–329.

105 Silberstein SD et al. The International Classification of Headache Disorders, 2nd edition (ICHD-II) – Revision of criteria for 8.2 Medication-overuse headache. Cephalalgia 2005; 25(6):460–465.

106 Kudrow L. Paradoxical effects of frequent analgesic use. Adv Neurol 1982; 33:335–341.

107 Ellner JJ, Bennett JE. Chronic meningitis. Medicine (Baltimore) 1976; 55(5):341–369.

108 Smith JE, Aksamit AJ, Jr. Outcome of chronic idiopathic meningitis. Mayo Clin Proc 1994; 69(6):548–556.

109 Coyle PK. Overview of acute and chronic meningitis. Neurol Clin 1999; 17(4):691–710.

110 Helbok R et al. Chronic meningitis. J Neurol 2009; 256(2):168–175.

111 Anderson NE, Willoughby WE. Chronic meningitis without predisposing illness – a review of 83 cases. Q J Med 1987; 63(240):283–295.

112 Ginsberg L, Kidd D. Chronic and recurrent meningitis. Pract Neurol 2008; 8(6):348–361.

113 Wall M. The headache profile of idiopathic intracranial hypertension. Cephalalgia 1990; 10(6):331–335.

114 Schoenen J, Sandor PS. Headache with focal neurological signs or symptoms: A complicated differential diagnosis. Lancet Neurol 2004; 3(4):237–245.

115 Suwanwela N, Phanthumchinda K, Kaoropthum S. Headache in brain tumor: A cross-sectional study. Headache 1994; 34(7):435–438.

116 The Childhood Brain Tumor Consortium. The epidemiology of headache among children with brain tumor. Headache in children with brain tumors. J Neurooncol 1991; 10(1):31–46.

117 Schankin CJ et al. Characteristics of brain tumour-associated headache. Cephalalgia 2007; 27(8):904–911.

118 Hamilton W, Kernick D. Clinical features of primary brain tumours: a case-control study using electronic primary care records. Br J Gen Pract 2007; 57(542):695–699.

119 Pfund Z et al. Headache in intracranial tumors. Cephalalgia 1999; 19(9):787–790:discussion 765.

120 American Academy of Neurology. Report of the Quality Standards Sub-Committee of the American Academy of Neurology. The utility of neuro imaging in the evaluation of headache in patients with normal neurological examinations. 2008. Available: www.aan.com/professionals/practice/pdfs/gl0088.pdf (17 Apr 2009).

121 Tew JMJ, Loveren H. Percutaneous rhizotomy in the treatment of intractable facial pain (trigeminal, glossopharyngeal, and vagal nerves). In: Operative neurosurgical techniques: Indications, methods, and results, 2nd edn. Schmidek HH, Sweet WH (eds). Orlando: Grune & Stratton; 1998:1111–1123.

122 Jannetta PJ. Arterial compression of the trigeminal nerve at the pons in patients with trigeminal neuralgia. J Neurosurg 1967; 26(1 Suppl):159–162.

123 Heir GM. Facial pain of dental origin – a review for physicians. Headache 1987; 27(10):540–547.

124 Evans KL. Recognition and management of sinusitis. Drugs 1998; 56(1):59–71.

125 Diaz I, Bamberger DM. Acute sinusitis. Semin Respir Infect 1995; 10(1):14–20.

126 Rushton JG, Stevens JC, Miller RH. Glossopharyngeal (vagoglossopharyngeal) neuralgia: A study of 217 cases. Arch Neurol 1981; 38(4):201–205.

127 Bruyn GW. Glossopharyngeal neuralgia. In: Handbook of clinical neurology. Headache. Vincken PJ, Bruyn GW, Klawans HL (eds). Amsterdam: Elsevier; 1986:487–494.

128 Siccoli MM, Bassetti CL, Sandor PS. Facial pain: Clinical differential diagnosis. Lancet Neurol 2006; 5(3):257–267.

129 Lascelles RG. Atypical facial pain and depression. Br J Psychiatry 1966; 112(488):651–659.

130 Feinmann C, Harris M, Cawley R. Psychogenic facial pain: presentation and treatment. BMJ (Clin Res Ed) 1984; 288(6415):436–438.

131 Oxman MN et al. A vaccine to prevent herpes zoster and postherpetic neuralgia in older adults. N Engl J Med 2005; 352(22):2271–2284.

132 Harpaz R, Ortega-Sanchez IR, Seward JF. Prevention of herpes zoster: Recommendations of the Advisory Committee on Immunization Practices (ACIP). MMWR Recomm Rep 2008; 57(RR-5):1–30:quiz CE2–4.

133 Wood MJ et al. Oral acyclovir therapy accelerates pain resolution in patients with herpes zoster: A meta-analysis of placebo-controlled trials. Clin Infect Dis 1996; 22(2):341–347.

134 Bowsher D. The effects of pre-emptive treatment of postherpetic neuralgia with amitriptyline: A randomized, double-blind, placebo-controlled trial. J Pain Symptom Manage 1997; 13(6):327–331.

135 Eaglstein WH, Katz R, Brown JA. The effects of early corticosteroid therapy on the skin eruption and pain of herpes zoster. JAMA 1970; 211(10):1681–1683.

136 Keczkes K, Basheer AM. Do corticosteroids prevent post-herpetic neuralgia? Br J Dermatol 1980; 102(5):551–555.

137 He L et al. Corticosteroids for preventing postherpetic neuralgia. Cochrane Database Syst Rev 2008:1:CD005582.

138 Lutt JR et al. Orbital inflammatory disease. Semin Arthritis Rheum 2008; 37(4):207–222.

139 Pascual J et al. Tolosa–Hunt syndrome: Focus on MRI diagnosis. Cephalalgia 1999; 19(Suppl 25):36–38.

140 Kline LB, Hoyt WF. The Tolosa–Hunt syndrome. J Neurol Neurosurg Psychiatry 2001; 71(5):577–582.

Cerebrovascular Disease

Cerebrovascular disease (CVD) is one of the commonest problems encountered in clinical neurology. Hippocrates (460–375 BCE) is credited with introducing the concept of apoplexy (derived from the Greek word for seizure, *apoplēxia, in the sense of being struck down)* to describe patients with stroke. He is also credited with the statement 'it is difficult to cure a mild case of apoplexy and impossible to cure a severe case'. This essentially is still the case today and thus the focus should be on **primary and secondary prevention**. The epidemiology of stroke is discussed in Appendix E.

MINOR STROKE OR TRANSIENT ISCHAEMIC ATTACK: DOES THE DEFINITION MATTER?

Patients with symptoms of cerebral ischaemia that have lasted less than 24 hours have been arbitrarily defined as suffering from a **transient ischaemic attack** (TIA) while patients with symptoms that last more than 24 hours have been designated as having had a stroke [1]. A term that has come and gone is the reversible ischaemic neurological deficit (RIND), which was defined as symptoms lasting more than 24 hours and less than 6 weeks. However, **cerebral infarction** can be demonstrated on diffusion-weighted MRI (dwMRI) in patients with symptoms lasting less than 24 hours [2, 3] and may predict the subsequent risk of stroke developing in patients who have had what is currently defined as a TIA [4]. This has led some authorities to recommend a change in the definition of TIA [5, 6].

There are essentially two types of patients with cerebral ischaemia:
- those with minor symptoms that may or may not resolve within a defined period
- those with cerebral ischaemia associated with a severe and disabling neurological deficit.

In the former group prompt assessment and institution of appropriate treatment provides an opportunity to prevent the severe stroke [7]. The risk of stroke after TIA or minor stroke is similar (see Table 10.1), once again suggesting that the separation between TIA and minor stroke is arbitrary and of little clinical value. Thus, all patients with minor symptoms of cerebral ischaemia, regardless of how long the symptoms last, should be treated as a matter of urgency.

Forty percent of patients who subsequently suffer a stroke after a TIA will do so within the first 7 days; in 17% the TIA will be on the day of the stroke while in 9% it will be on the day prior [8]. Unfortunately, many patients ignore minor symptoms and do not seek urgent medical advice. The opportunity to prevent stroke is lost. The subsequent risk of early stroke after minor cerebral ischaemia is greatest with severe carotid stenosis and in patients with repeated or crescendo TIAs, the 'capsular warning syndrome' [9, 10].

- All patients with minor cerebral isch-aemia should be evaluated as a matter of urgency.

- Recurrent stereotyped TIAs indicate a tight stenosis that could be either a large artery or a perforating vessel.

The principles of management of patients with CVD are simple and at the same time complex as many patients have more than one potential underly-ing pathological cause [12]. Patients can present with a cerebral infarct one time and an intracerebral haemorrhage the

TABLE 10.1   The subsequent risk of stroke after TIA and minor stroke (95% confidence intervals in brackets) [11]

	Subsequent risk of stroke (95% confidence interval)		
	7 days	**1 month**	**3 months**
TIA	8% (2.3% to 13.7%)	11.5% (4.8% to 18.2%)	17.3% (9.3% to 25.3%)
Minor stroke	11.5% (4.8% to 11.2%)	15.0% (7.5% to 22.5%)	18.5% (10.3% to 26.7%)

next [13, 14]. The symptoms and signs of a small intracerebral haemorrhage can be identical to a cerebral infarct of a similar size in the same area and many patients have coexistent medical problems that make the choice of subsequent therapy difficult.

This chapter will discuss the general principles of diagnosis, investigation and man-agement of the more common manifestations of CVD and as such is far from com-prehensive. For more detail the reader is referred to one of the many excellent books on the subject [15–20]. There are many websites that also help the clinician keep abreast of the latest developments (e.g. http://www.cochrane.org/reviews/en/topics/ 93_reviews.html, http://www.strokeassociation.org/presenter.jhtml?identifier=1200037, http://www.strokecenter.org/).

PRINCIPLES OF MANAGEMENT

The principles of management are shown in Figure 10.1. As treatment is currently largely disease-specific and different diseases affect different regions, accurate localisa-tion of the problem within the cerebral hemispheres, brainstem or cerebellum is essen-tial. A detailed knowledge of the basic principles of neuroanatomy, which were outlined in Chapter 1, 'Clinically oriented neuroanatomy', particularly the concept of the merid-ians of longitude and the parallels of latitude, is absolutely essential in this respect and a review of Chapter 1 and Chapter 4, in particular the 'Rule of 4' of the brainstem would be useful before reading further.

Carotid territory refers to cerebral ischaemia in the distribution of the main artery at the front of the neck: the carotid and its branches, the anterior and middle cerebral arteries. Vertebrobasilar territory refers to the arteries at the back of the neck: the two vertebral that coalesce to form the basilar arteries and the branches of the basilar artery, the posterior inferior cerebellar artery, the anterior inferior cerebellar artery, the superior cerebellar artery and the posterior cerebral arteries, and the small paramedian perforat-ing vessels that arise from the basilar artery.

It could be argued that modern diagnostic facilities (and yet to be developed tech-nology), such as CT scans, MRI scans, duplex carotid ultrasound, transthoracic and

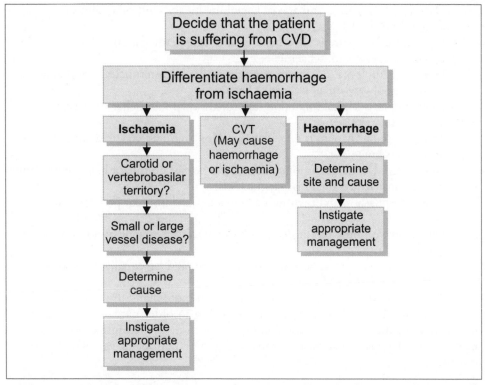

FIGURE 10.1   Principles of management of patients with cerebral vascular disease (CVD)

trans-oesophageal echocardiography, can readily establish if a patient has CVD, differentiate between haemorrhage and infarction, localise the exact site of the lesion, determined if it is lacunar infarction and most likely establish the aetiology. The difficulty with this approach is that not everybody has access to such facilities, the tests are not always positive in patients who are clinically suspected to have CVD (particularly patients with transient symptoms) and both asymptomatic cerebral infarction [21] and asymptomatic carotid stenosis are not uncommon. Therefore, a careful history and, in the presence of abnormal neurological signs, a detailed neurological examination remain the essential tools in management of patients with CVD.

DECIDING THE PROBLEM IS CEREBROVASCULAR DISEASE

Cerebral vascular disease should be suspected when a patient presents with the sudden or subacute onset of a focal neurological deficit *associated with loss of function*. The neurological deficit is usually of sudden onset within minutes if not quicker, particularly with an embolic source from the heart or from atherosclerotic vascular disease in one of the major extracranial vessels. Other modes of onset include stepwise stuttering (related to thrombosis rather than embolism) or fluctuating deficit [22, 23].

There *a number of common presentations* including:
- Vertebrobasilar territory ischaemia
  - Ataxia, nausea and vomiting with or without vertigo: cerebellar infarction or haemorrhage

- Dysphagia, dysarthria and ataxia: lateral medullary syndrome (almost always on an ischaemic basis)
- Pure motor hemiparesis affecting arm and leg: paramedian pontine syndrome (almost always on an ischaemic basis)
- Horizontal diplopia looking to one side: unilateral internuclear ophthalmoplegia (almost always on an ischaemic basis)
- Hemianopia: occipital infarction (almost always on an ischaemic basis)
- Carotid territory ischaemia
  - Transient or permanent monocular visual loss: retinal ischaemia (almost always on an ischaemic basis)
  - Non-fluent dysphasia and right-sided hemiparesis: dominant hemisphere frontal lobe (almost always on an ischaemic basis)
  - Fluent dysphasia with or without a hemianopia: dominant parietal or temporal lobe
  - Left-sided weakness and neglect, with or without hemianopia: non-dominant parietal lobe
  - Pure motor hemiparesis affecting the face, arm and leg equally: lacunar infarct deep within the cerebral hemisphere

  Note: The lacunar syndromes are ischaemic in more than 80% of cases.

There should be an increased level of suspicion in older patients when there are one or more of the risk factors listed above or when other manifestations of atherosclerotic vascular disease such as coronary artery or peripheral vascular disease are present.

Imaging in cerebrovascular disease

Apart from transient ischaemic attacks that last less than 3–4 hours, current imaging technology such as CT scanning and magnetic resonance imaging (MRI) can, in the great majority of patients, confirm the diagnosis of CVD, differentiate between haemorrhage and ischaemia and usually determine the exact site of the cerebral ischaemia within the central nervous system.

CT scan of the brain is often normal in the first 6 and sometimes up to 24 hours after cerebral infarction; MRI can detect changes as early as 1.5 hours after ischaemia [24]. Diffusion-weighted MRI (dwMRI; see Figure 10.2) has a sensitivity of > 90–95% for detecting early (within the first 6 hours after onset) ischaemic changes as opposed to CT scan with a sensitivity of only 70–75% [1, 25].

DwMRI should be performed within the first week after onset as the changes

It is important to remember that CVD can occur:

- at any age, even in childhood
- in patients without currently recognised risk factors for stroke
- with symptoms that do not always develop suddenly.

The longer the deficit takes to develop the less one can be certain clinically that the problem is CVD.

A normal dwMRI does not exclude cerebral ischaemia under the following circumstances:

- when performed in the first few hours
- for small lacunar infarcts in the brainstem, deep hemisphere or cortex [1].

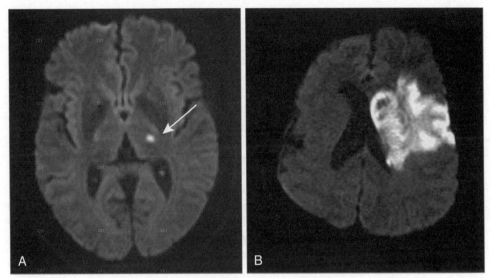

FIGURE 10.2   DwMRI showing lacunar **A** and larger artery infarction **B**

are transient and this helps to differentiate long-standing old 'asymptomatic' ischaemic changes from acute cerebral infarct.

DIFFERENTIATING BETWEEN HAEMORRHAGE AND ISCHAEMIA

- **Extradural haematoma** (due to rupture of an artery, usually the middle meningeal) and **acute subdural haematoma** (due to rupture of veins that cross the subdural space) are rarely confused with cerebral ischaemia; both present with the rapid onset of a depressed conscious state.
- A **chronic subdural haematoma,** on the other hand, can be confused with stroke as it often presents with a non-specific hemiparesis particularly in the elderly [26].
- **Subarachnoid haemorrhage** (SAH) presents in most patients with the sudden onset of a very severe headache, nausea and vomiting with or without depression of the conscious state. Although SAH is usually discussed under the heading of CVD it rarely presents with a stroke. Occasional patients will have a focal neurological deficit if bleeding occurs into the brain.
- A small **intracerebral haemorrhage** in the same location within the hemisphere or brainstem as an infarct will result in identical neurological symptoms and signs, and, very rarely, resembles lacunar syndromes [27].

Clues that may help differentiate haemorrhage from infarction
MORE IN KEEPING WITH HAEMORRHAGE
- *Early depression of the conscious state and vomiting.* Although these two clinical features can occur in brainstem infarction or haemorrhage, both can also reflect a rapid increase in intracranial pressure and should raise the suspicion of intracerebral haemorrhage within the hemisphere.
- *Headache* in a patient with a pure motor hemiparesis is more suggestive of haemorrhage [28].

- Neither vomiting nor early depression of the conscious state occur with a small haematoma mimicking a lacune. Although more than 80% of patients with pure motor hemiparesis or pure sensory stroke will have a lacunar infarct, a small percentage can be related to intracerebral haemorrhage [29, 30].

MORE IN KEEPING WITH ISCHAEMIA
- *Antecedent transient ischaemic attack(s)* with the same symptoms prior to the stroke would indicate ischaemia rather than haemorrhage. For example, repeated stereotyped episodes of weakness affecting the face, arm and leg are typical of the capsular warning syndrome, invariably on the basis of lacunar infarction [10, 31].
- *The neurological deficit gradually spreads* from one part of the body to the rest. For example, if it initially involves the arm and then spreads to the face and subsequently the leg, it is more likely to be ischaemic in origin.
- *Spontaneous improvement within the first few hours* favours ischaemia rather than haemorrhage.

HAEMORRHAGIC STROKE

Intracranial haemorrhage can occur into the extradural, subdural or subarachnoid spaces or be intracerebral or intraventricular (see Figure 10.3). Each site of haemorrhage is associated with a different symptom complex and results from different causes.

Extradural haematoma
Extradural haematoma results from a severe head injury and is almost invariably associated with a fractured skull.

The patient may be comatose from the start or deteriorate within minutes to hours with severe headache, vomiting, a hemiparesis and subsequent coma.

Treatment is essentially surgical evacuation but up-to-date recommendations regarding management of head injuries can be found on the National Neurotrauma Society website (http://www.neurotraumasociety.org/book.asp).

Subdural haematoma
Acute subdural haematoma usually results from trauma to the head although at times the trauma may appear trivial, for example striking one's head on the corner of a cupboard. On the other hand, almost half of patients with chronic subdural hematomas will not have a history of trauma. There is an increased risk of chronic subdural haematoma in patients on anticoagulants.

Subdural haematoma presents with headache, nausea, confusion and hemiparesis and, if acute, a depressed conscious state. In the elderly, hemiparesis may not be a feature [26]. A classic triad with a reduced conscious state, a dilated pupil ipsilateral to the haematoma (related to a 3rd nerve palsy) and a contralateral hemiparesis indicates life-threatening transtentorial herniation and is a surgical emergency. Occasionally, chronic subdural haematomas are bilateral and may present with an apraxic gait similar to the gait disturbance that occurs with frontal lobe pathology (see Chapter 5, 'The cerebral hemispheres and cerebellum').

Acute and large chronic subdural haematomas require surgical evacuation, but some chronic subdural haematomas resolve with conservative treatment. Hyperventilation and mannitol are used to reduce raised intracranial pressure.

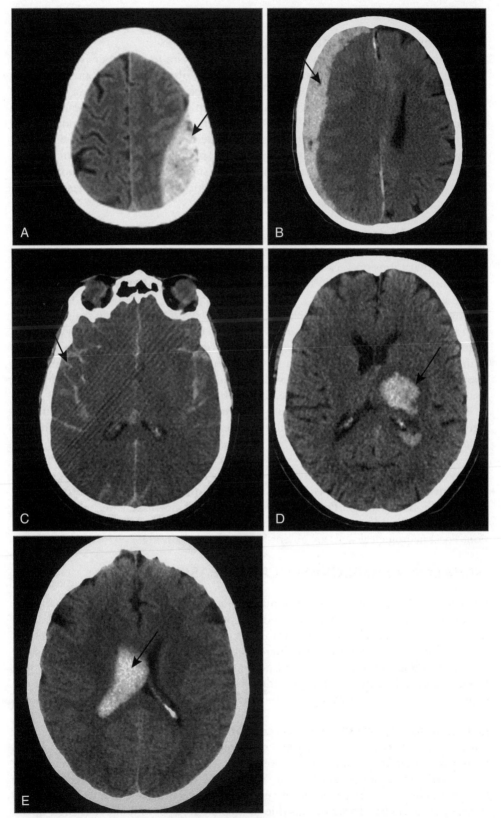

FIGURE 10.3 CT scans showing the different types of intracranial haemorrhages:
A extradural, **B** subdural, **C** subarachnoid, **D** intracerebral and **E** intraventricular

Subarachnoid haemorrhage

SAH is most often related to a ruptured berry aneurysm (a small out-pouching that looks like a berry and classically occurs at the point of bifurcation of an intracranial artery). Less often it is associated with: an arteriovenous malformation (a congenital disorder of blood vessels in the brain, brainstem or spinal cord that is characterised by a complex, tangled web of abnormal arteries and veins connected by one or more fistulas [abnormal communications]); a non-aneurysmal perimesencephalic haemorrhage [32] where the haemorrhage is centred anterior to the midbrain or pons, with or without extension of blood around the brainstem, into the suprasellar cistern or into the proximal sylvian fissures; or it may be traumatic in origin [33]. The clinical features have been described in Chapter 9, 'Headache and facial pain'.

Intracerebral haemorrhage

The commonest cause of intracerebral haemorrhage is rupture of a Charcot–Bouchard aneurysm that forms on very small intracerebral vessels in the setting of long-standing hypertension [34]. The haemorrhages occur in characteristic sites as shown in Figure 10.4 A and B.

Putaminal and basal ganglia haemorrhage are seen with hypertension and a ruptured Charcot–Bouchard aneurysm. Lobar haemorrhage occurs with cerebral amyloid angiopathy (also known as congophilic angiopathy or cerebrovascular amyloidosis, a disease of the small blood vessels in the brain in which deposits of amyloid protein occur in the vessel walls and lead to fragility of the wall and tendency to rupture), anticoagulants and less often vascular malformations or rarely aneurysms.

Classically seen with hypertension and a ruptured Charcot–Bouchard aneurysm, cerebellar haemorrhage is a not uncommon site in patients with anticoagulant-related haemorrhage.

Intraventricular haemorrhage

Intraventricular haemorrhage is usually secondary to rupture into the ventricles from intracerebral haemorrhage. Primary intraventricular haemorrhage is very rare and presents with a depressed conscious state or headache and vomiting with or without confusion. Focal neurological signs are absent [35].

ISCHAEMIC CEREBROVASCULAR DISEASE

Ischaemic stroke accounts for the great majority of patients with CVD. When managing a patient with ischaemic stroke one needs to consider whether the ischaemia relates to arterial or, much less likely, venous disease. In patients with cerebral ischaemia related to arterial disease it is important to differentiate between small vessel disease within the parenchyma due to occlusion of small perforating vessels and large artery disease that is most likely to be embolic in origin either from the heart, the arch of the aorta or the large arteries in the neck (see Figures 10.6 and 10.7).

Is it large artery, small vessel or cerebral venous disease?

Differentiating between large artery and small vessel disease can be very difficult. Access to diffusion-weighted MRI in the first week after stroke enables differentiation between large vessal and small vessel ischaemia. Small vessel disease is often referred to as the lacunar syndrome where occlusion of very small vessels is usually due to lipohyalinosis and that of slightly larger ones is due to atheromatous or embolic occlusion of the

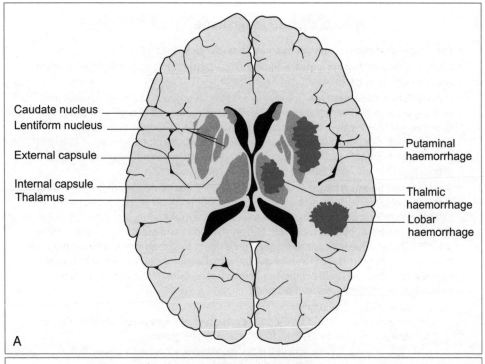

Caudate nucleus
Lentiform nucleus
External capsule
Internal capsule
Thalamus

Putaminal haemorrhage
Thalmic haemorrhage
Lobar haemorrhage

A

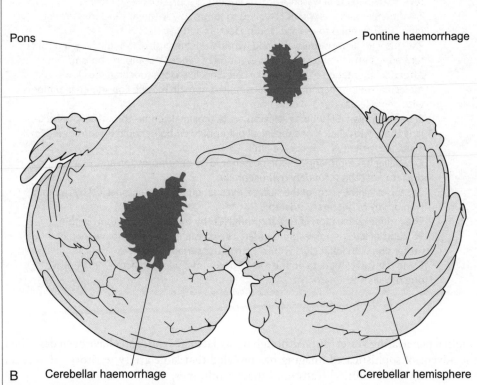

Pons
Pontine haemorrhage

B   Cerebellar haemorrhage
Cerebellar hemisphere

FIGURE 10.4 **A** Sites of intracerebral haemorrhage in the cerebral hemispheres
Reproduced with permission of HJM Barnett
B Sites of intracerebral haemorrhage in the brainstem and cerebellum
Reproduced with permission HJM Barnett

MANAGEMENT of INTRACRANIAL HAEMORRHAGE

- **Extradural and acute subdural haematomas.** Surgical evacuation.
- **Chronic subdural haematomas.** Can be treated conservatively, although many will require surgical evacuation.
- **Subarachnoid haemorrhage.** Transfer as a matter of urgency to a neurosurgical unit with expertise in the management of SAH. The management is complex and includes the timing of intervention, the method of occluding the aneurysm, with options of direct surgical clipping (the traditional method) or endovascular intervention [37], and the management of the cerebral vasospasm that occurs as a result of irritation by the subarachnoid blood and resulting secondary cerebral infarction.
- **Intracerebral haemorrhage** [38]. If the ICH is small it can be managed conservatively. Treatment of larger ICHs consists of ventilatory support, blood pressure control, reversal of any preexisting coagulopathy, intracranial pressure monitoring, osmotherapy, fever control, seizure prophylaxis, treatment of hyerglycaemia and nutritional supplementa-tion [39]. Despite these measures there is some doubt that mortality is reduced [40]. The only study of mannitol failed to show any benefit at 3 months [41]. The role of surgery is clearly established [42] with cerebellar haemorrhages, but the role of surgery in hemi-sphere haemorrhages is less well defined.

Current guidelines [37] recommend:

- Protamine sulfate should be used to reverse heparin-associated ICH, with the dose varying and related to the time from cessation of heparin.
- Patients with warfarin-associated ICH should receive intravenous vitamin K to reverse the effects of warfarin and treatment to replace clotting factors.
- Treatment of patients with ICH related to thrombolytic therapy includes urgent empirical therapies to replace clotting factors and platelets.
- Patients with acute primary ICH and hemiparesis/hemiplegia should have intermit-tent pneumatic compression for prevention of venous thromboembolism.
- After documentation of cessation of bleeding, low-dose subcutaneous low-molecular-weight heparin or unfractionated heparin may be considered in patients with hemiplegia after 3–4 days from onset.
- Patients with an ICH who develop an acute proximal venous thrombosis, particu-larly those with clinical or subclinical pulmonary emboli, should be considered for acute placement of a vena cava filter.
- Cerebellar haemorrhage > 3 cm, posterior fossa decompression and/or a ventricular drain to treat the secondary hydrocephalus.
- Lobar clots within 1 cm of the surface, evacuation of supratentorial ICH by standard craniotomy might be considered.
- The routine evacuation of supratentorial ICH by standard craniotomy within 96 hours of ictus is not recommended (see possible exception above for patients presenting with lobar clots within 1 cm of the surface).
- There is insufficient data on the role of decompressive craniectomy to improve outcome in ICH.

original penetrating vessel [36]. Although many lacunar syndromes have been described, the advent of sophisticated imaging has revealed that large artery territory infarcts can mimic many of the clinical features of these syndromes.

The most common and more likely features that reflect small vessel disease lacunar syndromes are pure motor hemiparesis and pure sensory loss affecting the contralateral face, arm and leg equally. This usually reflects involvement of the deep hemisphere, in particular the internal capsule and less likely the paramedian brainstem, although in this situation the face may not be affected if the infarct is below the mid pons.

The value of the lacunar syndromes is that they usually identify patients with small vessel disease. The pure motor hemiparesis is where the degree of weakness is similar in the face, arm and a leg and is not associated with any dysphasia, visual field loss or visual inattention; sensory symptoms or signs including sensory inattention; and the three parietal sensory signs described in Chapter 5, 'The cerebral hemispheres and cerebellum', stereognosis, graphaesthesia or 2-point discrimination. There are a number of other lacunar syndromes, such as ataxic hemiparesis (also referred to as crural paresis and homolateral ataxia), dysarthria clumsy hand syndrome and the sensorimotor stroke, but the same clinical features can occasionally be seen in large artery ischaemia. The advent of CT and MRI has allowed detection of many more lacunar infarcts and highlighted that the clinical features can be very varied, and these have been referred to as 'atypical lacunar syndromes' [43].

The risk factors associated with small vessel disease are virtually identical to those associated with large vessel disease, although lacunar infarcts are more common in patients with long-standing hypertension and diabetes. It is not uncommon for patients with a lacunar infarct to have multiple potential causes for ischaemia, such as an ipsilateral internal carotid artery stenosis or a cardiac source for embolism [12].

The presence of dysphasia, visual field disturbances and the cortical sensory signs as described in Chapter 5, 'The cerebral hemispheres and cerebellum', all indicate involvement of the cortex and, therefore, are related to large artery disease. An epileptic seizure associated with the stroke would also indicate cortical involvement and large artery disease.

Internuclear ophthalmoplegia (see Chapter 4, 'The cranial nerves and understanding the brainstem') can occur as an isolated phenomenon and can either be uni- or bilateral. It occurs with ischaemia of the median longitudinal fasciculus and usually in the setting of ostial atheroma affecting a paramedian pontine perforating artery, which may also be associated with more significant basilar artery atheroma.

CEREBRAL VEIN THROMBOSIS

Cerebral vein thrombosis is very rare. In the cerebral venous system blood drains from the cortical veins into the superior sagittal sinus and, together with the straight sinus, these drain into the torcular herepholi which then drains into the internal jugular veins via the lateral sinuses (see Figure 10.5).

The resultant clinical syndrome depends on which part of the venous system is affected [44].
- Lateral sinus usually results in intracranial hypertension, resembling idiopathic (IIH) or benign intracranial hypertension (BIH) with raised intracranial pressure causing headache and papilloedema.
- Superior sagittal sinus thrombosis may also result in idiopathic intracranial hypertension but more often it causes severe headache, focal or generalised convulsions and a focal neurological deficit, predominantly hemiparesis due to associated cortical vein thrombosis.
- Cavernous sinus thrombosis presents with unilateral periorbital pain, impaired ocular movements, proptosis (protruding eye) and chemosis (conjunctival oedema and erythema).
- The deep venous system (the straight sinus and its tributaries) is very rare and presents with headache, vomiting, fever and a depressed conscious state.

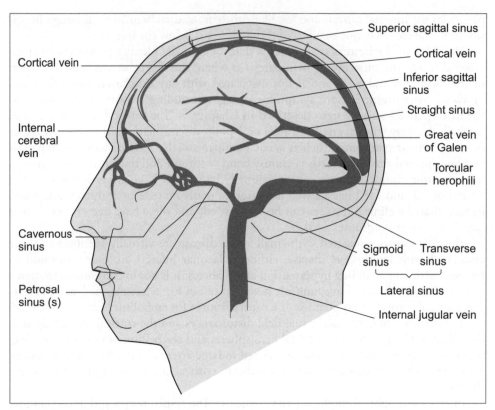

FIGURE 10.5   Cerebral venous system

Reproduced with permission from 'Cardiogenic stroke' by PC Gates, HJM Barnett, MD Silver, in *Stroke: Pathophysiology, Diagnosis and Management*, edited by HJM Barnett et al, 1986, Churchill Livingstone, Figure 35.1, p 732 [44]

IF IT IS A LARGE ARTERY DISEASE, WHAT IS THE VASCULAR TERRITORY OF THE CEREBRAL ISCHAEMIA?

The reason for differentiating between ischaemia in the carotid territory and ischaemia in the vertebrobasilar territory relates to the different management currently recommended for atherosclerotic vascular disease causing stenosis of the extracranial vessels. In addition, asymptomatic vascular disease is not uncommon and the risk of subsequent cerebral ischaemia is very different when the vascular disease is symptomatic compared to when it is asymptomatic.

At times it can be difficult to differentiate between anterior and posterior circulation ischaemia. As discussed in Chapter 2, 'The neurological history', many neurological symptoms and signs are non-specific in terms of their ability to localise a problem to a particular part of the nervous system, while others accurately identify the part of the nervous system affected. A hemiparesis affecting the arm and leg with or without the involvement of the ipsilateral side of the face; unilateral sensory abnormalities affecting the primary sensory modalities of pain, temperature, vibration and proprioception; and dysarthria are all non-specific symptoms with poor localising value, other than to say the lesion is in the CNS above the level of the uppermost signs. If the face, arm and leg are affected this clearly places the problem above the level of the 7th nerve nucleus in the pons but cannot localise it any more accurately. A hemiparesis affecting the arm and a leg in the absence of any other signs can occur with lesions in the contralateral brainstem or hemisphere.

Carotid territory ischaemia
Visual field defects and dysphasia, together with the parietal cortical signs discussed in Chapter 5, 'The cerebral hemispheres and cerebellum', would indicate the involvement of the cerebral hemispheres.

Vertebrobasilar territory ischaemia
The presence of bilateral weakness or sensory disturbance suggests that the brainstem is affected whereas diplopia or vertigo associated with a weakness or sensory disturbance clearly indicates that the problem is in the brainstem. Nausea, vomiting and an inability to stand are not pathognomonic for CVD, but when these symptoms are due to cerebral vascular disease it almost invariably points to cerebellar infarction or haemorrhage.

> Symptoms of cerebral ischaemia in two different vascular territories within a short period of time indicate that the likely source is proximal, either the heart or the arch of the aorta.

IF IT IS LARGE ARTERY DISEASE, WHAT IS THE UNDERLYING PATHOLOGY?
Cerebral ischaemia can result from multiple potential sources, some extremely rare. Figures 10.6 and 10.7 summarise the more common causes from the heart, arch of the aorta and the major extracranial and intracranial vessels. Very rarely, stroke may result from thrombosis within the cerebral venous system or a haematological abnormality. It is useful to consider these two diagrams when dealing with the patient with CVD and always ask where the embolic material has arisen from.

The commonest causes of large artery cerebral ischaemia are:
- embolism in patients with atrial fibrillation, less commonly thromboembolism from the left ventricle in the setting of myocardial infarction or a cardiomyopathy
- atheroma or thromboembolism from the arch of the aorta or the major extracranial vessels in patients suffering from atherosclerotic vascular disease.

The origin of the internal carotid artery is a common site for atherosclerotic vascular disease that can produce severe stenosis or even result in occlusion when superimposed thrombosis occurs. Cerebral ischaemia is rare in adults less than 40 years of age (unless they suffer from hypertension and diabetes when atherosclerotic vascular disease is the most likely cause of cerebral ischaemia); when it does occur extracranial arterial dissection needs to be considered. A patent foramen ovale is considered by some authorities to be a source of embolism and a cause of stroke in young adults [45, 46] and thrombus has been visualised traversing the patent foramen ovale [47], although coexistent deep venous thrombosis (DVT) is found in as few as 5% of patients with cerebral ischaemia and a patent foramen ovale.

A complete list of the causes of cerebral ischaemia is beyond the scope of this book and the interested reader is referred to more comprehensive texts. In many patients with cerebral ischaemia, particularly younger patients, current investigations are unable to elucidate the cause in as many as 30–40% [48]. In some patients with 'cryptogenic stroke' atrial fibrillation is subsequently detected [49].

There are the two common carotid arteries with their major branches, the internal and external carotid, with the anterior and middle cerebral arteries arising from the internal carotid and the two vertebral arteries joining intracranially to form the basilar

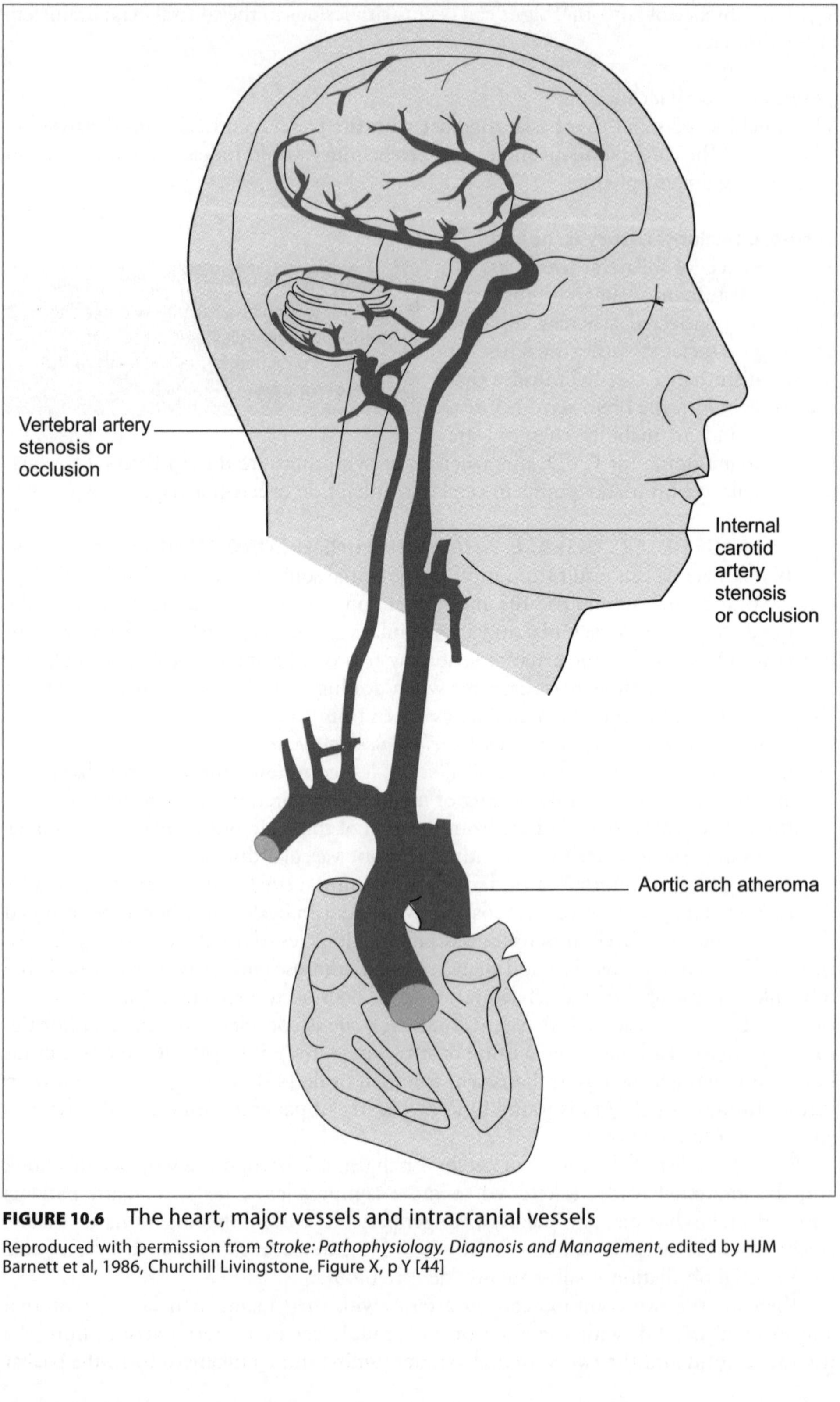

Vertebral artery stenosis or occlusion

Internal carotid artery stenosis or occlusion

Aortic arch atheroma

FIGURE 10.6 The heart, major vessels and intracranial vessels

Reproduced with permission from *Stroke: Pathophysiology, Diagnosis and Management*, edited by HJM Barnett et al, 1986, Churchill Livingstone, Figure X, p Y [44]

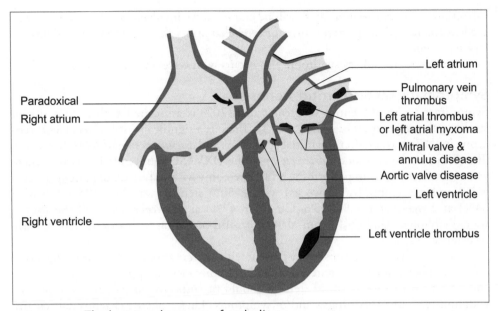

FIGURE 10.7   The heart and sources of emboli

Reproduced with permission from *Stroke: Pathophysiology, Diagnosis and Management*, edited by HJM Barnett et al, 1986, Churchill Livingstone, Figure 54.2, p 1088 [44]

artery. Major branches arise from the vertebral and basilar arteries to supply the lateral brainstem and cerebellum. These include the posterior inferior cerebellar artery (usually arises from the vertebral), the anterior inferior cerebellar artery, the superior cerebellar artery and the posterior cerebral arteries (all branches of the basilar).

The two commonest causes would be thromboembolism from the left atrium in the setting of atrial fibrillation and thromboembolism from the left ventricle related to either myocardial infarction or a cardiomyopathy. Once or twice a year most stroke units would see a patient with cerebral infarction related to infective endocarditis.

THREE STROKE SYNDROMES THAT SHOULD NOT BE MISSED

Cerebellar haemorrhage or infarction

Patients with cerebellar haemorrhage or infarction are at significant risk of brain stem compression and secondary hydrocephalus (dilatation of the 3rd and lateral ventricles) due to swelling of the cerebellar hemisphere. Prompt neurosurgical intervention can be life-saving.

Patients present in a variety of ways; in general, it is an inability to walk associated with nausea and vomiting with or without vertigo and headache. In some patients the vomiting is so severe it results in a Mallory–Weiss tear of the oesophagus and the patient presents with haematemesis. In patients with posterior inferior cerebellar artery territory infarcts, a triad of vertigo, headache and gait imbalance predominates at stroke onset. In patients with superior cerebellar artery infarcts, gait disturbance predominates at onset; vertigo and headache are significantly less common [50]. If the infarct also involves the lateral brainstem, in addition to the features resulting from infarction of the cerebellum, there will be cranial nerve involvement, for example with the involvement of the posterior inferior cerebellar artery there is often a lateral medullary syndrome.

Note: Lateral medullary syndrome also occurs with vertebral artery disease [51].

Symptomatic severe carotid stenosis

Symptomatic carotid stenosis of greater than 70% is associated with a 26% risk of stroke in the ensuing 18 months [52, 53]. There is a significant risk of recurrent ischaemia in the first week after the initial symptoms and *assessment should NOT be delayed*. The risk of stroke *prior to endarterectomy* in the OXVASC subpopulation (where there was a significant delay in performing endarterectomy with only 43% of patients undergoing endarterectomy by 12 weeks) with ≥ 50% stenosis was 21% (95% CI: 8 to 34%) at 2 weeks and 32% (95% CI: 17 to 47%) at 12 weeks, and half the strokes were disabling or fatal [54]. Contralateral carotid occlusion increases the risk of early recurrence [55].

Patients with carotid stenosis may present with a severe stroke without warning; however, a number will have an antecedent TIA that provides an opportunity to intervene and prevent the stroke. Carotid stenosis should be suspected in patients who present with unilateral **amaurosis fugax** and/or symptoms of hemisphere ischaemia particularly if there is an ipsilateral carotid bruit. Focal involvement of one limb or dysphasia with symptoms lasting longer than 1 hour are more likely to indicate the presence of a severe carotid stenosis than a lacunar syndrome [56–58]. Carotid stenosis is more common in patients with diabetes, those who smoke [59] and if there is coexistent coronary artery disease.

Basilar artery stenosis

The prognosis of basilar artery thrombosis is extremely poor and, although basilar artery occlusion may be the first presenting symptom, two-thirds of these patients experience in the weeks to months prior to the thrombosis a flurry of episodes of transient cerebral ischaemia that become more frequent just prior to infarction [60]. Tetraparesis is rare and occurs more frequently when the basilar artery syndrome is related to embolism rather than stenosis and superimposed thrombosis. Patients can present with any combination of symptoms reflecting involvement of the brainstem including a depressed conscious state, weakness, sensory abnormalities, vertigo, nausea and vomiting and diplopia [60]. Once again vertigo, diplopia and bilateral symptoms clearly indicate the involvement of the brainstem, but it is important to remember that not all patients with severe basilar artery stenosis will have symptoms that clearly indicate that the problem is in the brainstem. It is repeated stereotyped TIAs that should alert the clinician to the possibility of a tight stenosis and prompt urgent investigations.

THREE OF THE 'MORE COMMON' RARER CAUSES OF STROKE, PARTICULARLY IN THE YOUNG

Extracranial arterial dissection

Dissection of the carotid and vertebral arteries is one of the more common causes of stroke in young patients. In 50% of patients there will be not be any history of head or neck trauma; it can occur even during coughing or sneezing. This author has seen patients who developed arterial dissection by simply turning their head.

Essentially there are two presentations:

1 isolated carotid artery occlusion with ipsilateral pain in the head, face or neck with an isolated Horner's syndrome and a negligible risk of cerebral ischaemia [61]

2 focal cerebral ischaemia more often in the carotid rather than the vertebral artery territory.

Although an infarct may be the presenting event, it is more common for patients to have transient cerebral ischaemia beforehand and the onset may be some days or weeks after the onset of the headache. The headache characteristically is of sudden onset, severe and in more than 90% of cases it is ipsilateral to the dissection, affecting the neck, ear, face, temple or forehead. If the dissection extends intracranially (more common with vertebral artery dissection), rupture of the artery may occur resulting in SAH. Vertebral artery dissection may very rarely extend into the basilar artery. Recanalisation occurs in the majority of patients and the risk of recurrent events is negligible but not zero. This has led to considerable debate regarding the most appropriate treatment. There is no information from randomised controlled trials to guide therapy. This author has seen several cases of recurrent cerebral ischaemia, often when therapy was suboptimal where the ischaemia was in a more distal vessel than the original ischaemic symptoms, for example in patients with occipital lobe infarction when the initial presenting problem was lateral brainstem ischaemia. This suggests that, in part, recurrent ischaemial relates to throboembolism and supports the use of anticoagulants.

MANAGEMENT of ARTERIAL DISSECTION

The arterial dissection can be demonstrated on imaging studies such as MRI and MR angiography with fat saturation. Alternatively, CT angiography can be used if MRI is not available. The sensitivity of duplex carotid ultrasound (80–96% in the internal carotid artery and 70–86% in the vertebral arteries) is not high enough to exclude extracranial arterial dissection [62].

• For patients with ischaemic stroke or TIA and extracranial arterial dissection, either heparin followed by 3–6 months of warfarin or antiplatelet agents is recommended by most clinicians.

• Some clinicians keep patients on lifelong antiplatelet therapy despite the fact that the risk of recurrence is low.

• In the very rare patient who has recurrent ischaemia, despite adequate antithrombotic therapy and in the absence of any scientific proof of efficacy, some authorities would recommend endovascular stenting [63] or direct surgical intervention, despite the fact that surgery is associated with a high complication rate of stroke and death, in the order of 10–12% [64].

Patent foramen ovale

Patent foramen ovale (PFO) is present in up to 27% of the general population, and in 2% of the population is associated with an atrial septal aneurysm (ASA), which is a bulging of the atrial wall 1.2–15 cm into the left atrium. The presence of an ASA or a large right-to-left shunt has been reported to increase the risk of stroke. In a large French study [46] the risk of recurrent cerebral ischaemia was 2.3% with PFO alone and 15.2% if there was also an ASA. Other studies have failed to confirm the increased risk with an ASA [65]. Coexistent venous thrombus is seen in approximately 5–6%.

> **MANAGEMENT of CEREBRAL ISCHAEMIA WITH PFO**
>
> Current American Heart Association/American Stroke Association guidelines recommend antiplatelet therapy in patients with an ischaemic stroke or TIA associated with a PFO. Warfarin is reserved for high-risk patients who have other indications for oral anticoagulation such as those with an underlying hypercoagulable state or evidence of venous thrombosis. There is insufficient data to recommend PFO closure in patients with a first stroke [66].

Antiphospholipid antibody syndrome

Antiphospholipid (APL) antibodies were first described in 1906 [67] and are a heterogeneous group of autoantibodies directed against phospholipid-binding proteins. They can be broadly categorised into those antibodies that prolong phospholipid-dependent coagulation assays, known as lupus anticoagulants (LA), or anticardiolipin antibodies (aCL), which target a molecular congener of cardiolipin.

APL antibodies may cause various neurological diseases by vascular and immune mechanisms.

APL antibody syndrome is the presence of these antibodies in patients with arterial or venous thrombosis. The association between APL antibodies and stroke is strongest for young adults less than 50 years of age [68]. Recurrent thrombotic events are common despite treatment [69]. APL antibodies should be tested in all young patients, particularly if there is a combination of arterial and venous thrombosis and, although the association with stroke in the elderly is less convincing, in older patients with no apparent cause of stroke. Recurrent cerebral ischaemia is common and the risk is greatest with higher IgG anticardiolipin titres [70].

> **MANAGEMENT of THE ANTIPHOSPHOLIPID ANTIBODY SYNDROME**
>
> Current American Heart Association/American Stroke Association recommendations for patients with cryptogenic cerebral ischaemia in the setting of positive APL antibodies include antiplatelet therapy. Others [66] recommend oral anticoagulation with a target INR of 2–3 in patients with both arterial and venous occlusive disease in multiple organs, miscarriages and livedo reticularis who fulfill the criteria for the APL antibody syndrome. Lim et al [71] in a detailed review suggest moderate intensity aspirin in patients with first ischaemic stroke. The clinical relevance of transient or low titre APL antibodies remains uncertain.

MANAGEMENT OF ISCHAEMIC CEREBROVASCULAR DISEASE

The principles of management are discussed below. However, treatment will evolve rapidly and the reader should seek up-to-date information and guidelines from the American Heart Association stroke website and other websites dedicated to cerebral vascular disease such as the Cochrane collaboration and the stroke trials registry (http://www.americanheart.org/presenter.jhtml?identifier=3004586, http://www.strokecenter.org/trials/, http://www.cochrane.org/reviews/en/topics/93_reviews.html).

Essentially, the management of patients with cerebral ischaemia involves treatment at the time of the initial episode of cerebral ischaemia and secondary prevention through risk factor modification and cause-specific therapy adapted to the individual patient on the basis of their coexistent medical conditions, concurrent medications and social circumstances.

Many patients with CVD have multiple medical problems such as hypertension, diabetes, peptic ulcer and chronic obstructive airways, coronary artery or peripheral vascular disease that will influence the choice of therapy. They are often taking a large number of medications that may either contraindicate the introduction of new medications or result in adverse drug interactions. The presence or absence of a supportive family has a significant impact on management, as does the type of work that the patient is involved with and, of course, whether their house is suitable for someone who may have a residual neurological deficit resulting in some incapacity.

Initial management obviously depends on whether the patient presents with a minor episode of cerebral ischaemia such as a TIA or minor stroke or with a severe stroke.

MANAGEMENT OF ACUTE ISCHAEMIC STROKE

The American Heart Association Stroke Council has issued extensive guidelines for all aspects of the early management of patients with ischaemic stroke (which may be accessed on the AHA website, http://www.americanheart.org/presenter.jhtml?identif ier=3004586) [72].

Patients should be treated as a priority in the emergency department, preferably by a stroke team using organised protocols primarily to establish that the patient is suffering from cerebral ischaemia and whether they are suitable for thrombolytic therapy with tissue plasminogen activator (t-PA). The severity of the stroke should be assessed using the National Institute of Health Stroke Severity Scale (NIHSS). The patient should subsequently be admitted to a comprehensive specialised stroke unit.

Initial urgent bedside clinical assessment
- The pulse (looking for atrial fibrillation), temperature (that may indicate the presence of sepsis) and respiratory rate (that if elevated may indicate pneumonia) should be evaluated.
- The blood pressure should be measured (checking for the very rare case of hypertensive encephalopathy with a diastolic pressure > 120 mmHg and to determine if the blood pressure needs to be treated prior to considering thrombolysis).
- The heart should be auscultated to check for a cardiac murmur (that could be a potential case of infective endocarditis, < 1% of cases per year).
- An urgent ECG should be performed (to detect atrial fibrillation [AF] or the asymptomatic myocardial infarct, the latter particularly in patients with diabetes).

Investigations that should be performed immediately
- Non-contrast CT or MRI of the brain. In most instances CT is the only imaging modality available, but it can provide sufficient information to determine emergency management. The CT scan will rule out intracranial haemorrhage and other pathology such as tumours that may mimic a stroke.
- Full blood examination, platelet count, C-reactive protein (CRP) and ESR. Anaemia and an elevated ESR should alert the clinician to the possibility of endocarditis and an altered platelet count may indicate much rarer pathological processes such as thrombotic thombocytopaenic purpura (TTP) or essential thrombocytosis.
- Blood glucose. Asymptomatic diabetes is not uncommon and rarely hypoglycaemia may present with a focal deficit mimicking a stroke.

- Serum electrolytes and renal function tests. Many patients are on diuretics that may cause hyponatraemia or hypokalaemia, and impaired renal function will influence the choice of antihypertensive medication.
- Prothrombin time/international normalised ratio (PT INR). Particularly necessary in patients on warfarin.
- Activated partial thromboplastin time (APTT). In young patients as a screening test for the lupus anticoagulant (APPT is elevated).
- Oxygen saturation. Some patients may have suffered clinically unrecognised aspiration and also because many patients have been heavy smokers and have coexistent chronic obstructive airways disease.

Subsequent investigations

ASSESSING THE INTERNAL CAROTID ARTERY

The modality of choice for non-invasive carotid artery assessment depends largely on the clinical indications for imaging and the skills available in individual centres. Although digital subtraction angiography was the gold standard imaging technique used in the North American Symptomatic Carotid Endarterectomy Trial, currently most screening would be done with carotid duplex ultrasonography (DUS) that has a sensitivity of 98% and specificity of 88% for detecting > 50% ICA stenosis and 94% and 90%, respectively, for detecting > 70% ICA stenosis [73]. DUS can miss severe carotid stenosis. As imaging technology advances, it is possible that CT angiography or MR angiography may replace DUS. CT angiography and MR angiography are not suitable for all patients because of contraindications. CT angiography has a sensitivity and specificity for detecting carotid occlusion of 97% and 99%, respectively; however, the diagnostic accuracy is lower for severe stenosis in the range of 70–99% with a sensitivity of 85% and a specificity of 93%. The sensitivity and specificity of MR angiography is very dependent on the technique employed and currently is not adequate enough to replace the other imaging modalities.

A screening test and should be performed within the first 24 hours in patients with suspected large artery carotid territory ischaemia with an incomplete deficit (this term refers to an ischaemic stroke where there is some preservation of function that could be lost if further ischaemia were to occur) in order to detect carotid stenosis > 50%. In patients with small artery ischaemia and vertebrobasilar ischaemia, it can be delayed and performed as an outpatient.

LOOKING FOR A CARDIAC SOURCE OF EMBOLISM

In patients with large artery ischaemia and normal extracranial vessels, a more proximal source needs to be considered. A recent review [74] discusses the diagnostic yield of a 'cardiac workup'.

Cardiac monitoring

This is recommended in patients with large artery ischaemia who are not in AF, particularly if there is no significant stenosis in the major extracranial vessels. AF was found in 7% of 465 patients monitored for 54.55 ± 35.74 hours [75]. In one study of 36 patients with cryptogenic stroke where 20 underwent 30-day event monitoring, 4 (20%) were found to have previously undiagnosed AF [49]. AF is more likely to be present in patients ≥ 62 years of age, with an NIHSS ≥ 8, large artery ischaemia without extracranial large artery stenosis and a dilated left atrium as detected on transthoracic echocardiogram [76]. It is appropriate to monitor patients with large artery territory ischaemia with normal arteries to that territory for several days while there are other reasons for them to be an inpatient.

Echocardiography

Transthoracic echocardiography (TTE) will detect abnormalities of the left ventricle and enlargement of the left atrium, while transoesophageal (TOE) is more sensitive at detecting PFO, infective endocarditis vegetations and aortic arch atheroma. The latter is more invasive and may cause oesophageal rupture in elderly patients. At this point in time there is no consensus on who should have structural imaging of the heart, with some advocating all patients and others recommending a more restricted use. As there is no convincing evidence regarding the treatment of PFO or aortic arch atheroma while detection of a cardiomyopathy or dyskinetic anterior left ventricular wall would indicate the use of anticoagulation, it would seem reasonable to perform TTE in patients with large artery territory ischaemia and normal extracranial vessels, particularly if they have preexisting cardiac disease where the yield is higher. TOE should be performed in patients with suspected infective endocarditis and patients < 50 years of age to look for a PFO.

General supportive care and treatment of acute complications

- *Airway support and ventilator assistance* are recommended for patients with a decreased consciousness or who have bulbar dysfunction causing compromise of the airway.
- Hypoxic patients with stroke should receive *supplemental oxygen.*
- Patients should be *screened for dysphagia* and placed nil orally if they are unable to swallow. If swallowing does not improve a nasogastric tube may need to be inserted.
- The *management of arterial hypertension* remains controversial but it needs to be less than 185/110 mmHg if thrombolysis is contemplated.
- Hyperglycaemia and hypoglycaemia should be treated.
- *Prevention of DVT* with prompt initiation of subcutaneous anticoagulation on the day of admission should be undertaken in all patients.
- *Fever should prompt a septic workup.* Sources of fever should be treated and antipyretic medications should be administered to lower temperature in febrile patients.
- Patient's *chest and IV sites should be examined daily* as chest infections and aspiration pneumonia (even in patients who are nil orally and who have nasogastric tubes inserted) occur in the first few days after stroke.
- *Intravenous site and urinary tract infections are common complications* of patients with ischaemic stroke and require prompt attention and IV site infections or thrombosis of the vein are not uncommon.
- *Seizures* either focal or generalised may occur in a small percentage of patients with cortical cerebral ischaemia, usually within the first 24 hours.
- *Myocardial ischaemia* is seen in the occasional patient.
- *Pulmonary embolism* may occur despite prophylactic anticoagulants.

Dysphagia screen

Many patients with stroke develop dysphagia that predisposes them to potential aspiration pneumonia. The dysphagia is often transient but it may persist for some days to weeks and patients will require nasogastric feeding. In some patients swallowing does not recover and these patients require long-term feeding with a percutaneous endoscopic gastrostomy (PEG) tube. Although controversial [77], the risk of aspiration may be reduced with dysphagia screening [78]. Most stroke units would perform a dysphagia screen on all patients and, if the patient fails the screen, they are placed nil orally until a speech therapist undertakes a formal assessment of swallowing as soon as possible.As dysphagia is often temporary, it is not unreasonable to defer insertion of a nasogastric tube until it is clear that improvement is not occurring.

Note: The Barwon Health Stroke unit has a speech therapist 7 day per week. The Barwon Health Dysphagia Screen is shown in Appendix G.

Intravenous therapy
Intravenous therapy is often required in the first 24–48 hours in patients who fail a dysphagia screen. Normal saline should be used, not 5% glucose as the latter enters the intracellular space and will exacerbate cerebral oedema.

Thrombolytic therapy
Intravenous thrombolysis with t-PA (0.9 mg/kg with a maximum dose of 90 mg) is recommended in patients with cerebral ischaemia who meet very stringent inclusion and exclusion criteria (see Appendix F) [72, 79–81]. Although the time window has been extended beyond the original 3 hours [82], IV t-PA should be administered as soon as possible after the onset of stroke. Refer to Appendix E for details.

Symptomatic intracerebral haemorrhage including fatal haemorrhage is the most dreaded complication of this therapy and occurs in 1.7–7.3% of patients (depending on how symptomatic intracerebral haemorrhage is defined) [79, 83].

The very stringent inclusion and exclusion criteria, in particular the narrow time window, imply that only a small percentage of patients will benefit from thrombolytic therapy. Similarly, clot retrieval devices [84, 85], stenting [86] and intra-arterial t-PA [87] require massive resources, are confined to large academic centres and are unlikely to become gold standard treatments in the near future. It is hoped that one day neuroprotection will allow a longer period before recanalisation is attempted with thrombolytic therapy.

Antiplatelet agents
The International Stroke Trial (IST) [88] and the Chinese Acute Stroke Trial (CAST) [89] have both demonstrated a non-significant trend towards a better outcome with antiplatelet agents. A combined analysis of both trials demonstrated a statistically significant benefit in terms of reduced incidence of recurrent stroke with aspirin given in the first 24–48 hours of acute stroke. It should not be given in the first 24 hours to patients undergoing thrombolysis. The recommended dose is aspirin 160–300mg [90]. Ticlopidine, clopidogrel and dipyridamole have not been evaluated in acute stroke.

Anticoagulants
Apart from prophylaxis for DVT anticoagulants are not recommended in acute completed (maximum deficit already present at time patient presents) ischaemic stroke [91].

URGENT MANAGEMENT OF SUSPECTED TIA OR MINOR ISCHAEMIC STROKE

One of the most challenging aspects is the urgent management of minor ischaemic stroke or TIA. A number of patients do not recognise that minor neurological symptoms may represent a warning of a more severe stroke and do not seek medical attention. In other patients the interval between the initial symptom and the subsequent severe cerebral infarct is brief and therefore the time to intervene is limited. At times it is impossible to be certain clinically whether the symptoms represent cerebral ischaemia and thus prompt emergency investigations or whether it is a less urgent problem when investigations could wait. Finally, having decided the patient has cerebral ischaemia the question arises as to whether one can gain access to the urgent imaging required or should the patient be admitted to hospital. All these questions are not readily answered.

Patients with suspected minor cerebral ischaemia should be assessed as a matter of urgency. The urgent bedside assessment is the same as for more severe ischaemic stroke (see 'Initial urgent bedside clinical assessment' under 'Management of acute ischaemic stroke') and includes pulse, blood pressure, respiratory rate, temperature, an urgent ECG, CT of the brain and, if carotid territory ischaemia, imaging (if there is uncertainty about whether it is carotid territory then err on the safe side and obtain urgent imaging because the consequences of missing a severe symptomatic internal carotid stenosis are potentially disastrous). The earliest risk of recurrence is in patients with large artery atherosclerotic vascular disease, accounting for more than one-third of recurrent cerebral ischaemia within the first 7 days [9]. Carotid territory should be imaged on the same day as half of all recurrent strokes during the 7 days after a TIA occur in the first 24 hours [92].

A vexed question is whether to admit the patient to hospital. Although currently proven therapy can be administered on an outpatient basis, some would argue that in the high risk group admission to hospital provides an excellent opportunity for the urgent detection of subsequent cerebral infarction and prompt administration of thrombolytic therapy. In recent years a scoring system, referred to as the ABCD2 score (see Table 10.2), based on five factors has been advocated as a technique to detect patients who require admission because of a greater likelihood of early recurrence of cerebral ischaemia [93]. Admission is advised if the score is 4 or more, while those with a score of less than 4 can be investigated as outpatients. However, in a recent study of 1176 patients in the SOS_TIA registry, the ABCD2 score < 4 would have missed 20% of patients requiring urgent treatment for carotid stenosis > 50%, intracranial stenosis, AF and other major cardiac causes of embolism [94]. Those authors advocate a DSU as part of the emergency assessment. Patients with recurrent TIAs should be admitted, as should patients with severe carotid stenosis with a view to urgent endarterectomy.

TABLE 10.2 The ABCD2 score for prediction of 2-day stroke risk [93]	
Factor	**Points**
Age ≥ 60 years	1
Blood pressure ≥ 140/90 mmHg	1
Unilateral weakness	2
Speech impairment without weakness	1
Duration of event ≥ 60 min	2
Duration of event = 10–59 min	1
Diabetes	1

SECONDARY PREVENTION

The epidemiology and primary prevention of stroke are discussed in Appendix E. The same principles apply in secondary prevention (treatment after the onset of symptoms of cerebral vascular disease). Risk factor modification, such as treatment of hypertension, atrial fibrillation, asymptomatic carotid stenosis, hyperlipidaemia, diabetes, obesity and smoking, is just as relevant.

This section discusses antiplatelet therapy, anticoagulation, carotid endarterectomy and carotid stenting.

Antiplatelet, anticoagulant and surgical therapy for secondary prevention

ANTIPLATELET THERAPY

Unless there are contraindications, all patients with cerebral ischaemia in the absence of the specific cardiac causes discussed below should receive aspirin. There is considerable debate about the actual dose that should be prescribed. The early trials [95, 96] used large doses in the order of 1200 mg/day. The addition of dipyridamole to aspirin was found to be superior to aspirin alone [97].

Current recommendations as first-line treatment from the American Heart Association/American Stroke Association Council on stroke [66] include:

- aspirin 50–325 mg/day combined with dipyridamole [97, 98], or
- clopidogrel 75 mg/day [99, 100].

Clopidogrel has been shown to be equivalent to aspirin/dipyridamole [99], but combination therapy with aspirin and clopidogrel is not recommended because of an increased risk of haemorrhage [101]. The problem with dipyridamole is that a number of patients cannot tolerate it because of headache. The headache may resolve if the drug is introduced at a small dose and increased gradually and the patient can persevere for a few days to weeks despite the headache [102].

There is an increased risk of intracranial haemorrhage complicating head trauma with clopidogrel, which is not seen with aspirin [103].

Although warfarin is often prescribed in patients with recurrent events on antiplatelet therapy, it has not been shown to be more beneficial than aspirin in patients with atherosclerotic vascular disease [104].

ENDARTERECTOMY FOR SYMPTOMATIC CAROTID STENOSIS

The North American Symptomatic Carotid Endarterectomy Trial (NASCET) [105] and the European Carotid Surgery Trial (ECST) [106] both demonstrated a very significant benefit (absolute risk reduction of 17% and 14%, respectively) of carotid endarterectomy in patients with a 70% or more stenosis of the internal carotid artery. The benefit for patients with a symptomatic 50–69% stenosis was modest, with an absolute risk reduction of only 1% [107].

The European Society of Vascular Surgeons (ESVS) published guidelines recommend [108]:

- carotid endarterectomy (CEA) in symptomatic patients with > 50% stenosis if the perioperative stroke/death rate is < 6%, preferably within 2 weeks of the patient's last symptoms
- aspirin at a dose of 75–325 mg daily and statins given before, during and following CEA.

The complications rates for endarterectomy have varied enormously from one institution to another, from as low as 0% to as high as 21% [109, 110]. An acceptable complication rate for patients with symptomatic stenosis is < 6%.

It is irrelevant what the results of treatment (in this case endarterectomy) are in the literature. It is ABSOLUTELY essential that the risk is known in the institution that is treating your patient, as any benefit is lost if the complication rate is too high.

The only complication rate, however, that is relevant is that of the surgeon performing the operation on your patient!

CAROTID ARTERY STENTING
Symptomatic carotid stenosis

The ESVS published guidelines [108] recommend that carotid artery stenting (CAS) should be performed only in patients at high-risk for CEA, in high-volume centres with documented low perioperative stroke and death rates or inside a randomised controlled trial. CAS should be performed under dual antiplatelet treatment with aspirin and clopidogrel.

In one trial of less than 350 patients with severe carotid artery stenosis and increased surgical risk, no significant difference could be shown in long-term outcomes between patients who underwent CAS with an emboli-protection device and those who underwent endarterectomy [111]. In a larger trial [112] of 1214 patients, carotid angioplasty with stenting was not shown to be inferior to CEA in terms of the number of subsequent events of cerebral ischaemia after a short follow-up of only 2 years. Although there is some uncertainty regarding the accuracy of DSU in determining the degree of stenosis in patients with an in situ stent, the re-stenosis rate was higher in the stent group.

Others would argue that CAS, despite the attraction of its less invasive nature, has not been shown to be as effective in the long term as CEA in patients who are not at increased surgical risk and that CAS should be reserved for patients with medical or surgical contraindications to CEA until such time that it has been proven to be as effective in both the short and long term [113]. The results of the International Carotid Stenting Study presented recently have shown that endarterectomy is superior to stenting [114]. The 30-day periprocedural stroke rate was 58 (6.7%) in the stenting group versus 27 (3.2%) in the endarterectomy group. This risk was not influenced by the use of protection devices. The 120-day risk of stroke, myocardial infarction or death was 8.3% versus 5.1%, respectively.

A recent meta-analysis [115] has concluded that carotid endarterectomy is superior to CAS for short-term outcomes, mainly due to an increase in non-disabling strokes in stented patients. An accompanying editorial [116] concluded that CAS is not yet ready to replace endarterectomy.

Intracranial stenosis

Although intracranial stenting appears to be feasible, adverse events vary widely, there is a high rate of re-stenoses and no clear impact of new stent devices on outcome. A recent review concluded that the widespread application of intracranial stenting outside the setting of randomised trials and in inexperienced centres currently does not seem to be justified [86].

Ischaemic stroke or TIA related to cardiac disease [66]
ATRIAL FIBRILLATION

The recommendations apply to both persistent and paroxysmal (intermittent) AF:
- Anticoagulation with adjusted-dose warfarin (target INR, 2.5; range, 2.0–3.0)
- Patients unable to take oral anticoagulants, aspirin 325 mg/day

ACUTE MYOCARDIAL INFARCTION (MI) WITH LEFT VENTRICULAR (LV) MURAL THROMBUS

- Oral anticoagulation aiming for a PT INR of 2.0–3.0 for at least 3 months and up to 1 year.
- Aspirin should be used concurrently for ischaemic coronary artery disease during oral anticoagulant therapy in doses up to 162 mg/day.

DILATED CARDIOMYOPATHY

- Either warfarin (INR, 2.0–3.0) or antiplatelet therapy.

VALVULAR HEART DISEASE

Rheumatic mitral valve disease

- Whether or not AF is present, long-term warfarin therapy with a target INR of 2.5 (range, 2.0–3.0).
- Add aspirin if recurrent emboli on warfarin.

Mitral valve prolapse

- Antiplatelet therapy.

Mitral annular calcification

- Antiplatelet therapy.

Prosthetic heart valves

- Modern mechanical prosthetic heart valves.
- Anticoagulants with an INR target of 3.0 (range, 2.5–3.5)
- Add aspirin 75–100 mg/day if ischaemic stroke or systemic embolism despite adequate therapy with oral anticoagulants.

MANAGEMENT OF PATIENTS WITH ANTICOAGULATION-ASSOCIATED INTRACRANIAL HAEMORRHAGE

There is a little scientific evidence in the literature to provide guidance in the management of this situation. Temporary interruption of anticoagulation therapy seems safe for patients with intracranial haemorrhage and mechanical heart valves without previous evidence of systemic embolisation. For most patients, discontinuation for 1–2 weeks should be sufficient to observe the evolution of a parenchymal haematoma, to clip or coil a ruptured aneurysm or to evacuate an acute subdural haematoma [115]. Others have argued for a 6-month cessation of anticoagulation [116]. Some would recommend heparin during the period of warfarin withdrawal [117].

The most sensible approach would appear to be to reverse the anticoagulant immediately with either vitamin K or fresh frozen plasma and withhold anticoagulation for at least 1–2 weeks. The decision to resume anticoagulation after 3–4 weeks would depend on the underlying risk for thromboembolism, but it is recommended that patients be monitored more carefully and the PT INR be kept at the lower end of the therapeutic range [66]. (*Note*: If the intracranial haemorrhage is SAH related to rupture of an aneurysm, the anticoagulation should not be resumed until the aneurysm is secured.) In patients with artificial heart valves, the risk is so high that anticoagulation must be recommended and, in patients with AF and a high CHADS$_2$ score, the benefits would outweigh the risks. Anticoagulation can be safely resumed in patients with intracerebral haemorrhage.

REFERENCES

1 *Ad hoc* committee established by the Advisory Council for the National Institute of Neurological and Communicative Disorders and Stroke, National Institutes of Health. A classification and outline of cerebrovascular diseases. II. Stroke 1975; 6(5):564–616.

2 Engelter ST et al. The clinical significance of diffusion-weighted MR imaging in stroke and TIA patients. Swiss Med Wkly 2008; 138(49–50):729–740.

3 Kidwell CS et al. Diffusion MRI in patients with transient ischemic attacks. Stroke 1999; 30(6): 1174–1180.

4 Purroy F et al. Higher risk of further vascular events among transient ischemic attack patients with diffusion-weighted imaging acute ischemic lesions. Stroke 2004; 35(10):2313–2319.

5 Easton JD et al. Definition and evaluation of transient ischemic attack: A scientific statement for healthcare professionals from the American Heart Association/American Stroke Association Stroke Council; Council on Cardiovascular Surgery and Anesthesia; Council on Cardiovascular Radiology and Intervention; Council on Cardiovascular Nursing; and the Interdisciplinary Council on Peripheral Vascular Disease. The American Academy of Neurology affirms the value of this statement as an educational tool for neurologists. Stroke 2009; 40(6):2276–2293.

6 Albers GW et al. Transient ischemic attack – proposal for a new definition. N Engl J Med 2002; 347(21):1713–1716.

7 Rothwell PM et al. Effect of urgent treatment of transient ischaemic attack and minor stroke on early recurrent stroke (EXPRESS study): A prospective population-based sequential comparison. Lancet 2007; 370(9596):1432–1442.

8 Rothwell PM, Warlow CP. Timing of TIAs preceding stroke: Time window for prevention is very short. Neurology 2005; 64(5):817–820.

9 Lovett JK, Coull AJ, Rothwell PM. Early risk of recurrence by subtype of ischemic stroke in population-based incidence studies. Neurology 2004; 62(4):569–573.

10 Rothrock JF et al. 'Crescendo' transient ischemic attacks: Clinical and angiographic correlations. Neurology 1988; 38(2):198–201.

11 Coull AJ, Lovett JK, Rothwell PM. Population based study of early risk of stroke after transient ischaemic attack or minor stroke: Implications for public education and organisation of services. BMJ 2004; 328(7435):326.

12 Moncayo J et al. Coexisting causes of ischemic stroke. Arch Neurol 2000; 57(8):1139–1144.

13 Wang HC et al. Risk factors for acute symptomatic cerebral infarctions after spontaneous supratentorial intra-cerebral hemorrhage. J Neurol 2009; 256(8):1281–1287.

14 Ariesen MJ et al. Predictors of risk of intracerebral haemorrhage in patients with a history of TIA or minor ischaemic stroke. J Neurol Neurosurg Psychiatry 2006; 77(1):92–94.

15 Caplan LR. Posterior circulation disease: Clinical findings, diagnosis, and management, vol 1. Boston: Blackwell Science; 1996.

16 Vinken PJ, Bruyn GW, Klawans HL (eds). Vascular diseases: Handbook of clinical neurology, vol. 53–55. Elsevier Science Publishers; 1988.

17 Bogousslavsky J, Caplan LR. Uncommon causes of stroke. Cambridge: Cambridge University Press; 2001.

18 Bogousslavsky J, Caplan LR. Stroke syndromes, 2nd edn. Cambridge: Cambridge University Press; 2001.

19 Barnett HJM et al. Stroke, pathophysiology, diagnosis and management, 3rd edn. New York: Churchill Livingstone; 1998.

20 Warlow CP et al. Stroke: A practical guide to management. Oxford: Blackwell Science; 2001.

21 Kempster PA, Gerraty RP, Gates PC. Asymptomatic cerebral infarction in patients with chronic atrial fibrillation. Stroke 1988; 19(8):955–957.

22 Bogousslavsky J, Van Melle G, Regli F. The Lausanne Stroke Registry: Analysis of 1,000 consecutive patients with first stroke. Stroke 1988; 19(9):1083–1092.

23 Mohr JP et al. The Harvard Cooperative Stroke Registry: A prospective registry. Neurology 1978; 28(8):754–762.

24 Kucinski T et al. Correlation of apparent diffusion coefficient and computed tomography density in acute ischemic stroke. Stroke 2002; 33(7):1786–1791.

25 Saur D et al. Sensitivity and interrater agreement of CT and diffusion-weighted MR imaging in hyperacute stroke. AJNR Am J Neuroradiol 2003; 24(5):878–885.

26 Patrick D, Gates PC. Chronic subdural haematoma in the elderly. Age Ageing 1984; 13(6):367–369.

27 Mori E, Tabuchi M, Yamadori A. Lacunar syndrome due to intracerebral hemorrhage. Stroke 1985; 16(3):454–459.

28 Arboix A et al. Haemorrhagic pure motor stroke. Eur J Neurol 2007; 14(2):219–223.

29 Arboix A et al. Clinical study of 99 patients with pure sensory stroke. J Neurol 2005; 252(2):156–162.

30 Arboix A et al. Clinical study of 222 patients with pure motor stroke. J Neurol Neurosurg Psychiatry 2001; 71(2):239–242.

31 Donnan GA et al. The capsular warning syndrome: Pathogenesis and clinical features. Neurology 1993; 43(5):957–962.

32 Schwartz TH, Solomon RA. Perimesencephalic nonaneurysmal subarachnoid hemorrhage: Review of the literature. Neurosurgery 1996; 39(3):433–440;discussion 440.

33 van Gijn J, Rinkel GJ. Subarachnoid haemorrhage: Diagnosis, causes and management. Brain 2001; 124 (Pt 2):249–278.

34 Sutherland GR, Auer RN. Primary intracerebral hemorrhage. J Clin Neurosci 2006; 13(5):511–517.

35 Gates PC et al. Primary intraventricular hemorrhage in adults. Stroke 1986; 17:872–877.

36 Fisher CM. Lacunar strokes and infarcts: A review. Neurology 1982; 32(8):871–876.

37 Derdeyn CP et al. The International Subarachnoid Aneurysm Trial (ISAT): A position statement from the Executive Committee of the American Society of Interventional and Therapeutic Neuroradiology and the American Society of Neuroradiology. Am J Neuroradiol 2003; 24(7):1404–1408.

38 Broderick J et al. Guidelines for the management of spontaneous intracerebral hemorrhage in adults: 2007 update: A guideline from the American Heart Association/American Stroke Association Stroke Council, High Blood Pressure Research Council, and the Quality of Care and Outcomes in Research Interdisciplinary Working Group. Stroke 2007; 38(6):2001–2023.

39 Rincon F, Mayer SA. Clinical review: Critical care management of spontaneous intracerebral hemorrhage. Crit Care 2008; 12(6):237.

40 Qureshi AI, Mendelow AD, Hanley DF. Intracerebral haemorrhage. Lancet 2009; 373(9675):1632–1644.

41 Misra UK et al. Mannitol in intracerebral hemorrhage: A randomized controlled study. J Neurol Sci 2005; 234:41–45.

42 Elijovich L, Patel PV, Hemphill JC, 3rd. Intracerebral hemorrhage. Semin Neurol 2008; 28(5):657–667.

43 Arboix A et al. Clinical study of 39 patients with atypical lacunar syndrome. J Neurol Neurosurg Psychiatry 2006; 77(3):381–384.

44 Gates PC, Barnett HJM, Silver MD. Cardiogenic Stroke. In: Barnett HJM et al (eds). Stroke: pathophysiology, diagnosis and management. New York: Churchill Livingstone; 1986:1085–1110.

45 Lechat P et al. Prevalence of patent foramen ovale in patients with stroke. N Engl J Med 1988; 318(18):1148–1152.

46 Mas JL et al. Recurrent cerebrovascular events associated with patent foramen ovale, atrial septal aneurysm, or both. N Engl J Med 2001; 345(24):1740–1746.

47 Srivastava TN, Payment MF. Images in clinical medicine: Paradoxical embolism–thrombus in transit through a patent foramen ovale. N Engl J Med 1997; 337(10):681.

48 Guercini F et al. Cryptogenic stroke: Time to determine aetiology. J Thromb Haemost 2008; 6(4): 549–554.

49 Elijovich L et al. Intermittent atrial fibrillation may account for a large proportion of otherwise cryptogenic stroke: A study of 30-day cardiac event monitors. J Stroke Cerebrovasc Dis 2009; 18(3):185–189.

50 Kase CS et al. Cerebellar infarction. Clinical and anatomic observations in 66 cases. Stroke 1993; 24(1): 76–83.

51 Kim JS. Pure lateral medullary infarction: Clinical-radiological correlation of 130 acute, consecutive patients. Brain 2003; 126(Pt 8):1864–1872.

52 European Carotid Surgery Trialists' Collaborative Group. MRC European Carotid Surgery Trial: Interim results for symptomatic patients with severe (70–99%) or with mild (0–29%) carotid stenosis. Lancet 1991; 337(8752):1235–1243.

53 North American Symptomatic Carotid Endarterectomy Trial Collaborators. Beneficial effect of carotid endarterectomy in symptomatic patients with high-grade carotid stenosis. N Engl J Med 1991; 325(7): 445–453.

54 Fairhead JF, Mehta Z, Rothwell PM. Population-based study of delays in carotid imaging and surgery and the risk of recurrent stroke. Neurology 2005; 65(3):371–375.

55 Kastrup A et al. Risk factors for early recurrent cerebral ischemia before treatment of symptomatic carotid stenosis. Stroke 2006; 37(12):3032–3034.

56 Harrison MJ, Marshall J. Indications for angiography and surgery in carotid artery disease. BMJ 1975; 1(5958):616–618.

57 Harrison MJ, Marshall J, Thomas DJ. Relevance of duration of transient ischaemic attacks in carotid territory. BMJ 1978; 1(6127):1578–1579.

58 Harrison MJ, Iansek R, Marshall J. Clinical identification of TIAs due to carotid stenosis. Stroke 1986; 17(3):391–392.

59 Mast H et al. Cigarette smoking as a determinant of high-grade carotid artery stenosis in Hispanic, black, and white patients with stroke or transient ischemic attack. Stroke 1998; 29(5):908–912.

60 Voetsch B et al. Basilar artery occlusive disease in the New England Medical Center Posterior Circulation Registry. Arch Neurol 2004; 61(4):496–504.

61 West TE, Davies RJ, Kelly RE. Horner's syndrome and headache due to carotid artery disease. BMJ 1976; 1(6013):818–820.

62 Nebelsieck J et al. Sensitivity of neurovascular ultrasound for the detection of spontaneous cervical artery dissection. J Clin Neurosci 2009; 16(1):79–82.

63 Malek AM et al. Endovascular management of extracranial carotid artery dissection achieved using stent angioplasty. Am J Neuroradiol 2000; 21(7):1280–1292.

64 Muller BT et al. Surgical treatment of 50 carotid dissections: Indications and results. J Vasc Surg 2000; 31(5):980–988.

65 Homma S et al. Effect of medical treatment in stroke patients with patent foramen ovale: Patent foramen ovale in Cryptogenic Stroke Study. Circulation 2002; 105(22):2625–2631.

66 Sacco RL et al. Guidelines for prevention of stroke in patients with ischemic stroke or transient ischemic attack: A statement for healthcare professionals from the American Heart Association/American Stroke Association Council on Stroke: Co-sponsored by the Council on Cardiovascular Radiology and Intervention: The American Academy of Neurology affirms the value of this guideline. Circulation 2006; 113(10):e409–e449.

67 Wassermann A, Neisser A, Bruck C. Eine serodiagnostische Reaction bei Syphilis [German]. Dtsch Med Wochenschr 1906; 32:745–746.

68 The Antiphospholipid Antibodies in Stroke Study (APASS) Group. Anticardiolipin antibodies are an independent risk factor for first ischemic stroke. Neurology 1993; 43(10):2069–2073.

69 Cervera R et al. Morbidity and mortality in the antiphospholipid syndrome during a 5-year period: A multicentre prospective study of 1000 patients. Ann Rheum Dis 2009; 68(9):1428–1432.

70 Levine SR et al. Recurrent stroke and thrombo-occlusive events in the antiphospholipid syndrome. Ann Neurol 1995; 38(1):119–124.

71 Lim W, Crowther MA, Eikelboom JW. Management of antiphospholipid antibody syndrome: A systematic review. JAMA 2006; 295(9):1050–1057.

72 Adams HP, Jr et al. Guidelines for the early management of adults with ischemic stroke: A guideline from the American Heart Association/American Stroke Association Stroke Council, Clinical Cardiology Council, Cardiovascular Radiology and Intervention Council, and the Atherosclerotic Peripheral Vascular Disease and Quality of Care Outcomes in Research Interdisciplinary Working Groups: The American Academy of Neurology affirms the value of this guideline as an educational tool for neurologists. Stroke 2007; 38(5):1655–1711.

73 Jahromi AS et al. Sensitivity and specificity of color duplex ultrasound measurement in the estimation of internal carotid artery stenosis: A systematic review and meta-analysis. J Vasc Surg 2005; 41(6):962–972.

74 Morris JG, Duffis EJ, Fisher M. Cardiac workup of ischemic stroke: Can we improve our diagnostic yield? Stroke 2009; 40(8):2893–2898.

75 Vivanco Hidalgo RM et al. Cardiac monitoring in stroke units: Importance of diagnosing atrial fibrillation in acute ischemic stroke. Rev Esp Cardiol 2009; 62(5):564–567.

76 Suissa L et al. Score for the targeting of atrial fibrillation (STAF): A new approach to the detection of atrial fibrillation in the secondary prevention of ischemic stroke. Stroke 2009; 40(8):2866–2868.

77. Perry L, Hamilton S, Williams J. Formal dysphagia screening protocols prevent pneumonia. Stroke 2006; 37(3):765.

78 Hinchey JA et al. Formal dysphagia screening protocols prevent pneumonia. Stroke 2005; 36(9):1972–1976.

79 The National Institute of Neurological Disorders and Stroke rt-PA Stroke Study Group. Tissue plasminogen activator for acute ischemic stroke. N Engl J Med 1995; 333(24):1581–1587.

80 Clark WM et al. Recombinant tissue-type plasminogen activator (Alteplase) for ischemic stroke 3 to 5 hours after symptom onset. The ATLANTIS Study: A randomized controlled trial. Alteplase Thrombolysis for Acute Noninterventional Therapy in Ischemic Stroke. JAMA 1999; 282(21):2019–2026.

81 Del Zoppo GJ et al. Expansion of the time window for treatment of acute ischemic stroke with intravenous tissue plasminogen activator: A Science Advisory from the American Heart Association/American Stroke Association. Stroke 2009; 40(8):2945–2948.

82 Hacke W et al. Thrombolysis with alteplase 3 to 4.5 hours after acute ischemic stroke. N Engl J Med 2008; 359(13):1317–1329.

83 Wahlgren N et al. Thrombolysis with alteplase for acute ischaemic stroke in the Safe Implementation of Thrombolysis in Stroke-Monitoring Study (SITS-MOST): An observational study. Lancet 2007; 369(9558):275–282.

84 Smith WS et al. Safety and efficacy of mechanical embolectomy in acute ischemic stroke: Results of the MERCI trial. Stroke 2005; 36(7):1432–1438.

85 Smith WS et al. Mechanical thrombectomy for acute ischemic stroke: Final results of the Multi MERCI trial. Stroke 2008; 39(4):1205–1212.

86 Groschel K et al. A systematic review on outcome after stenting for intracranial atherosclerosis. Stroke 2009; 40(5):e340–e347.

87 IMS II Trial Investigators. The Interventional Management of Stroke (IMS) II Study. Stroke 2007; 38(7):2127–2135.

88 International Stroke Trial Collaborative Group. The International Stroke Trial (IST): A randomised trial of aspirin, subcutaneous heparin, both, or neither among 19435 patients with acute ischaemic stroke. Lancet 1997; 349(9065):1569–1581.

89 CAST (Chinese Acute Stroke Trial) Collaborative Group. CAST: Randomised placebo-controlled trial of early aspirin use in 20,000 patients with acute ischaemic stroke. Lancet 1997; 349(9066):1641–1649.

90 Sandercock PA et al. Antiplatelet therapy for acute ischaemic stroke. Cochrane Database Syst Rev 2008(3):CD000029.

91 Gubitz G, Sandercock P, Counsell C. Anticoagulants for acute ischaemic stroke. Cochrane Database Syst Rev 2004(3):CD000024.

92 Chandratheva A et al. Population-based study of risk and predictors of stroke in the first few hours after a TIA. Neurology 2009; 72(22):1941–1947.

93 Johnston SC et al. Validation and refinement of scores to predict very early stroke risk after transient ischaemic attack. Lancet 2007; 369(9558):283–292.

94 Amarenco P et al. Does ABCD2 score below 4 allow more time to evaluate patients with a transient ischemic attack? Stroke 2009; 40(9):3091–3095.

95 Bousser MG et al. "AICLA" controlled trial of aspirin and dipyridamole in the secondary prevention of athero-thrombotic cerebral ischemia. Stroke 1983; 14(1):5–14.

96 The Canadian Cooperative Study Group. A randomized trial of aspirin and sulfinpyrazone in threatened stroke. N Engl J Med 1978; 299(2):53–59.

97 Diener HC et al. European Stroke Prevention Study. 2: Dipyridamole and acetylsalicylic acid in the secondary prevention of stroke. J Neurol Sci 1996; 143(1–2):1–13.

98 The ESPS Group. The European Stroke Prevention Study (ESPS). Principal end-points. Lancet 1987; 2(8572):1351–1354.

99 Diener HC et al. Effects of aspirin plus extended-release dipyridamole versus clopidogrel and telmisartan on disability and cognitive function after recurrent stroke in patients with ischaemic stroke in the Prevention Regimen for Effectively Avoiding Second Strokes (PRoFESS) trial: A double-blind, active and placebo-controlled study. Lancet Neurol 2008; 7(10):875–884.

100 CAPRIE Steering Committee. A randomised, blinded, trial of clopidogrel versus aspirin in patients at risk of ischaemic events (CAPRIE). Lancet 1996; 348(9038):1329–1339.

101 Diener HC et al. Aspirin and clopidogrel compared with clopidogrel alone after recent ischaemic stroke or transient ischaemic attack in high-risk patients (MATCH): Randomised, double-blind, placebo-controlled trial. Lancet 2004; 364(9431):331–337.

102 Theis JG, Deichsel G, Marshall S. Rapid development of tolerance to dipyridamole-associated headaches. Br J Clin Pharmacol 1999; 48(5):750–755.

103 Wong DK, Lurie F, Wong LL. The effects of clopidogrel on elderly traumatic brain injured patients. J Trauma 2008; 65(6):1303–1308.

104 Sacco RL et al. Comparison of warfarin versus aspirin for the prevention of recurrent stroke or death: Subgroup analyses from the Warfarin-Aspirin Recurrent Stroke Study. Cerebrovasc Dis 2006; 22(1):4–12.

105 North American Symptomatic Carotid Endarterectomy Trial Collaborators. Beneficial effect of carotid endarterectomy in symptomatic patients with high-grade carotid stenosis. N Engl J Med 1991; 325(7):445–453.

106 European Carotid Surgery Trialists' Collaborative Group. MRC European Carotid Surgery Trial: Iinterim results for symptomatic patients with severe (70–99%) or with mild (0–29%) carotid stenosis. Lancet 1991; 337(8752):1235–1243.

107 Chaturvedi S et al. Carotid endarterectomy – an evidence-based review: Report of the Therapeutics and Technology Assessment Subcommittee of the American Academy of Neurology. Neurology 2005; 65(6):794–801.

108 Liapis CD et al. ESVS guidelines. Invasive treatment for carotid stenosis: Indications, techniques. Eur J Vasc Endovasc Surg 2009; 37(4 Suppl):1–19.

109 Fode NC et al. Multicenter retrospective review of results and complications of carotid endarterectomy in 1981. Stroke 1986; 17(3):370–376.

110 Brott T, Thalinger K. The practice of carotid endarterectomy in a large metropolitan area. Stroke 1984; 15(6):950–955.

111 Gurm HS et al. Long-term results of carotid stenting versus endarterectomy in high-risk patients. N Engl J Med 2008; 358(15):1572–1579.

112 Eckstein HH et al. Results of the Stent-Protected Angioplasty versus Carotid Endarterectomy (SPACE) study to treat symptomatic stenoses at 2 years: A multinational, prospective, randomised trial. Lancet Neurol 2008; 7(10):893–902.

113 Gates PC et al. Symptomatic and asymptomatic carotid stenosis: Just when we thought we had all the answers. Intern Med J 2006; 36(7):445–451.

114 Wacher K. Carotid endartercectomy deemed safer than stenting. World Neurology 2010; 25(1):15.

115 Meier P, Knapp G, Tamhane V et al. Short-term and intermediate-term comparison of endarterectomy versus stenting for carotid artery stenosis: Systematic review and meta-analysis of randomised controlled clinical trials. BMJ 2010; 340:c467.
116 Norris JW, Halliday A. Carotid artery stenosis: Carotid artery stenting is not yet ready to replace endarterectomy. BMJ 2010; 340:c748.
117 Wijdicks EF et al. The dilemma of discontinuation of anticoagulation therapy for patients with intracranial hemorrhage and mechanical heart valves. Neurosurgery 1998; 42(4):769–773.
118 Ananthasubramaniam K et al. How safely and for how long can warfarin therapy be withheld in prosthetic heart valve patients hospitalized with a major hemorrhage? Chest 2001; 119(2):478–484.
119 Bertram M et al. Managing the therapeutic dilemma: Patients with spontaneous intracerebral hemorrhage and urgent need for anticoagulation. J Neurol 2000; 247(3):209–214.

Common Neck, Arm and Upper Back Problems

Neck and arm pain and sensory disturbance with or without weakness in the arm are very common complaints. This chapter will discuss the more frequently encountered peripheral nervous system (lower motor neuron)[1] problems and the non-neurological conditions seen in everyday clinical practice. It will emphasise those features that help differentiate one problem from another. The chapter will be divided into three sections reflecting the regions of complaints most often seen in clinical practice:

1 the neck
2 the shoulder and upper arm
3 the forearm and hand.

A few very rare conditions (including suprascapular nerve entrapment, thoracic outlet syndrome, radial tunnel syndrome or posterior interosseous nerve entrapment and complex regional pain syndrome) are discussed because a delay in diagnosis may result in long-term disability.

Essentially there are *only four neurological symptoms* that can develop in a limb:

1 pain
2 weakness (with or without wasting)
3 altered sensation
4 incoordination.

When a patient presents complaining of problems in the arm, for example, the important thing to establish is whether the symptoms relate to a non-neurological or a neurological problem and whether, if the latter, it is a peripheral ('lower motor neuron') or central ('upper motor neuron') problem. Remember the peripheral nervous system in the upper limb consists of the anterior horn cell in the spinal cord, the motor and sensory nerve roots, brachial plexus, peripheral nerves, neuromuscular junctions and muscle. A central nervous system problem is anything above the level of the anterior horn cell, i.e. in the spinal cord, brainstem, deep cerebral hemisphere or cortex (see Figure 1.1). The pattern of weakness and sensory disturbance together with the reflexes will help determine whether the problem is central or peripheral. Finally, it is important to establish whether the symptoms are intermittent or persistent as different conditions present with either paroxysmal or persistent symptoms. Pain in the arm is only occasionally related to the nervous system but, when it is, it almost invariably indicates a problem in the peripheral nervous system as central causes of pain are very rare.

---

1 See Chapters 1 and 3 for a discussion of upper versus lower motor neuron problems.

Symptoms arising from peripheral nerve lesions can arise as a result of three mechanisms:

- direct trauma, in which case the neurological symptoms will be present from the moment of trauma
- compression of the nerve (referred to as entrapment syndromes), in which case the symptoms will be persistent and, as the compression worsens, the severity of the symptoms (in terms of intensity and the extent of involvement of the muscles or area of sensation supplied by the particular nerve or nerve root) will increase
- irritation, which is also seen with entrapment syndromes, where the symptoms are initially intermittent and often provoked by certain activities; with repeated and prolonged irritation damage may result in persistent weakness and/or sensory loss.

- Most patients with pain in the arm have a non-neurological problem.
- Although there are rare central nervous system causes of pain, the great majority of patients with neurological symptoms in the arm associated with pain will have a problem in the peripheral nervous system.

NECK PAIN

Although pain in the neck is common, symptoms arising in the neck are often poorly localised and a precise diagnosis is not always possible.

Acute spasm of the neck muscles

One of the more common causes of neck pain is acute spasm of the neck muscles. The exact cause of the spasm is uncertain but it appears to be related to bad posture. Patients often awake with severe neck pain, with the neck twisted to one side, and pain that is aggravated by attempts to turn the head.

The most common form is *torticollis*, often referred to as a '*wry neck*'. It is a self-limiting condition, resolving within days. More severe and disabling but very rare forms of congenital and acquired spasmodic torticollis occur [1] but are beyond the scope of this book.

Non-specific neck pain

A number of patients are encountered with *non-specific neck pain* in the centre and/or to the side of the neck that is constant and present most days but fluctuates in severity. The pain is usually bilateral, often associated with stiffness in the neck, and is aggravated by neck movement. There are no associated neurological symptoms in the limbs and no sensory symptoms in the neck to suggest the pain is of radicular origin. Occasionally, the pain radiates to the base of the skull. The trapezius and sternocleidomastoid muscles are often tense and tender to palpate, but the relationship of this finding to the neck discomfort is not clear.

The aetiology of this entity is uncertain but it is often encountered in patients with psychological problems such as anxiety or depression [2].

Whiplash

Another common cause of neck pain is *whiplash*. This is a syndrome that follows sudden flexion and extension of the neck and is often the result of motor vehicle collisions. A variety of symptoms develop and not all patients experience all symptoms.

- Within the hours to first day or up to a few days after whiplash injury the patient complains of neck pain and stiffness, with or without a decreased a range of motion of the neck. Tenderness on palpation of the neck muscles and even the spinal processes is common. The pain may radiate into the shoulders or down the spine to the thoracic region.

- Headache frequently occurs together with insomnia, complaints of poor memory and difficulty concentrating [3].
- A small percentage of patients will develop non-specific and diffuse arm pain with or without subjective weakness and/or sensory symptoms in the arm that are clearly beyond the distribution of a single nerve or nerve root and are not related to nerve root compression. The pain and neurological symptoms in the arm, unlike cervical nerve root compression, are often aggravated by movement of both the arm and the neck while nerve root compression may be aggravated by movement of the neck but not the arm.
- Imaging is usually normal although in older patients degenerative disease may be seen and is often incorrectly invoked as the cause of the symptoms.
- The duration of symptoms varies from a few weeks to months or even years (the late whiplash syndrome, a controversial entity [4]), although 90–95% of patients experience only pain that settles within weeks.

The aetiology of whiplash is unknown and, curiously, it is not seen at all in Lithuania where there is little awareness of the syndrome and no accident compensation scheme [5, 6].

Cervical spondylosis

Cervical spondylosis (degenerative changes) in the cervical spine is very common and is often asymptomatic, particularly in the elderly. Thus, although neck pain aggravated by neck movement may occur, it is important to consider the possibility that the *neck pain may not relate to the spondylosis* and other possible causes should be considered. On the other hand, if neck pain is aggravated by movement of the neck and is associated with pain radiating into the shoulder or arm in a radicular distribution, particularly if associated with weakness and/or sensory disturbance in the limb, it is likely to be related to cervical spondylitic **radiculopathy**.

MANAGEMENT of NECK INJURIES RESULTING IN WHIPLASH SYNDROME

This section discusses the management of minor neck injuries that result in the whiplash syndrome, not the initial assessment of patients with trauma in whom serious underlying cervical spine injuries could be present. The Canadian C-spine rule [8] is currently recommended for the acute assessment of the latter patients.

Imaging is not justified in patients with mild symptoms or those under the age of 65 [3]. In more severe cases plain X-rays, CT or MRI scans are often performed but rarely demonstrate any abnormality. Most patients with mild pain can be reassured and advised to lead a normal life without restrictions [3].

With more severe pain a period of abstinence from intense training and sporting activities is recommended. Simple analgesia or a non-steroidal anti-inflammatory drug (NSAID) can be prescribed. In patients with severe pain it is important to advise them that recovery is very likely to occur but may take months and, in these cases, lifestyle including work is often restricted.

The role of physical therapy is controversial. The Bone and Joint Decade 2000–2010 Task Force on Neck Pain and its Associated Disorders concluded that 'best evidence suggests that therapies involving manual therapy and exercise are more effective than alternative strategies for patients with neck pain' [9].

Management of cervical nerve root compression is discussed in the section 'Pain with or without focal neurological symptoms in the shoulder and upper arm' in this chapter.

Cervical radiculopathy

Cervical radiculopathy arising from the 3rd and 4th cervical nerve roots is very rare. *Unilateral pain* in the suboccipital region, extending to the back of the ear, and in the dorsal or lateral aspect of the neck occurs with radiculopathy of the 3rd cervical nerve root. C4 radiculopathy results in *unilateral pain* that may radiate to the posterior neck and trapezius region and to the anterior chest but does not typically radiate into the upper extremity [7]. Neither is associated with any discernible weakness although neurological symptoms may occur with sensory symptoms in the distribution of the C3 or C4 nerve root and, in the *very rare* occurrence when a radiculopathy is associated with spinal cord compression, an upper motor neuron pattern of weakness in all four or just the lower limbs with or without sensory symptoms and a possible sensory level may result. The term 'sensory level' refers to the level within the central nervous system that the spinothalamic dermatomal sensory loss extends up to on the trunk or in the limbs.

PROBLEMS AROUND THE SHOULDER AND UPPER ARM

This section discusses common neurological and non-neurological conditions affecting the shoulder and upper arm that can result in pain with or without focal neurological symptoms or focal neurological symptoms in the absence of pain.

Pain with or without focal neurological symptoms in the shoulder and upper arm

There are a number of conditions, both neurological and non-neurological, that can cause pain in and around the shoulder. These include:
* nerve root compression of the 4th, 5th and 6th cervical nerve roots
* brachial neuritis
* suprascapular nerve entrapment syndrome
* arthritis of the shoulder joint
* adhesive capsulitis
* bursitis
* rotator cuff pathology.

Pain in the shoulder and upper arm most often relates to diseases of the joints, ligaments or bones where pain occurs in the absence of neurological symptoms and is aggravated by movement of the affected joint or there is localised tenderness at the site of the pain. The presence of joint swelling and/or tenderness is another clue that the pain is not of neurological origin.

Figure 11.1 lists the common causes of pain in the region of the shoulder.

NEUROLOGICAL CAUSES

Radicular pain

Pain from nerve root compression, if associated with weakness and/or sensory disturbance in the distribution of the nerve root, is readily diagnosed. However, pain may occur in the absence of or precede neurological symptoms by days or even weeks. Although radicular pain may affect the upper (C4–C5) arm, it is more common in the lower (C6–8) arm.

Numbness and/or localised shoulder pain not influenced by movement of the shoulder suggests a possible C5 nerve root problem. Where neurological symptoms and signs develop, the numbness is located over the top of the shoulder along its mid-portion and

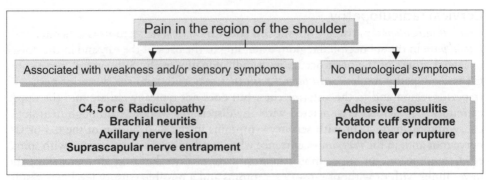

FIGURE 11.1   Painful conditions affecting the shoulder region

extends laterally to the upper arm but not into the forearm. There may be weakness of the supraspinatus, infraspinatus and deltoid muscles [7].

Brachial neuritis or neuralgic amyotrophy

The diagnosis should be suspected when *severe shoulder pain aggravated by movement of the shoulder is associated with weakness and sensory disturbance in the arm.* Van Alfen et al [10] have described the clinical details in a large series of patients. As there is no 'gold standard' diagnostic test for brachial neuritis, the clinical features of neuralgic **amyotrophy** are likely to evolve.

SYMPTOMS

The classic symptoms begin with the subacute onset over weeks of increasingly severe constant unilateral pain predominantly in the shoulder girdle; less commonly, the pain may come on rapidly. Rarely, bilateral cases occur but one side is usually affected for some hours or up to 2 days before the other side is involved [11]. This con-

- Ascertain whether the arm pain is aggravated by movement of the arm, suggesting local pathology in the arm, or aggravated by movement of the neck, indicating possible referred pain from nerve root compression.
- Pain occurring simultaneously with neurological symptoms is very likely to be related to a neurological cause. The pain may not be neurological in origin when it occurs in the absence of neurological symptoms.
- If testing the strength of muscles around a joint evokes marked pain, this may cause the patient not to exert a full effort and give the incorrect impression that there may be associated weakness when it is the pain that is limiting the effort, not the weakness.

stant pain persists on average for approximately 3–4 weeks but may last as little as a few days or up to 60 days or more. In many patients it may be followed by a movement-evoked severe stabbing pain that can persist for months. In a small proportion of cases the pain can radiate from the shoulder to the arm, the cervical spine or neck down into the arm, the scapular or dorsal region to the chest wall and/or arm, or be confined to a lower plexus distribution (e.g. medial arm and/or hand, axilla).

The *shoulder pain is aggravated by movement of the shoulder, not the neck,* but here there are neurological symptoms such as weakness and sensory disturbance in the arm that indicate a neurological cause for the pain. Although local heat to the shoulder region occasionally provides some relief from the pain, this is non-specific and cannot be used in diagnosis. Individual nerves can be affected in brachial neuritis, in particular the suprascapular, axillary, musculocutaneous, long thoracic and radial nerves [11].

Progressive weakness developing over days may commence within 24 hours after the onset of the pain or may be delayed for up to 4 weeks [11]. Although any part of the plexus can be involved, the upper brachial plexus is more commonly affected in males whereas the middle and lower brachial plexus is more commonly affected in females. Wasting may occur with prolonged symptoms. Recovery can take months or even years. Sensory involvement is common and sensory symptoms can be very diffuse and non-localising.

Recurrence is rare but can occur and familial cases, termed hereditary neuralgic amyotrophy, have been described. Hereditary neuropathy with pressure palsy can also cause neuralgic amyotrophy and is related to a defect in the peripheral myelin protein 22 and is regarded as a distinct disorder [12].

Axillary nerve lesion

Axillary nerve lesions are usually related to traumatic dislocation of the shoulder joint as a result of either a sporting injury or secondary to a tonic–clonic seizure. Less commonly they occur with a fracture of the neck of the humerus or following shoulder surgery. As with all single nerve (mononeuritis) lesions, some are idiopathic (unknown cause).

EXAMINATION

There is weakness of shoulder abduction beyond the first 30° (the initial 30° is supplied by the supraspinatus muscle) due to weakness of the deltoid muscle (see Figure 11.2). There may be a small patch of numbness over the lower aspect of the deltoid muscle. When the lesion relates to dislocation, there is often pain in the shoulder aggravated by movement of the shoulder. The presence of pain and weakness with a history of

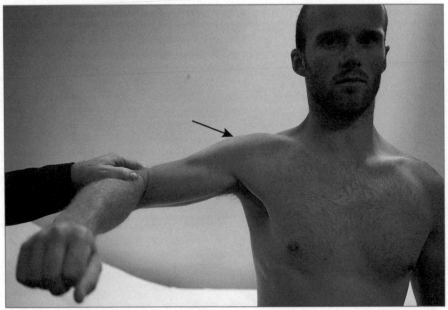

FIGURE 11.2 Testing the deltoid muscle (the arrow points to the deltoid muscle/ axillary nerve)

trauma to the shoulder is a strong pointer to the diagnosis. The prognosis for recovery is variable [13].

Suprascapular nerve entrapment

The suprascapular nerve arises from the junction of the 5th and 6th cervical nerve roots and traverses an oblique course across the supraspinatus fossa, relatively fixed on the floor of the fossa and tethered underneath the transverse scapular ligament, to the scapular notch and supplies the supraspinatus and infraspinatus muscles. Most often the suprascapular entrapment syndrome relates to local compression by the suprascapular ligament although it may be idiopathic in origin or due to rarer causes [14]. Although very rare, it is a diagnosis not to be missed as prompt treatment is more likely to result in resolution of the problem.

SYMPTOMS

The pain is deep and diffuse, localised to the posterior and lateral aspects of the shoulder and may be referred into the arm, neck or upper anterior chest wall. Certain scapular motions may be painful, causing the patient to restict shoulder movement. Adduction of the arm across the body tenses the nerve and may increase the pain. Occasionally, the patient may complain of burning, aching or crushing pain.

EXAMINATION

It is important to test the supraspinatus and infraspinatus muscles, looking for weakness confined to those muscles. Remember, pain may give the appearance of weakness with the patient not exerting a full effort as a result of the pain. The clue that the weakness relates to pain from the shoulder is that, in addition to the supraspinatus and infraspinatus appearing weak, the deltoid and subscapularis muscles will also appear weak. Severe suprascapular nerve entrapment results in atrophy and permanent weakness of the supraspinatus and infraspinatus muscles (see Figure 11.3).

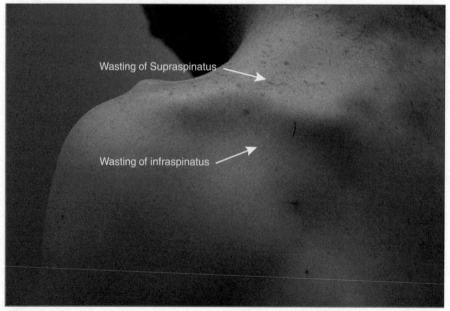

FIGURE 11.3   Suprascapular entrapment with marked wasting of the supraspinatus and infraspinatus muscles

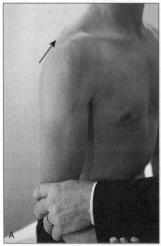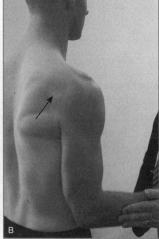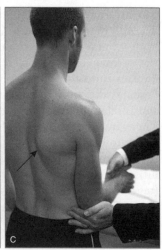

FIGURE 11.4 **A** Method of testing the supraspinatus. The arm is abducted approximately 20–30° away from the chest wall while the examiner pushes on the elbow, trying to force the arm back against the chest wall.
B Method of testing the infraspinatus. The elbow is kept next to the chest wall and the semi-flexed forearm is externally rotated against resistance.
C Method of testing the subscapularis. The arm is bent at a right angle at the elbow and the forearm is semi-pronated. The elbow is kept at the side and the patient is asked to rotate the forearm in towards the body while the examiner tries to prevent this by pushing the forearm in the opposite direction.

TREATMENT of SUPRASCAPULAR NERVE ENTRAPMENT

Confirmation of the diagnosis depends on the electromyogram. Some authorities [15] feel that a normal result of an electromyogram is consistent with the diagnosis of suprascapular nerve entrapment, whereas others [16] think that a positive result of an electromyogram is essential in confirming the diagnosis. The diagnostic finding is a prolonged latency from stimulation at **Erb's point** to the recording needle in either the supraspinatus or infraspinatus muscle. Treatment is surgical decompression [14].

NON-NEUROLOGICAL CAUSES OF SHOULDER PAIN

The following section may seem out of place but neurologists are frequently asked to see patients with pain of non-neurological origin when the patient would more appropriately be referred to a rheumatologist or orthopaedic surgeon. It is hoped that a detail discussion will aid the non-neurologist to sort out the neurological and non-neurological causes of pain.

> Pain that radiates past the elbow to the hand is usually not related to shoulder pathology.
> Ascertain whether the arm pain is aggravated by:
> - movement of the arm, suggesting local pathology in the arm
> - movement of the neck, indicating possible referred pain from nerve root compression.

Adhesive capsulitis

Adhesive capsulitis or the 'frozen shoulder' results in a gradual onset of pain and stiffness that leads to a restricted range of movement at the shoulder joint. It is usually seen in patients over the age of 40. A normal range of movement of the shoulder is incompatible with the diagnosis and X-rays are usually normal. The aetiology of this condition is unclear but it is not uncommon in the setting of a hemiplegia.

Rotator cuff syndrome

Probably the commonest cause of pain affecting the shoulder joint is non-neurological and is related to rotator cuff syndrome, also referred to as impingement syndrome. There are four tendons in the rotator cuff and these tendons are related individually to the following muscles: teres minor, subscapularis, infraspinatus and supraspinatus. The rotator cuff is compressed against the acromium causing bursitis, tendinitis and eventually a rotator cuff tear. Partial or complete tears or inflammation (tendinitis, tendinosis, calcific tendinitis) associated with rotator cuff injury occur in the region near where these tendon/muscle complexes attach to the humerus [17]. Other causes of pain in the shoulder joint include adhesive capsulitis and arthritis.

SYMPTOMS

Symptoms are generally those of pain, initially after and then during activity. The pain can often be relieved by rest. Patients over 40 years of age are more susceptible to rotator cuff tendinosis with overuse. In this age group the most prominent complaint is pain with overhead use and athletic activities. Night pain and an inability to lie on that side are also common [17]. Although the pain may radiate into the arm and the neck it is clearly related to movement of the shoulder and not the neck, indicating local shoulder pathology and not radicular pain. Pain in the shoulder between 60° and 180° of elevation is typical of a rotator cuff problem and is termed the painful arc syndrome (see Figure 11.5).

MANAGEMENT of ROTATOR CUFF SYNDROME

Plain X-rays can be helpful to diagnose calcific tendinitis, acromial spur, humeral head cysts or superior migration of the humeral head, but in most cases are typically normal. Arthrography, ultrasound, CT and MRI are the definitive tests in the diagnosis of rotator cuff injury. Arthrography and ultrasound of the shoulder can help determine whether or not there is a full tear in the rotator cuff. An MRI can detect a full or partial tear, chronic tendinosis or other cause of the shoulder pain [18].

- Physiotherapy is superior to NSAIDs alone [19]. Physical therapy in the form of stretching exercises will lead to improvement in the majority of patients but the pain may take several months to subside [20].
- Subacromial corticosteroid injections are recommended for non-responders [21]; however, these injections are difficult to give and the needle is not always placed accurately [22]. Corticosteroid injections may, however, increase the subsequent risk of tendon rupture and repeated injections are associated with a higher failure rate for surgical repair of ruptured tendons [23]. Corticosteroid injection is the preferred and definitive treatment for trochanteric bursitis [24].
- Surgery is recommended for patients who fail to respond to non-surgical measures after 3 months. Subacromial decompression has been recommended for the impingement syndrome but has not been shown in randomised trials to be more beneficial than physical therapy [25, 26]. Surgical repair of rotator cuff tears can result in less pain and increased strength and movement but recovery can take up to 6 months [27].

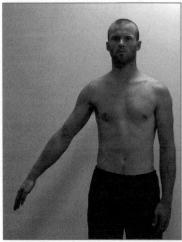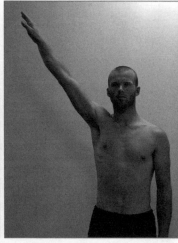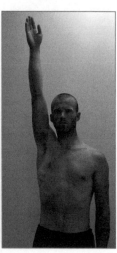

FIGURE 11.5 Testing of the painful arc and the impingement test

Painless weakness affecting the shoulder region and upper arm

The two conditions that cause painless weakness around the shoulder and upper arm are nerve root compression and winging of the scapula. Rarely, axillary nerve palsy can result in painless weakness of the deltoid muscle.

CERVICAL NERVE ROOT COMPRESSION

Cervical nerve root compression more commonly affects the lower cervical nerve roots (C7–T1), but rarely compression of the C5 and/or C6 nerve root or an upper cord brachial plexus problem [28] can result in painless weakness in the shoulder and upper arm region [29, 30]. The weakness will affect all C5 and C6 innervated muscles around the shoulder: supraspinatus, infraspinatus, subscapularis, deltoid, biceps and brachialis. If C6 is the major component, brachioradialis will also be weak. In general, a radiculopathy is more likely to be associated with pain.

WINGING OF THE SCAPULA

Most patients with a mononeuritis of the long thoracic nerve to the serratus anterior muscle are not aware of the problem until someone points out that their shoulder blade is protruding (see Figure 11.6). Occasional patients notice difficulty reaching up to high places with the affected arm with or without mild shoulder pain [31]. Most patients recover spontaneously but this may take up to 2 years.

Examination

This test is performed by having the patient's arm horizontal to the floor and pushing against the examiner's hand while the examiner looks to see if the scapular comes off the chest wall, indicating weakness of the serratus anterior muscle.

Painless numbness affecting the shoulder and upper arm

Sensation over the lower aspect of the neck, shoulder and upper arm is supplied via the 3rd to 5th cervical nerve roots. As degenerative disease predominantly affects the lower aspect of the cervical spine (C6, C7, C8 and T1), it is uncommon to see isolated sensory loss in the distribution of these nerve roots. If it does occur the sensory loss will be in a dermatome pattern as shown in Figures 1.12 and 1.13.

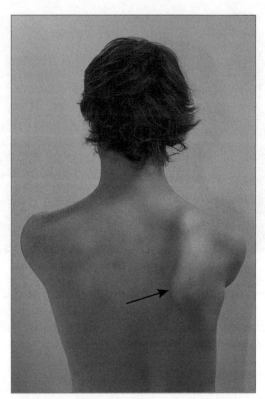

FIGURE 11.6   Winging of the scapula due to weakness of the serratus anterior muscle

PROBLEMS IN THE FOREARMS AND HANDS
Numbness in the hand, forearm or both
The commonest problems are carpal tunnel syndrome (CTS) at the wrist and an ulnar nerve lesion at the elbow (tardy ulnar palsy). Median nerve lesions are sometimes confused with a C6 radiculopathy and an ulnar nerve lesion may be confused with a C8–T1 radiculopathy or a lower cord brachial plexus lesion.

CARPAL TUNNEL SYNDROME
Carpal tunnel syndrome is one of the most common neurological conditions encountered in clinical practice. The annual incidence is approximately 3–4 per 1000 patients. It is more common during pregnancy and may resolve spontaneously after delivery. It is also more common in patients who gain excessive weight and may resolve with weight loss. It is important to exclude hypothyroidism. There is a high incidence of CTS in patients with diabetes, although it is rarely the presenting symptom of that diagnosis.

Symptoms
Carpal tunnel syndrome presents in two ways.
1 In most patients the symptoms arise as a result of irritation and compression of the median nerve at the wrist by the flexor retinaculum of the carpal tunnel. Patients experience paraesthesia (numbness, pins and needles or tingling) or dysaesthesia (an unpleasant sensation). The sensory branches of the median nerve innervate the lateral 3½ digits, but many patients find it difficult to localise the sensory symptoms and

often describe sensory disturbance well beyond the lateral 3½ digits [32]. The duration of altered sensation varies from a few minutes up to 30 minutes or rarely longer.

2 A second presentation is usually encountered in older patients who present with either persistent altered sensation within the median nerve distribution in the hand or marked wasting of the thenar eminence (the muscles at the base of the thumb), with little in the way of nocturnal sensory symptoms.

The characteristic and almost pathognomonic (diagnostic for a particular disease) complaint is waking in the middle of the night or in the morning with altered sensation in one or particularly both hands (other than CTS little else causes paroxysmal numbness in both hands simultaneously) that is relieved by shaking, moving or hanging the arm and hand out of the side of the bed. Other activities that may precipitate the symptoms include driving, knitting, reading, mowing the lawn or using hand tools.

Some patients complain of pain in the hand and at times up the arm even as far as the shoulder [33]. If the pain occurs only when the patient is experiencing sensory symptoms, it is reasonable to accept that the pain may be related to CTS. On the other hand, if the patient experiences pain at times when there are no sensory symptoms, this pain is less likely to be related to CTS and the patient may have two conditions, e.g. arthritis or occupational overuse syndrome. Patients should be advised that this pain may not be due to CTS and therefore may not resolve with appropriate treatment of CTS. The presence of pain, swelling and tenderness is not typical of CTS and suggests that either the CTS is secondary to the development of rheumatoid arthritis or the patient is not suffering from CTS.

Examination

In young patients there is usually no wasting or sensory loss, and the only abnormalities that may be found are a positive Tinel's and/or Phalen's sign (see Figure 11.7A–C). Tinel's sign[2] is the precipitation of a fleeting pain or sensory symptoms radiating into the palm and fingers when the median nerve is tapped at the wrist. Phalen's sign [35] is the presence of altered sensation in some or all of the lateral 3½ digits precipitated by forced flexion of the wrist. The wrist may need to be flexed for up to 60 seconds. Occasionally, patients with a negative Phalen's sign may develop the sensory symptoms when the wrists are extended.

The sensitivity of clinical examination by a neurologist for the diagnosis of this syndrome is 84% with a specificity of 72%. The sensitivity and specificity of Tinel's sign were 0.60 and 0.67, respectively, and of Phalen's sign were 0.75 and 0.47, respectively [36].

The electrophysiological diagnosis is discussed in Appendix H, 'Nerve conduction studies and electromyography'.

CARPAL TUNNEL SYNDROME VERSUS C6 RADICULOPATHY

Carpal tunnel syndrome is far more common than a C6 radiculopathy. Both may result in paraesthesia affecting the lateral aspect of the hand and both may result in pain in the hand and arm, although pain radiating down the arm is more in keeping with a C6 radiculopathy. Figure 11.8 highlights the difference between these two entities.

ULNAR NERVE LESIONS

Ulnar nerve lesions at the elbow present with *unilateral* symptoms (bilateral cases are extremely rare). Intermittent symptoms can occur if the patient leans the elbow on a desk or the arm of a chair. Isolated sensory symptoms may precede weakness for

---

2 Tinel described a tingling sensation when the proximal stump of an injured nerve was tapped [34].

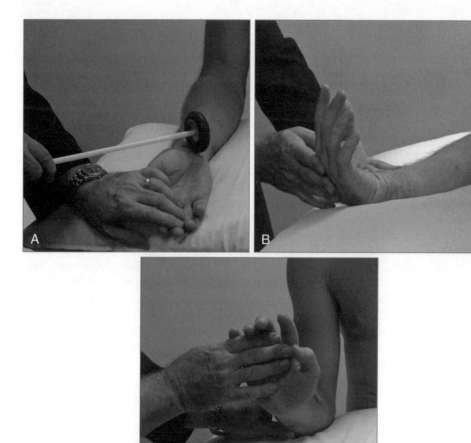

FIGURE 11.7 **A** Tinel's sign. The median nerve is tapped using the tendon hammer several times from the proximal portion of the hand across the wrist for 2–3 cm. **B, C** Phalen's sign. The classic description is that the wrist is flexed (B) for up to 60 seconds and, if positive, the patient will experience transient altered sensation in the fingers and hand within the distribution of the median nerve. Some patients do not experience paraesthesia in the hands with wrist flexion but may with wrist extension (**C**).

months or even years but this is unusual. The more common presentation is the gradual onset of numbness and/or pins and needles affecting the medial 1½ digits and the medial aspect of the hand on both the palmar and dorsal surfaces. Pins and needles or numbness is the initial symptom in most patients with ongoing compression weakness and eventually wasting of the hypothenar eminence

- Abnormalities consistent with the diagnosis of CTS demonstrated on nerve conduction studies (NCS) do not imply that some or all of the patient's symptoms are related to CTS. Asymptomatic median nerve compression detected by NCS is not uncommon.
- Normal NCS do not exclude a mild CTS.

(base of the 4th and 5th digits) and the interossei and medial two lumbricals (the small muscles between the digits). An ulnar nerve lesion at the elbow is sometimes referred to

THERAPEUTIC OPTIONS FOR TREATING CARPAL TUNNEL SYNDROME

If the symptoms are not too severe and the patient is tolerating them a conservative approach can be taken, and in some patients the symptoms will resolve, particularly after pregnancy or with weight loss.

- Splinting the wrists at night can provide symptomatic benefit [37]. In a randomised controlled trial surgery was better than splinting [38].
- Corticosteroid injection into the wrist is beneficial in some patients, although long-term benefit is unproven [39]. Repeat injections (8 weeks after the first) are of no value [40]. In an open randomised study surgical carpal tunnel release resulted in better symptomatic and neurophysiological outcome than corticosteroid injections [41] and was more cost effective [42].
- Surgery provides long-term benefit and is recommended in patients with more severe symptoms, regardless of the severity of the NCS abnormalities. Nocturnal or day time paraesthesiae resolve completely in more than 90% of patients [41]. Surgery is also recommended in patients with severe NCS abnormalities regardless of the severity of the symptoms. The results of surgery in elderly patients who present with permanent wasting and sensory disturbance with no sensory response on NCS are less favourable [43]. Some authors state that surgical carpal tunnel decompression has a significant failure rate [44]. This was based on a retrospective questionnaire where patients stated whether they were better, unchanged or worse after surgery. NCS can predict the response to surgery, with patients who have mid-range severity abnormalities having better results than those with either very severe or no abnormality [44]. Response to surgery has been assessed using the Global Symptom Score (GSS). This is a scoring system that rates symptoms on a scale of 0 (no symptoms) to 10 (severe) in five categories: pain, numbness, paraesthesia, weakness/clumsiness and nocturnal awakening. The sum of the scores in each category is the GSS [45].

Note: For an explanation of NCS, see Appendix H, 'Nerve conduction studies and electromyography'.

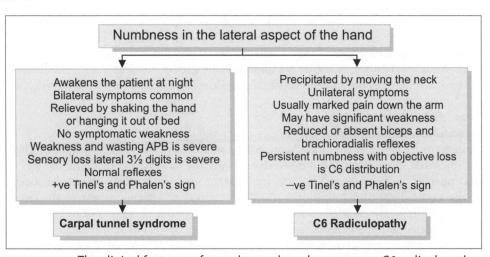

FIGURE 11.8 The clinical features of carpal tunnel syndrome versus C6 radiculopathy

as 'tardy ulnar palsy'. Compression of the ulnar nerve at the level of the wrist will affect the deep branch of the ulnar nerve and will not produce any sensory disturbance.

IDIOPATHIC SENSORY DISTURBANCE
A number of patients complain of intermittent paraesthesia, fluctuating in severity with variable intensity and distribution predominantly affecting the medial aspect of the forearm and hand. The paraesthesia is never associated with any weakness or objective loss of sensation and, despite extensive investigations, its cause cannot be established. The cause of this problem is unclear; it can mimic the symptoms of an ulnar nerve lesion, a lower cord brachial plexus problem or a C8–T1 radiculopathy.

Weakness with or without numbness in the hand and forearm
The commonest condition affecting the hand is CTS. Weakness is not usually a feature of CTS as it is only the abductor pollicus brevis muscle that is affected and patients are usually not aware of any weakness. Ulnar nerve lesions at the elbow and a C8–T1 radiculopathy produce almost identical symptoms and signs but there are subtle differences that enable a diagnosis at the bedside. Weakness of the extensor muscles of the wrist and hand can result from radial nerve lesions or a C7 radiculopathy and, once again, there are subtle differences that enable the diagnosis to be established at the bedside.

ULNAR NERVE LESIONS
Occasionally, patients with compression of the ulnar nerve at the elbow will present with progressive weakness in the hand with little in the way of sensory disturbance. Compression of the deep branch of the ulnar nerve at the wrist will result in weakness of the abductor digiti minimi (abduction of the little finger), the small interosseous muscles (abduction and adduction of the digits) and the 3rd and 4th lumbricals (flexion of the metacarpophalangeal joints). Sensory symptoms are absent.

ULNAR NERVE LESION AT THE ELBOW VERSUS C8–T1 RADICULOPATHY
Both conditions can present with a gradual onset of weakness of the hand associated with altered sensation affecting the medial two digits and the medial aspect of the forearm, although often with ulnar nerve lesions the numbness is confined to the fingers and hand. The hand weakness is usually more marked with a radiculopathy as more muscles used to grip objects are affected. In neither will there be any change in the reflexes. Figure 11.9 lists the differences between these two entities. Figures 11.10 and 11.11 show how to test the long flexors of the distal phalanges of the medial four digits. Very rarely, the lower cord of the brachial plexus may be affected, e.g. with a tumour in the apex of the lung, and in this situation the sympathetic ganglion may also be affected resulting in an ipsilateral Horner's syndrome.

Examination
A careful examination of *the pattern of weakness will differentiate these two entities*. With an ulnar nerve lesion at the elbow there will be weakness of the abductor digiti minimi, the interossei, the medial two lumbricals and only the long flexors (bending the tips of the fingers at the distal interphalangeal joint) of the medial two digits (the medial aspect of the flexor digitorum profundus). Both the medial and lateral aspect of the flexor digitorum profundus is affected with C8–T1 radiculopathy. A nerve root or lower cord brachial plexus lesion will result in weakness of the long flexors of the medial four digits.

The fingers are prevented from flexing at the proximal phalangeal joint (supplied by the median nerve to the flexor digitorum superficialis) and the examiner asks the patient

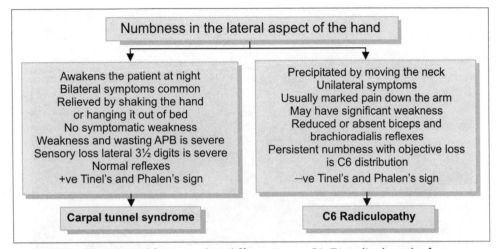

Numbness in the lateral aspect of the hand

Awakens the patient at night
Bilateral symptoms common
Relieved by shaking the hand
or hanging it out of bed
No symptomatic weakness
Weakness and wasting APB is severe
Sensory loss lateral 3½ digits is severe
Normal reflexes
+ve Tinel's and Phalen's sign

Precipitated by moving the neck
Unilateral symptoms
Usually marked pain down the arm
May have significant weakness
Reduced or absent biceps and
brachioradialis reflexes
Persistent numbness with objective loss
is C6 distribution
−ve Tinel's and Phalen's sign

Carpal tunnel syndrome

C6 Radiculopathy

FIGURE 11.9 The clinical features that differentiate a C8–T1 radiculopathy from an ulnar nerve lesion at the elbow

*A C8–T1 radiculopathy can be painless.

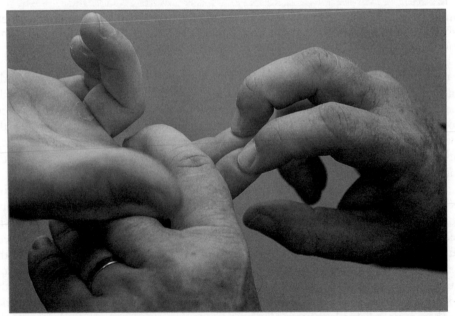

FIGURE 11.10 Testing the long flexors of the lateral two digits. The examiner's other hand is used to prevent the patient from flexing the fingers at the proximal interphalangeal joint by flexor digitorum superficialis that is supplied by the median nerve

to bend the tips of their fingers while the examiner attempts to straighten them. The lateral two (Figure 11.10) are supplied by the median nerve and the medial two (Figure 11.11) by the ulnar nerve.

THORACIC OUTLET SYNDROME

The reason for discussing thoracic outlet syndrome (TOS) [48] is that it is frequently suspected by non-neurologists in patients with paraesthesia affecting the medial aspect

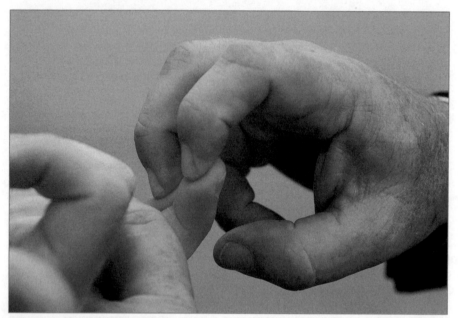

FIGURE 11.11 Testing the long flexors of the medial two digits. The examiner's other hand is used to prevent the patient from flexing the fingers at the proximal interphalangeal joint by flexor digitorum superficialis that is supplied by the median nerve

of the forearm and hand in the absence of an ulnar nerve lesion [49]. Thoracic outlet syndrome is a controversial entity. It can occur in children and young adults [50, 51]. There are three types: arterial, venous and neurogenic. Neurogenic TOS is the commonest but in itself is exceedingly rare. It relates to brachial plexus compression, usually from scarred scalene muscles secondary to neck trauma. Compression can also occur with a cervical rib; however, the absence of a cervical rib on X-ray does not exclude the diagnosis as compression may be due to a fibrous band.

The most frequent neurological symptom is aching pain in the side or back of the neck extending across the shoulder and down the arm. Tingling and numbness are common in the forearm and hand in the ulnar (C8–T1) distribution. Paraesthaesia in the medial forearm and hand is a common complaint (90%), with the little finger involved four times as often as the thumb. One clue to the diagnosis is the precipitation of the paraesthesia with overhead activity or carrying heavy objects [52]. Objective sensory loss is uncommon and muscle weakness and wasting are late signs; once they develop the prognosis for recovery is poor. Sensory signs can occur without weakness and vice versa.

There is no reliable laboratory diagnostic test to confirm or exclude the diagnosis. The presence of a cervical rib is not proof as this is a common incidental finding in asymptomatic individuals.

RADIAL NERVE PALSY (SATURDAY NIGHT PALSY)
The term 'Saturday night palsy' refers to the intoxicated patient who falls asleep in the chair and awakens with a wrist drop due to radial nerve compression in the radial groove of the humerus in the upper arm. The typical story is a patient awakening with a painless wrist drop with an inability to extend the wrist and fingers occasionally associated with mild sensory loss at the base of the first and second digits on the dorsal surface (see Figure 1.14).

Classical teaching has recommended a conservative approach with a wrist splint while the patient makes a complete recovery within days to weeks. *Alternative pathology should be considered in patients who present with radial nerve palsy but who have not 'slept on their arm'.* In two cases the author has seen alternate pathology was present. In the first, a fibrous band caused progressive weakness over several weeks and surgery led to a complete resolution. In the second, the radial nerve weakness was of sudden onset during the day and was due to torsion of the nerve. A delay in the diagnosis resulted in a poor outcome despite surgery.

Symptoms
- The patient will have weakness of the supinator (turning the forearm from the hand pointing to the ground to pointing to the ceiling), brachioradialis (flexing the elbow with the forearm semi-pronated) and the extensors of the wrist, fingers and thumb.
- The apparent weakness of the small muscles of the hand is due to the wrist drop. Strength in the adductor and abductor muscles of the fingers is normal when tested with the hand flat on a hard surface eliminating the wrist drop (see Figure 11.13F).
- The triceps reflex is preserved.
- The brachioradialis reflex is reduced or absent.
- The degree of weakness of wrist and finger extension is severe, resulting in the wrist drop.

RADIAL NERVE PALSY VERSUS A C7 RADICULOPATHY
Patients with a C7 radiculopathy may also present with weakness of wrist and finger extension but it is usually less severe and radicular arm pain is more prominent.

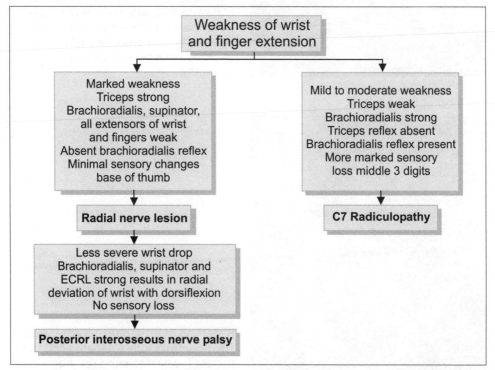

FIGURE 11.12 Differentiating between a C7 radiculopathy and a radial nerve lesion

Figure 11.12 lists the differences between a C7 radiculopathy and a radial nerve lesion. Figure 11.13 shows how to determine on clinical examination if it is a radial nerve palsy and how to test finger abduction when the finger and wrist extension are very weak.

RADIAL TUNNEL SYNDROME OR POSTERIOR INTEROSSEOUS NERVE ENTRAPMENT

Radial tunnel syndrome is an extremely rare cause of weakness affecting the extensor muscles of the wrist and hand. Once again, a delay in recognition is more likely to result in a poor outcome with treatment. It is due to a compressive neuropathy of the posterior interosseous nerve (a branch of the radial nerve). The posterior interosseous nerve is compressed in an aponeurotic (deep fascia attached to muscle) cleft in the supinator muscle.

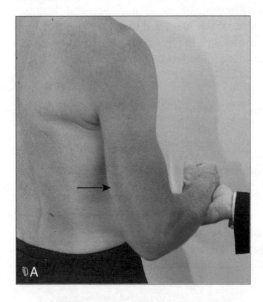

Figure 11.13
A Method of testing the triceps. Ask the patient to extend the elbow from 90° of flexion. It is important NOT to fully bend the elbow when testing the triceps as this will produce a false positive weakness of elbow extension (normal strength).

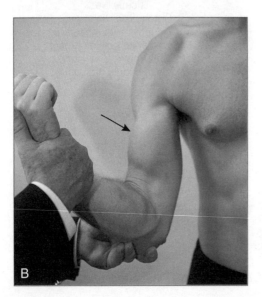

B Method of testing the biceps (arrow). The forearm is fully supinated and the patient is asked to bend the elbow (normal strength).

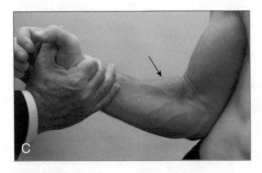

Figure 11.13—cont'd
C Method of testing the brachioradialis. The arm is semi-pronated and flexed at the elbow, and the patient is asked to bend the arm at the elbow (weak).

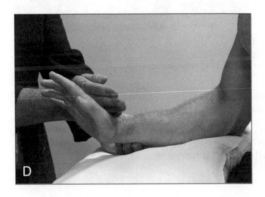

D Method of testing the extensor muscles of the wrist. The patient is asked to extend the wrist and the back of the examiner's hand is placed over the back of the patient's hand and both exert a full effort (weak).

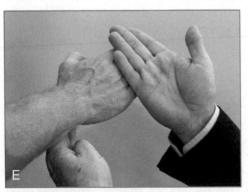

E Method of testing the extensor muscles of the fingers. The examiner places the metacarpophalangeal (MCP) joints across the patient's 5th digit, and the patient's MCP joints are placed across the examiner's 5th digit so that both the patient and the examiner are using the same muscles to test finger extension. Both should push as hard as possible. If the strength is normal, neither the patient nor the examiner can overcome finger extension. A common method used by many is pushing down on the extended fingers with the ulnar border of the hand, but it is hard to be sure how hard the examiner should push (weak).

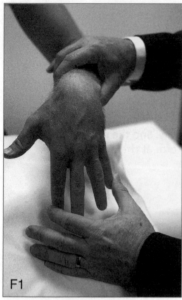
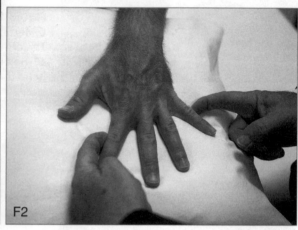

Figure 11.13—cont'd
F1, F2 Method of testing finger abduction and adduction in the presence of wrist drop. A wrist drop can give the false impression of weakness of the ulnar innervated muscles that abduct and adduct the fingers. Ask the patient to place the palm on a firm surface so that the fingers are touching the surface and then test adduction and abduction. The strength will be normal with a radial nerve lesion.

The pain of radial tunnel syndrome is similar to the pain of tennis elbow and is located 3–4 cm distal to the lateral epicondyle on the dorsal aspect of the forearm. With more prolonged compression, progressive weakness and wasting of the extensor muscles occurs (excluding the extensor carpi radialis, a muscle that deviates the wrist laterally with extension) in the absence of any sensory symptoms.

Pain in the forearm

Forearm pain is most often unrelated to any neurological cause but is more often due to lateral epicondylitis (tennis elbow), tenosynovitis or occupational overuse syndrome. If the pain is of neurological origin it is likely to be a C6, C7 or C8 radiculopathy. Although the ulnar and radial nerves innervate the muscles and skin of the forearm, lesions of these nerves rarely if ever cause pain.

TENNIS ELBOW OR LATERAL EPICONDYLITIS

Although referred to as tennis elbow, this condition is not confined to tennis players. It produces pain and tenderness over the lateral aspect of the elbow, radiating into the proximal forearm extensor muscles. The pain is aggravated by the patient clenching the fist, e.g. while lifting heavy objects. There is no sensory disturbance or weakness, although the pain may limit the patient's ability to exert a full effort giving the impression of weakness. It is an overuse injury involving the extensor radialis brevis muscle, which originates on the lateral epicondylar region of the distal humerus.

> **TREATMENT of LATERAL EPICONDYLITIS**
>
> Although many treatments for lateral epicondylitis have been advocated, there is little clear consensus on which modality (conservative or operative) works best. Rest, use of counterforce supportive forearm bracing and non-steroidal anti-inflammatory drugs (NSAIDs) often provide relief of symptoms. Wrist splinting is sometimes necessary but efficacy is uncertain. In many patients the problem eventually resolves spontaneously.

OCCUPATIONAL OVERUSE SYNDROME

Repetition strain injury (RSI) or occupational overuse syndrome (OOS) is a controversial entity and describes a range of conditions characterised by discomfort or persistent pain in muscles, tendons and other soft tissues with or without physical manifestations. RSI is caused or aggravated by repetitive movement, sustained constrained postures and/or forceful movements. This condition occurs among workers performing tasks involving either frequent repetitive and/or forceful movements of the limb, for example keyboard operators, machinists etc.

Pain is the predominant symptom and is diffuse occurring in the hand, wrist, forearm, elbow, shoulder, scapular region and neck, clearly beyond the distribution of any single nerve or nerve root. There is also diffuse tenderness of muscles, joints and ligaments in the forearm and less commonly the upper arm [53].

The aetiology is uncertain and treatment limited.

TENDINOSIS OR TENOSYNOVITIS

Tendinosis is a term preferred by some as it does not imply an inflammatory aetiology; tendonitis and tenosynovitis (inflammation of the tendon sheath) are terms used by others. There is pain aggravated by movement of the tendon, with swelling and crepitus on palpation of the affected tendons or tendon sheath. The most commonly affected tendons are the dorsal extensors of the wrist. Pain occurs in the absence of any sensory disturbance or actual weakness, although the pain can be severe enough to prevent the patient from exerting a full effort when testing strength.

FOREARM PAIN RELATED TO CERVICAL RADICULOPATHY

Forearm pain can occur with C7 and C8 radiculopathies. The site of pain can indicate the likely nerve root involved.

Relationship between symptoms and nerve root involvement

Sensory symptoms, if present, will be in the distribution of the nerve roots (see Figures 1.12 and 1.13).

The particular nerve root involved will influence the pattern of weakness.

- In the forearm pain occurs along the lateral border (radial side) of the forearm with C6 lesions.
- Pain involving the whole arm radiating into the 3rd digit suggests C7 (as the C7 nerve root supplies the periosteum of bone, the pain is more diffuse affecting the whole limb).
- Pain on the medial (ulnar side) indicates C8 nerve root pathology.
- Upper arm or shoulder pain may also occur with a C6, C7 or C8 radiculopathy. Suprascapular pain (C5 or C6), interscapular pain (C7 or C8) or scapular pain (C8).

Cervical radiculopathy may be acute or chronic:
- Acute cervical radiculopathy with significant pain is more common in younger patients and is usually the result of a tear in the annulus fibrosis and subsequent prolapse of the nucleus pulposus (jelly-like substance in the middle of the spinal disc) or the disc itself.
- Subacute radiculopathy occurs in patients with preexisting cervical spondylosis. These patients experience occasional neck pain and develop insidious symptoms, which are often polyradicular in nature.
- Chronic radiculopathies occur either spontaneously or when acute or subacute radiculopathies fail to respond to treatment. The gradual onset of wasting and weakness of the small muscles of the hand and forearm, sometimes associated with fasciculations is seen in the elderly and this sometimes leads to the suspicion of motor neuron disease.

Radicular pain is often accentuated by activities that stretch the involved nerve root, such as coughing, sneezing, Valsalva and certain cervical movements or positions. It is NOT influenced by movement of the arm. C7 nerve root compression is the commonest while C6 is the second most common. Very rarely, the radiculopathy is due to malignancy or benign neural tumours such as neurofibroma or meningioma.

The clue to the diagnosis, although not always present, is that in most patients the arm pain is NOT influenced by moving the arm but is exacerbated by turning the neck in certain but not in all directions.

It is important to remember that the first seven cervical nerve roots emerge above the corresponding vertebra and the 8th below the 7th cervical vertebrae. Thus, C6 nerve root compression will occur between the 5th and 6th cervical vertebrae.

Confirming the diagnosis of cervical nerve root compression
- A plain X-ray of the cervical spine with anteroposterior, lateral and oblique views will often demonstrate narrowing of the disc space or degenerative changes causing the problem. It is *important to request oblique views* to see the foramen through which the nerve roots emerge.
- If the pain does not settle with conservative (non-surgical) treatment, an MRI scan can usually identify the underlying pathology.
- A plain CT scan (i.e. without myelography) only occasionally identifies the underlying pathology and is not recommended in this situation.
- When the main complaint is arm pain, surgery almost invariably relieves the pain. The weakness and sensory loss may take some months to resolve and in some cases never resolve.

COMPLEX REGIONAL PAIN SYNDROME
Although this condition is extremely rare it is one of those diagnoses THAT MUST NOT BE MISSED. The consequences of a delay in diagnosis are often severe and prolonged problems.

Symptoms can recur once or many times months or even years later.

A variety of terms have been used to describe this entity, including causalgia, shoulder–hand syndrome, reflex sympathetic dystrophy and Sudeck's atrophy. The current nomenclature refers to complex regional pain syndrome (CRPS) types I and II, where the only difference between types I and II is the presence of a nerve lesion in type II with the

---

PRINCIPLES of MANAGEMENT FOR CERVICAL NERVE ROOT COMPRESSION

Treatment will be determined by the patient's ability to tolerate pain. Motor and sensory symptoms in isolation are not indications for surgery, as one cannot guarantee resolution of such symptoms.

- Some patients who have little tolerance of pain request surgery as soon as possible. If patients can be persuaded to tolerate the pain it often resolves within 4–6 weeks.
- If moving the neck aggravates the pain a collar that immobilises the neck can provide symptomatic benefit until the pain resolves.
- Analgesics and precise fluoroscopically guided transforaminal placement of corticosteroids close to the disc–nerve root interface and near the dorsal root ganglia have been shown to be of benefit [54].
- Despite the lack of scientific evidence of benefit some patients appear to settle with oral corticosteroids (50 mg per day of prednisolone for 10 days) with some relapsing when the steroids are withdrawn.[3]

Pain improves faster with surgery than with conservative treatment but at 1 year there is no difference [55]. A Cochrane review concluded that data from the reviewed trials were inadequate to provide reliable conclusions on the balance of risk and benefit from cervical spine surgery for spondylotic radiculopathy or myelopathy [56].

---

latter termed causlagia[4] [Greek: kausos(heat) + algos (pain)]. Causalgia is burning pain, allodynia (pain evoked by innocuous stimulatio of the skin) and hyperpathia (an abnormal exaggerated response to a painful stimulus), usually in the hand or foot after partial injury of a nerve or one of its major branches. Pain is more severe in type II.

Clinical features

The problem may appear after a trivial injury and sometimes complicates minor surgery, e.g. for carpal tunnel. The essential clinical features include:

- *persistent pain* developing within days to weeks after the injury or surgery and pain that is not clearly confined to the distribution of a single nerve or nerve root
- initially increased temperature, then fluctuating between a sense of increased heat or coldness and subsequently persistent coldness
- swelling in the region of the pain
- changes in the colour of the skin, often described as mottled
- less frequently, excessive or reduced sweating [59].

Figure 11.14 lists the clinical features of some of the problems affecting the forearm and hands. It separates them into those that cause paroxysmal and those that cause persistent symptoms. Occasionally pain is absent and the patient presents with the other clinical features after an injury such as isolated coldness or altered sweating [54].

---

3 Personal unproven observation.
4 Diagnostic criteria recommended to the author early in his training by a senior neurosurgeon for complex regional pain syndrome type I [57] (not all authors agree with this nomenclature [58]):
  1 The presence of an initiating noxious event or a cause of immobilisation.
  2 Continuing pain, allodynia or hyperalgesia with which the pain is disproportionate to any inciting event.
  3 Evidence at some time of oedema, changes in skin blood flow or abnormal sudomotor activity in the region of the pain.
  4 This diagnosis is excluded by the existence of a condition that otherwise would account for the degree of pain and dysfunction.

MANAGEMENT of COMPLEX REGIONAL PAIN SYNDROME

A variety of treatments have been advocated for CRPS type 1 but evidence to support these treatments is lacking [60, 61]. These include:

- corticosteroids [62] in the form of oral prednisolone 40 mg/day for 14 days, followed by 10 mg/week taper
- intravenous guanethidine [63, 64]
- chemical and surgical sympathectomy, although a Cochrane review concluded that there was no evidence of benefit [61].

Some have argued that, with so little to offer therapeutically, it seems not unreasonable to consider one or two sympatholytic procedures on an empirical basis [58]. Drug treatment is based, not unreasonably, on experience gained in the treatment of neuropathic pain in general. Drugs such as opioids, gabapentin and tricyclic antidepressants are recommended but have not yet been shown in randomised controlled trials to be effective in CRPS. Bisphosphonates, including pamidronate, clodronate and alendronate, have been advocated by some authorities [65]. Phenoxybenzamine (intravenous [66] and oral [67]) has also been reported to result in *resolution of early CPRS type I*. (It is important to warn men of the side effect of retrograde ejaculation.)

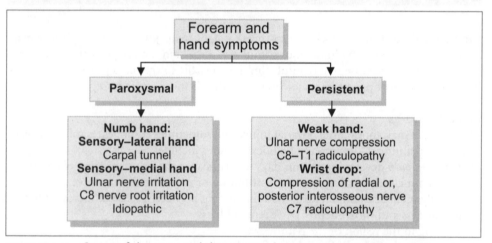

FIGURE 11.14 Some of the essential diagnostic clues in patients with symptoms in the forearms and hands

REFERENCES

1 Dauer WT et al. Current concepts on the clinical features, aetiology and management of idiopathic cervical dystonia. Brain 1998; 121(Pt 4):547–560.

2 Linton SJ. A review of psychological risk factors in back and neck pain. Spine 2000; 25(9):1148–1156.

3 Jansen GB et al. Whiplash injuries: Diagnosis and early management. The Swedish Society of Medicine and the Whiplash Commission Medical Task Force. Eur Spine J 2008; 17(Suppl 3):S355–S417.

4 Radanov BP, Sturzenegger M, Di Stefano G. Long-term outcome after whiplash injury: A 2-year follow-up considering features of injury mechanism and somatic, radiologic, and psychosocial findings. Medicine (Baltimore) 1995; 74(5):281–297.

5 Obelieniene D et al. Pain after whiplash: A prospective controlled inception cohort study. J Neurol Neurosurg Psychiatry 1999; 66(3):279–283.

6 Schrader H et al. Natural evolution of late whiplash syndrome outside the medicolegal context. Lancet 1996; 347(9010):1207–1211.

7 Harrop JS et al. Neurological manifestations of cervical spondylosis: An overview of signs, symptoms, and pathophysiology. Neurosurgery 2007; 60(Suppl 1):S14–S20.

8   Stiell IG et al. The Canadian C-spine rule versus the NEXUS low-risk criteria in patients with trauma. N Engl J Med 2003; 349(26):2510–2518.

9   Hurwitz EL et al. Treatment of neck pain: Noninvasive interventions. Results of the Bone and Joint Decade 2000–2010 Task Force on Neck Pain and Its Associated Disorders. J Manipulative Physiol Ther 2009; 32 (2 Suppl):S141–S175.

10 van Alfen N, van Engelen BG. The clinical spectrum of neuralgic amyotrophy in 246 cases. Brain 2006; 129(2):438–450.

11 Cruz-Martinez A, Barrio M, Arpa J. Neuralgic amyotrophy: Variable expression in 40 patients. J Periph Nerv Syst 2002; 7(3):198–204.

12 Chance PF. Inherited focal, episodic neuropathies: Hereditary neuropathy with liability to pressure palsies and hereditary neuralgic amyotrophy. Neuromol Med 2006; 8(1–2):159–174.

13 Perlmutter GS. Axillary nerve injury. Clin Orthop Relat Res 1999; 368:28–36.

14 Post M. Diagnosis and treatment of suprascapular nerve entrapment. Clin Orthop Relat Res 1999; 368:92–100.

15 Zoltan JD. Injury to the suprascapular nerve associated with anterior dislocation of the shoulder: Case report and review of the literature. J Trauma 1979; 19(3):203–206.

16 Solheim LF, Roaas A. Compression of the suprascapular nerve after fracture of the scapular notch. Acta Orthop Scand 1978; 49(4):338–340.

17 Rodgers JA, Crosby LA. Rotator cuff disorders. Am Fam Physician 1996; 54(1):127–134.

18 Lewis JS. Rotator cuff tendinopathy/subacromial impingement syndrome: Is it time for a new method of assessment? Br J Sports Med 2009; 43(4):259–264.

19 Pajareya K et al. Effectiveness of physical therapy for patients with adhesive capsulitis: A randomized controlled trial. J Med Assoc Thai 2004; 87(5):473–480.

20 Hawkins RH, Dunlop R. Nonoperative treatment of rotator cuff tears. Clin Orthop Relat Res 1995; 321:178–188.

21 Blair B et al. Efficacy of injections of corticosteroids for subacromial impingement syndrome. J Bone Joint Surg Am 1996; 78(11):1685–1689.

22 Yamakado K. The targeting accuracy of subacromial injection to the shoulder: An arthrographic evaluation. Arthroscopy 2002; 18(8):887–891.

23 Watson M. Major ruptures of the rotator cuff: The results of surgical repair in 89 patients. J Bone Joint Surg Br 1985; 67(4):618–624.

24 Stephens MB, Beutler AI, O'Connor FG. Musculoskeletal injections: A review of the evidence. Am Fam Physician 2008; 78(8):971–976.

25 Haahr JP, Andersen JH. Exercises may be as efficient as subacromial decompression in patients with subacromial stage II impingement: 4–8-years' follow-up in a prospective, randomized study. Scand J Rheumatol 2006; 35(3):224–228.

26 Gartsman GM, O'Connor PD. Arthroscopic rotator cuff repair with and without arthroscopic subacromial decompression: A prospective, randomized study of one-year outcomes. J Shoulder Elbow Surg 2004; 13(4):424–426.

27 Codsi MJ. The painful shoulder: When to inject and when to refer. Cleve Clin J Med 2007; 74(7): 473–474:477–478, 480–482 passim.

28 Schott GD. A chronic and painless form of idiopathic brachial plexus neuropathy. J Neurol Neurosurg Psychiatry 1983; 46(6):555–557.

29 Shimizu S et al. Radiculopathy at the C5/6 intervertebral foramen resulting in isolated atrophy of the deltoid: An aberrant innervation complicating diagnosis. Report of two cases. Eur Spine J 2008; 17 (Suppl 2):S338–S341.

30 Yoss RE et al. Significance of symptoms and signs in localization of involved root in cervical disk protrusion. Neurology 1957; 7(10):673–683.

31 Wiater JM, Flatow EL. Long thoracic nerve injury. Clin Orthop Relat Res 1999; 368:17–27.

32 Caliandro P et al. Distribution of paresthesias in carpal tunnel syndrome reflects the degree of nerve damage at wrist. Clin Neurophysiol 2006; 117(1):228–231.

33 Bland JD. Treatment of carpal tunnel syndrome. Muscle Nerve 2007; 36(2):167–171.

34 Tinel J. Presse Medicale 1915; 47:388.

35 Phalen GS. The birth of a syndrome, or carpal tunnel revisited. J Hand Surg Am 1981; 6(2):109–110.

36 Katz JN et al. The carpal tunnel syndrome: Diagnostic utility of the history and physical examination findings. Ann Intern Med 1990; 112(5):321–327.

37 O'Connor D, Marshall S, Massy-Westropp N. Non-surgical treatment (other than steroid injection) for carpal tunnel syndrome. Cochrane Database Syst Rev 2003(1):CD003219.

38 Gerritsen AA et al. Splinting vs surgery in the treatment of carpal tunnel syndrome: A randomized controlled trial. JAMA 2002; 288(10):1245–1251.

39 Marshall S, Tardif G, Ashworth N. Local corticosteroid injection for carpal tunnel syndrome. Cochrane Database Syst Rev 2007(2):CD001554.

40 Wong SM et al. Single vs two steroid injections for carpal tunnel syndrome: A randomised clinical trial. Int J Clin Pract 2005; 59(12):1417–1421.

41 Hui AC et al. A randomized controlled trial of surgery vs steroid injection for carpal tunnel syndrome. Neurology 2005; 64(12):2074–2078.

42 Korthals-de Bos IB et al. Surgery is more cost-effective than splinting for carpal tunnel syndrome in the Netherlands: Results of an economic evaluation alongside a randomized controlled trial. BMC Musculoskelet Disord 2006; 7:86.

43 Iida J et al. Carpal tunnel syndrome: Electrophysiological grading and surgical results by minimum incision open carpal tunnel release. Neurol Med Chir (Tokyo) 2008; 48(12):554–559.

44 Bland JD. Do nerve conduction studies predict the outcome of carpal tunnel decompression? Muscle Nerve 2001; 24(7):935–940.

45 Herskovitz S, Berger AR, Lipton RB. Low-dose, short-term oral prednisone in the treatment of carpal tunnel syndrome. Neurology 1995; 45(10):1923–1925.

46 Weber RA, Rude MJ. Clinical outcomes of carpal tunnel release in patients 65 and older. J Hand Surg Am 2005; 30(1):75–80.

47 Leit ME, Weiser RW, Tomaino MM. Patient-reported outcome after carpal tunnel release for advanced disease: A prospective and longitudinal assessment in patients older than age 70. J Hand Surg Am 2004; 29(3):379–383.

48 Peet RM et al. Thoracic-outlet syndrome: Evaluation of a therapeutic exercise program. Proc Staff Meet Mayo Clin 1956; 31(9):281–287.

49 Sanders RJ, Hammond SL, Rao NM. Diagnosis of thoracic outlet syndrome. J Vasc Surg 2007; 46(3): 601–604.

50 Maru S et al. Thoracic outlet syndrome in children and young adults. Eur J Vasc Endovasc Surg 2009; 38(5):560–564.

51 Gunther T et al. Late outcome of surgical treatment of the nonspecific neurogenic thoracic outlet syndrome. Neurol Res 2009;[vol]:[pages].

52 Leffert RD, Perlmutter GS. Thoracic outlet syndrome: Results of 282 transaxillary first rib resections. Clin Orthop Relat Res 1999; 368:66–79.

53 Dennett X, Fry HJ. Overuse syndrome: A muscle biopsy study. Lancet 1988; 1(8591):905–908.

54 Slipman CW, Chow DW. Therapeutic spinal corticosteroid injections for the management of radiculopathies. Phys Med Rehabil Clin N Am 2002; 13(3):697–711.

55 Persson LC, Lilja A. Pain, coping, emotional state and physical function in patients with chronic radicular neck pain. A comparison between patients treated with surgery, physiotherapy or neck collar – a blinded, prospective randomized study. Disabil Rehabil 2001; 23(8):325–335.

56 Fouyas IP, Statham PF, Sandercock PA. Cochrane review on the role of surgery in cervical spondylotic radiculomyelopathy. Spine (Phila Pa 1976) 2002; 27(7):736–747.

57 Stanton-Hicks M et al. Reflex sympathetic dystrophy: Changing concepts and taxonomy. Pain 1995; 63(1):127–133.

58 Schott GD. Complex? Regional? Pain? Syndrome? Pract Neurol 2007; 7(3):145–157.

59 Veldman PH et al. Signs and symptoms of reflex sympathetic dystrophy: Prospective study of 829 patients. Lancet 1993; 342(8878):1012–1016.

60 Cepeda MS, Carr DB, Lau J. Local anesthetic sympathetic blockade for complex regional pain syndrome. Cochrane Database Syst Rev 2005(4):CD004598.

61 Mailis A, Furlan A. Sympathectomy for neuropathic pain. Cochrane Database Syst Rev 2003(2):CD002918.

62 Christensen K, Jensen EM, Noer I. The reflex dystrophy syndrome response to treatment with systemic corticosteroids. Acta Chir Scand 1982; 148(8):653–655.

63 Hannington-Kiff JG. Intravenous regional sympathetic block with guanethidine. Lancet 1974; 1(7865):1019–1020.

64 Bonelli S et al. Regional intravenous guanethidine vs stellate ganglion block in reflex sympathetic dystrophies: A randomized trial. Pain 1983; 16(3):297–307.

65 Robinson JN, Sandom J, Chapman PT. Efficacy of pamidronate in complex regional pain syndrome type I. Pain Med 2004; 5(3):276–280.

66 Malik VK et al. Intravenous regional phenoxybenzamine in the treatment of reflex sympathetic dystrophy. Anesthesiology 1998; 88(3):823–827.

67 Inchiosa MA, Jr, Kizelshteyn G. Treatment of complex regional pain syndrome type I with oral phenoxybenzamine: Rationale and case reports. Pain Pract 2008; 8(2):125–132.

chapter 12

Back Pain and Common Leg Problems With or Without Difficulty Walking

Patients experience difficulty walking as a result of pain in their legs, and the commonest cause of pain is arthritis of the joints in the lower limbs. In the absence of pain, altered strength (which may be due to a lower motor or upper motor neuron problem) or sensation (particularly proprioception) in the lower limbs or impaired balance resulting from either a cerebellar disturbance or vestibular problem may cause difficulty walking. In the absence of pain, weakness or altered sensation, patients may experience difficulty walking related to Parkinson's syndrome or a condition often confused with Parkinson's that is termed apraxia of gait.

In this chapter there is a discussion of back pain but only to highlight that the most important thing to ascertain is whether the pain is in the lumbar or thoracic region. After a brief discussion of back pain, there is a description of the clinical features of the various neurological disorders affecting the peripheral nervous system and the non-neurological conditions in the upper and lower leg and foot that may or may not result in difficulty walking. A few very rare conditions (including akathisia, painful legs and moving toes and erythromelalgia) are also discussed.

Difficulty walking that is related to central nervous system problems will be discussed in Chapter 13, 'Abnormal movements and difficulty walking due to central nervous system problems'.

BACK PAIN

Almost every person will at some stage in life experience a bout of back pain. A search of the Internet using Entrez PubMed yields in excess of 30,000 articles, Google scholar more than 2 million and Google more than 47 million articles! Despite the explosion of information only a few principles will be discussed here.

The first is principle is to establish exactly where in the back the pain is:
- Most *low back (lumbar) pain* is non-specific and relates to problems affecting soft tissues or is related to degenerative disease of the lumbosacral spine.
  A word of warning: degenerative disease of the lumbosacral spine is very common, particularly in the elderly or obese patient, and may not necessarily be the cause of the back pain or problems in the legs.
- On the other hand thoracic back pain may be more sinister:
  - Patients who subsequently develop malignant cord compression often experience thoracic back pain for days or weeks prior to the onset of the neurological symptoms.
  - Pain related to osteoporotic vertebral fractures is commonly in the thoracic region.

- Rarely, thoracic back pain may be the presenting symptom of a ruptured aortic aneurysm.
- If there is an associated **radiculopathy** (sciatica), the degenerative disease or lumbar disc disease may be the cause.
- Routine imaging early on in the course of low back pain is of no benefit [1]. An MRI scan can detect spinal metastases in patients with normal plain X-rays or CT scan [2]. A nuclear bone scan can also detect metastases in the vertebral column before cord compression but MRI is superior [3].
- In most patients with low back pain, symptoms resolve without surgical intervention:
- Physical therapy and non-steroidal anti-inflammatory drugs (NSAIDs) are the cornerstones of non-surgical treatment [4].
- Superficial heat is the only therapy with good evidence of efficacy for treatment of acute low back pain.
- Bed rest is often advocated for the treatment of acute low back pain but continuing ordinary activity may lead to a more rapid recovery [5].
- There is conflicting evidence of efficacy for spinal manipulation in low back pain [6, 7].
- Massage and acupuncture are better than no treatment but have not been compared to conventional treatment.

TREATMENT OF CHRONIC BACK PAIN

Chronic back pain can be very difficult to treat. Although there is limited evidence for the efficacy of aquatic exercises [8], this author[1] has seen numerous patients return to a normal life once they began swimming on a regular basis, at least three times per week and 20 minutes at a time.

Note: A randomised study detected higher ambulation rates in patients with malignant spinal cord compression (MSCC) who received high-dose dexamethasone before radiotherapy (RT) compared with patients who did not receive corticosteroids before RT (81% v 63% at 3 months, respectively; P = 0.046).

PROBLEMS IN THE UPPER LEG
Painless numbness

MERALGIA PARAESTHETICA
Meralgia paraesthetica is very common, particularly in patients who are overweight. It is essentially about the only cause of numbness in the thigh or upper leg because compression of the sensory nerve roots in the upper lumbar (L2–3) spine is very rare.

Symptoms
- Symptoms may be intermittent initially, but subsequently the patient may develop permanently altered sensation.
- Symptoms vary from a mildly altered sensation over the anterolateral aspect of the thigh, often only noticed when the patient touches the thigh or clothes brush up against the thigh, to a more marked alteration in sensation with persistent numbness within the distribution of the lateral cutaneous nerve of the thigh but not always involving the entire extent.
- Some patients complain of pain and others may experience dysaesthesia, an unpleasant sensation when the skin is touched. This condition is due to

---

1 Personal observations.

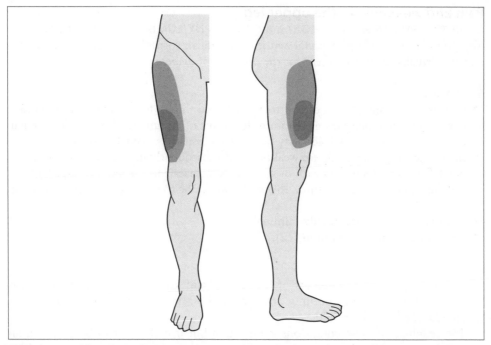

FIGURE 12.1   The area of sensation supplied by the lateral cutaneous nerve of the thigh

Reproduced from *Aids to the Examination of the Peripheral Nervous System*. 4th edn, *Brain*, 2000, WB Saunders, Figure 78. p 50.

compression of the lateral cutaneous nerve of the thigh beneath the inguinal ligament just medial to the anterior superior iliac spine and pressure over this point is often associated with tenderness.
* The presence of weakness or an altered knee reflex excludes the diagnosis.
* The condition may be unilateral or bilateral.

Examination
The simplest test is to stroke the skin over the lateral aspect of the thigh and, if there is altered sensation, test in all directions, mapping out the exact pattern and sensory loss. The patient is then shown Figure 12.1 and immediately identifies the problem.

Another diagnostic test is to inject local anaesthetic in the region of the lateral cutaneous nerve beneath the inguinal ligament; a transient resolution of symptoms is considered diagnostic [9].

MANAGEMENT of MERALGIA PARAESTHETICA

Once the benign nature of the condition is explained, the great majority of patients do not request any specific treatment. In a number of patients the problem may resolve spontaneously [9]. Patients with pain or dysaesthesia may respond to a corticosteroid injection and, if that fails, decompression of the nerve or avulsion of the nerve (neurectomy) [10]. This latter procedure will replace dysaesthesia with permanent numbness. Regardless of the treatment chosen most patients remain free of symptoms following treatment [9, 11].

Pain and weakness in the upper leg
DIABETIC AMYOTROPHY/FEMORAL AMYOTROPHY/LUMBOSACRAL NEURITIS
The clinical features of lumbosacral neuritis, femoral amyotrophy and diabetic amyotrophy are virtually identical, except for the presence of diabetes.

Symptoms
- Increasingly severe pain in the buttocks, hips and thighs developing over hours to days is the initial presenting symptom. It is most often unilateral but, as in brachial neuritis, the contralateral side may be involved, usually within 1–2 weeks.
- In addition to the pain, severe weakness and subsequently marked wasting of the quadriceps muscles occurs with or without parasthaesia in the anterior aspect of the thigh and at times the shin. The weakness can be so severe to render the patient unable to walk.
- Sensory symptoms are usually minimal.
- Weight loss is not uncommon [12].

Examination
The examination reveals weakness of hip flexion and knee extension with an absent knee-jerk. Although it may occur at any age, lumbosacral neuritis is more common in the middle-aged to elderly [13].

The aetiology of these conditions is uncertain but it is thought to be based on an inflammatory vasculitis [12, 14].

**MANAGEMENT of DIABETIC AMYOTROPHY/FEMORAL AMYOTROPHY/
LUMBOSACRAL NEURITIS**

Although the condition may resolve spontaneously after many months or years, immuno-modulatory therapy, including corticosteroids or even cytotoxic drugs, may shorten the duration of the illness. Intravenous immunoglobulin has also been recommended and several case reports describe apparent dramatic responses [15, 16].

At this point in time there are no randomised controlled trials to guide therapy but, in the absence of specific therapy, significant disability persists for months or years.

POLYMYALGIA RHEUMATICA
Polymyalgia rheumatica is a condition seen in middle-aged to elderly patients.

Symptoms
It presents with aching and stiffness predominantly affecting the shoulders but in 50–70% of cases may also affect the hips [17]. The condition is thought to relate to synovitis of the proximal joints and extra-articular synovial structures.

> In both lumbosacral neuritis and polymyalgia rheumatica there is constant pain. The worsening of pain with movement of the hips is seen only in polymyalgia and the presence of severe weakness and sensory disturbance occurs only in lumbosacral neuritis.

The pain is constant day and night, as opposed to osteoarthritis of the hips where the pain mainly occurs on weight bearing. It often radiates to the knee and is exacerbated by movement of the hip joints. Although initially it may be unilateral, almost invariably patients develop bilateral symptoms.

A low-grade fever, fatigue and anorexia may occur in as many as 40% of patients and the presence of high spiking fevers should alert the clinician to the possibility of an associated giant-cell arteritis affecting the aorta and major branches. This can result in constant headaches, scalp tenderness and jaw claudication (see Chapter 9, 'Headache and facial pain', for further discussion).

Examination
The examination reveals restricted active and passive movement of the hips but in the absence of any joint swelling.

MANAGEMENT of POLYMYALGIA RHEUMATICA

In patients with polymyalgia rheumatica the erythrocyte sedimentation rate is invariably raised and corticosteroids are the treatment of choice. Doses as little as 10–20 mg/day almost invariably lead to a rapid resolution of the aching and stiffness within days and a rapid response at this low dose is considered diagnostic.

Occasional patients may require higher doses for longer periods [17]. If the patient fails to respond to 30 mg of prednisolone within 1 week the diagnosis should be questioned.

Early cessation of steroids may lead to a relapse and treatment at a low dose should be continued for 1–2 years [18]. Methotrexate has been shown in a randomised controlled trial to be an effective steroid-sparing agent.

Unfortunately, side effects of steroids in this group are common.

DRUG-INDUCED MUSCLE PAIN AND/OR WEAKNESS
A large number of pharmaceutical agents, including lipid lowering agents, NSAIDs, antineoplastic drugs and even over-the-counter essential amino acids, such as L-tryptophan, can result in myalgia or even myositis causing muscle pain, cramps, swelling, tenderness and weakness [19, 20]. This list is almost certain to enlarge with the advent of new therapeutic agents.

In any patient presenting with myalgia or muscle weakness a detailed list of drugs used should be obtained and each drug should be checked to see if it has been reported to cause myalgia or myositis. Some drugs produce a pure muscle disorder; others are associated with a neuropathy. The pharmacy department of the public hospital is a very useful resource, as is the patient's own pharmacist.

Weakness in the upper leg
POLYMYOSITIS/DERMATOMYOSITIS
Inflammatory disorders of muscle, including polymyositis, dermatomyositis and inclusion body myositis, are extremely rare and most general practitioners are unlikely to encounter a case during their working career.

Patients present with the insidious onset of proximal weakness in the legs in the absence of sensory disturbance. The weakness is bilateral but may be asymmetrical. Pain in the muscles occurs in approximately 50% of cases but, as opposed to the above two conditions, is rarely severe. Dysphagia, neck weakness and impaired respiratory function may occur [21]. Inclusion body myositis affects the long flexors of the fingers and, in the lower limbs, the extensor muscles of the knees and hip flexors, resulting in significant proximal weakness. In this latter condition the knee reflex is often absent, whereas in polymyositis and dermatomyositis the reflexes are preserved.

> ## MANAGEMENT of MYOSITIS
>
> Most patients will have an elevated creatinine phosphate kinase (CPK), but a normal CPK does not exclude the diagnosis. The nerve conduction studies (NCS) should be normal, but electromyography may demonstrate a typical myopathic pattern associated with fibrillation potentials and positive sharp waves indicating an inflammatory muscle disorder. Magnetic resonance imaging, contrast-enhanced ultrasound and positron emission tomography can demonstrate abnormalities in muscles in patients with inflammatory myositis and can help determine the site for the definitive diagnostic test, a muscle biopsy [22].
>
> Corticosteroids are the cornerstone of treatment, unfortunately often associated with significant side effects. Other immunomodulatory drugs, such as azathioprine, methotrexate, cyclosporine, cyclophosphamide, interferon, intravenous immunoglobulin and plasma exchange, are often used as steroid-sparing agents despite the lack of good evidence regarding the effectiveness of any of these treatments [23]. Apart from exercise there is no specific treatment for inclusion body myositis at the time of writing this text.

MUSCLE WEAKNESS DUE TO ENDOCRINE DYSFUNCTION

Hyperthyroidism, hypothyroidism and Addison's disease may all present with muscle weakness. Usually there are associated manifestations to point to the underlying endocrine disorder. Hyperthyroidism may also present with periodic paralysis [24] or rhabdomyolysis [25] and hypothyroidism may present with muscle hypertrophy [26].

The weakness will resolve with correction of the endocrine disturbance.

PERIPHERAL NEUROPATHY

Certain peripheral neuropathies such acute and chronic inflammatory demyelinating peripheral neuropathy and the IgG- and IgA-related peripheral neuropathies can result in significant proximal weakness in the lower limbs. However, this rarely occurs in isolation and these patients usually present with generalised weakness affecting the proximal lower limbs and the distal upper limbs and neck weakness with or without respiratory muscle weakness. Peripheral neuropathy is discussed in more detail later in this chapter.

PROBLEMS IN THE LOWER LEGS AND FEET

Unpleasant sensations in the feet

In the lower leg and feet patients can experience unpleasant sensations at rest that can cause difficulty walking or unpleasant sensation at rest improved by walking or, in fact, that can be improved by walking. Figure 12.2 shows an approach to patients with discomfort or unpleasant sensation in their feet. Erythromelalgia and painful legs moving toes are extremely rare.

There are many non-neurological causes of pain in the feet where pain is either exacerbated or precipitated by weight bearing and/or walking. These include osteoarthritis in the ankle or joints of the feet, a calcaneal spur and plantar fasciitis. The neurological causes of pain in the feet that can result in difficulty walking due to pain include Morton's neuroma or metatarsalgia and tarsal tunnel syndrome. All will have pain with weight bearing, but there are subtle differences in the nature of the pain and the presence of altered sensation that occurs with the neurological causes to help differentiate the various entities.

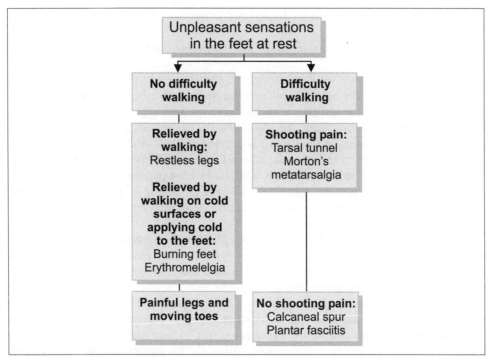

FIGURE 12.2 Suggested approach to pain in the feet

UNPLEASANT SENSATIONS AT REST THAT DO NOT CAUSE DIFFICULTY WALKING
Restless legs syndrome (RLS) and burning feet are the two common conditions that cause unpleasant sensations in the feet and lower legs. They do not interfere with walking; in fact, the symptoms improve with walking with RLS and walking on a cold surface with burning feet.

Restless legs syndrome
Restless legs syndrome [27–31] is common, affecting 5% of the population. However, many patients complain that most doctors do not seem to be aware of the entity or know much about it. A more appropriate term is restless limbs syndrome because in more severe cases it can also affect the upper limbs and, rarely, symptoms may be confined to the upper limbs.

The essential features of RLS are:
- Patients develop symptoms when they are not moving, such as prolonged sitting at the dinner table, on an aeroplane or in a lecture or movie.
- Symptoms are particularly severe in bed at night.
- Patients find it very difficult to describe the nature of the symptoms except to say that they are unpleasant.[2]
- Patients cannot keep their limbs still because of this unpleasant sensation that feels deep inside the limb, not over the surface or affecting just the skin.
- The pain is in the feet, shins, calves and often seems to cross joints but is not confined to the joints.

---

2 One patient described it as one leg boxing the other all night! Others describe aching, gnawing sensations.

- Symptoms persist on and off for hours until patients are forced to be up and about.
- Both legs are usually affected although the symptoms can be either confined to or more severe in one leg.
- Patients invariably pace the floor at night to obtain relief but, unlike burning feet syndrome, they do not need to walk on cold surfaces and the symptoms are not relieved by moving the feet to where the sheets are colder.
- There are no symptoms during the day unless the patient sits down.
- Sleep is disturbed whether the patient is sleeping at night or during the day.
- The neurological examination of the affected limbs should be completely normal, although sometimes this condition is associated with a peripheral neuropathy, so patients should be examined specifically looking for absent ankle reflexes, weakness of dorsiflexion of the toes and feet and possible peripheral sensory loss affecting the toes and distal aspect of the feet.

The condition can occur at any age although most patients will have experienced their first symptom before the age of 30. The symptoms are more marked in the presence of renal failure, iron deficiency and pregnancy. It is important to test for iron deficiency and impaired renal function.

The aetiology of RLS is unclear although there is a genetic factor with autosomal dominant and autosomal recessive inheritance. As it is predominantly inherited as an autosomal dominant condition, a positive family history can be obtained in up to 90% of patients with detailed questioning, although the patient may not be aware of the specific name but can recall their parents or grandparents pacing the floor at night. Other patients will initially say that there is no other family member affected but, when sent away to enquire, discover one or more relatives who have the condition. In many but not all patients there is involuntary jerking of the limbs referred to as myoclonus. The symptoms of RLS increase in severity with increasing age and duration of the disease.

Conditions that may be confused with restless leg syndrome include peripheral vascular disease (PVD) and *two very rare conditions, akathisia* and a curious entity called *painful legs and moving toes.*

MANAGEMENT of RESTLESS LEGS SYNDROME

Exclude iron deficiency and renal failure.
    Abstinence from alcohol, caffeine, nicotine and drugs that may exacerbate the problem is advocated [32].
    A number of treatments have been recommended:

- Some patients can minimise their symptoms by either exercising just before retiring to bed or by running several kilometres each day. In most patients such exercise is not practical and drug therapy is necessary [30].
- Levodopa is considered the treatment of choice [30, 33].
- Other medications include benzodiazepines such as clonazepam [34], the dopamine agonists pramipexol [35] and ropinerole [36], rotigotine transdermal patches [37], in severe cases opiates such as oxycodone [38] and in very severe cases methadone [39]. *Note:* Methadone has not been studied in randomised controlled trials; the evidence is based on a case series.[3]

The characteristic feature of PVD is exercise-induced leg pain relieved by rest but occasionally it can cause pain at rest. The symptoms are confined to the lower limbs and upper limb symptoms would exclude this diagnosis. The pain is usually in the feet and calves; very rarely, buttock pain can occur due to involvement of the internal iliac artery. The peripheral pulses will be difficult to palpate with PVD.

Akathisia

Akathisia consists of an inner sense of restlessness with a desire to move not just the limbs but the entire body. It is only seen in patients who have been exposed to dopamine antagonists. Whereas the unpleasant sensations associated with RLS are alleviated by walking or moving the limbs, patients with akathisia cannot obtain relief with movement.

Painful legs and moving toes

Painful legs and moving toes may develop in the setting of spinal cord and cauda equina trauma, lumbar root lesions, injuries to bony or soft tissues of the feet and peripheral neuropathy; in some patients it is idiopathic [40]. It is not familial and is not thought to be related to RLS.

It consists of continuous or semi-continuous involuntary writhing movements of the toes associated with pain in the affected extremity [41]. Symptoms may begin on one side and become bilateral; movements may be momentarily suppressed by voluntary action or exacerbated by changing posture [40]. Pain preceding the movements was most commonly burning in nature. Movements consisted of flexion/extension, abduction/adduction and fanning or clawing of toes/fingers and sometimes the foot or hand [42]. Surface electromyography (EMG) showed movements suggestive of both chorea and dystonia. Movements are partially suppressible and diminished but still apparent during light sleep.

Gamma-aminobutyric acid (GABAergic) agents are most effective in controlling the pain and the movements [42].

Burning feet syndrome

Patients complain of an unpleasant burning sensation involving mainly the soles of the feet and occasionally the dorsal aspect of the feet and the legs below the knees that predominantly occurs in bed at night. They prefer to remove the bed covers, move their feet to where the sheets are colder or walk on cold surfaces to obtain some relief.

This differs from RLS where relief is obtained simply by walking on any surface. In some patients burning feet occurs in the setting of a distal sensory peripheral neuropathy; in most patients, the examination does not reveal any abnormality in the peripheral pulses or the skin and there are no abnormal neurological signs.

The aetiology of the syndrome is thought to be a small fibre neuropathy, and reduced intraepidermal nerve fibre density has been demonstrated on skin biopsy [43]. It has been reported in:

- diabetes mellitus or impaired glucose tolerance detected by oral glucose tolerance testing [44]
- hypothyroidism [45]
- HIV [46]
- vitamin B deficiency such as thiamine (B1), riboflavin (B2), nicotinic acid (B3), pantothenic acid (B5) and cyanocobalamin (B12)

---

3 Personal observations in several patients suffering from very severe restless legs syndrome is that methadone has provided significant benefit, although tachyphylaxis has occurred, requiring increased doses. Methadone is approved for the treatment of severe RLS by the Australian Pharmaceutical Benefits Scheme on an authority preseription.

Note: Vitamin B deficiency may cause burning feet syndrome that will respond to replacement therapy, but the evidence for this is poor [47].

MANAGEMENT of BURNING FEET SYNDROME

Cold soaks

One of the most effective treatments for significant burning, prickling and tingling in the feet that is present mainly at night is to use cold foot soaks [47].

- Use cold tap water in a basin and leave the feet in it for 20 minutes.
- Take them out and dry them very thoroughly and use a lotion such as Vaseline Intensive Care massaged into the feet. Often this is needed a couple of times a day to gain good relief.
- In addition a tricyclic antidepressant, such as amitriptyline or nortriptyline, at night can be used [48], starting with a small dosage and gradually building up to 50–75 mg.

    With a combination of foot soaking and amitriptyline you can get the vast majority of patients under control.

Aspirin lotion[4]

Ingredients: 1 x 300-mL pump pack of sorbolene cream; 1 x 100-tablet pack of soluble aspirin (e.g. Disprin)

    To make soluble aspirin lotion for skin application:

1 Pump 20 mL (1½ teaspoons) of sorbolene cream into a wide-mouthed glass receptacle or cup.

2 In a spoon dissolve two soluble aspirin in a few drops of water.

3 When the fizzing stops, mix very thoroughly into the sorbolene using a spoon handle in a stirring/beating motion.

4 Apply and rub this cream into the affected skin 3 times a day.

    Every morning make up a similar quantity freshly for each day's use. Alternatively, aspirin tablets may be crushed to a powder and thoroughly mixed with the cream.

Erythromelalgia

Erythromelalgia is a rare condition, of uncertain aetiology, characterised by *episodic* erythema, intense burning pain and warmth of the hands and/or feet. When chronic, it is associated with significant disability [50]. Severe erythromelalgia may spread up the legs and arms and even affect the ears and face. It may be unilateral or bilateral. Symptoms flare up late in the day and continue overnight.

This may not be a disease entity at all, but a syndrome of dysfunctional vascular dynamics [51]. Exposure to warmth can trigger flaring and increase its severity; symptoms are relieved by cooling in ice water. Sometimes the condition may be precipitated by immersing the affected area in hot water for 10–30 minutes [51]. Many patients have either small or large fibre neuropathy (quoted as unpublished data in the article by Kuhnert et al [52]).

Erythromelalgia can be primary or secondary. Primary erythromelalgia begins spontaneously at any age. Secondary erythromelalgia has been reported with many disorders but most often with polycythemia, thrombocythemia, neuropathies and autoimmune diseases.

---

4 Aspirin lotion has been shown to be superior to oral aspirin for the burning pain of acute herpes zoster [49]. This recipe was found some years ago by the author who can no longer find the reference. It is an innocuous treatment with no side effects and has been used with apparent good effect in patients with burning feet.

UNPLEASANT SENSATIONS IN THE FEET AT REST THAT CAUSE DIFFICULTY WALKING

Tarsal tunnel syndrome

Tarsal tunnel syndrome (TTS) is a controversial entity in which the posterior tibial nerve is compressed under the flexor retinaculum in the tarsal tunnel, inferior and posterior to the medial malleolus. This is much rarer than most medical practitioners think.

The symptoms consist of:

- Tingling and numbness on the sole of the foot. If paraesthesia occurs it MUST be confined to the sole of the foot and within the distribution of either the medial and/or lateral plantar nerves (see Figure 1.21). *Paraesthesia on the top of the foot excludes the diagnosis.*
- Burning paraesthesia and pain described as sharp, shooting, shock-like or electric radiating either proximally or distally.
- The symptoms worsen after prolonged standing or walking [53].
- The symptoms are more intense at the end of the day.
- Symptoms do not awaken the patient from sleep and are unlike carpal tunnel.
- Rarely, pain confined to the soles of the foot may also occur at rest and in non-weight-bearing positions [54]. A positive Tinel's sign with tapping of the nerve behind the medial malleolus producing tingling into the sole(s) would be diagnostic but is very rare. Altered sensation within the distribution of the medial and/or lateral plantar nerves is also rarely seen.

The diagnosis of TTS may be difficult as the symptoms are often vague, as are the physical findings and signs. Bilateral cases are seen occasionally. There is often a long delay in diagnosis of up to 2½ years [55].

MANAGEMENT of TARSAL TUNNEL SYNDROME

The entrapment neuropathy of TTS and its treatment are controversial. Nerve conduction studies are of uncertain value due to the lack of definitive studies [56]. Their value is in excluding peripheral neuropathy. Symptoms and signs, operative findings and response to therapy define most cases of TTS reported in the literature [56]. A variety of pathologies have been reported with MRI scans [57], although most are idiopathic in origin.

Surgery consisting of neurolysis of the tibial nerve in the tarsal tunnel and the medial, lateral plantar, calcaneal nerves in their own tunnels and immediate postoperative mobilisation of the posterior tibial nerve through ambulation can achieve a good or excellent outcome in >90% of cases [58].

Morton's neuroma or metatarsalgia

Morton's neuroma is entrapment of the interdigital nerve, most commonly between the 3rd and 4th and less commonly the 2nd and 3rd toes.

- Patients complain that it feels like there is a stone or pebble in their shoe.
- There is the gradual onset of pain while walking with sudden attacks of throbbing burning pain and paraesthesia, on the *plantar surface of the foot* localised to the web space that radiates to the corresponding toes.
- As opposed to pain of neurological origin it is not burning, shooting or associated with altered sensation.
- Pain is minimal or absent when sitting or lying as opposed to a calcaneal spur and plantar fasciitis.

- The clue to the diagnosis is that the pain is aggravated by wearing tight shoes and may be relieved by massage to the forefoot and toes [59].
- There is a localised area of reproducible tenderness between the metatarsal heads.

It occurs most commonly in middle-aged women. Bilateral cases are seen occasionally. If the pain is severe it can create difficulties walking because of the pain, referred to as the antalgic gait. A characteristic limp, characterised by a very short stance phase, may be adopted so as to avoid pain on weight-bearing structures.

MANAGEMENT of MORTON'S NEUROMA

In patients with suspected Morton's neuroma an ultrasound may detect an ovoid, hypoechoic mass located just proximal to the metatarsal heads in the intermetatarsal space, most often between the 2nd and 3rd or 3rd and 4th metatarsals in >90% of patients [60].

Patients should be advised about suitable footwear and possibly be given orthoses to control abnormal pronation.

Injections of local anaesthetic and hydrocortisone around the nerve or surgical excision are recommended [59] although there are no randomised trial results to support this [61].

Calcaneal spur

A calcaneal spur causes:

- sharp, stabbing chronic *heel pain,* particularly in overweight patients [62]
- pain that is characteristically worse in the morning
- tenderness to firm palpation at the distal aspect of the heel where the tendon inserts into the calcaneus bone.

Calcaneal spurs are seen in some patients with plantar fasciitis.

Plantar fasciitis

Plantar fasciitis is the most common cause of plantar heel pain.

SYMPTOMS

- Pain is felt in the sole of the foot.
- Pain is worse when standing after periods of rest or on taking the first steps in the morning.
- The pain improves only to worsen again later in the day after prolonged weight bearing.
- Nocturnal pain is *not* a feature of plantar fasciitis.
- The pain is searing, throbbing or piercing *not* burning or shooting.
- There is tenderness over the origin of the plantar fascia and the anteromedial aspect of the heel.

TREATMENT for PLANTAR FASCIITIS

A variety of treatment regimens have been recommended, but there is no scientific evidence to help guide choice of a particular therapy.

- First-line treatment consists of the combination of a viscous-elastic heel pad, a stretching program, NSAIDS and a tension night splint [64].
- Extracorporeal shockwave therapy is also recommended [65].
- Combined local corticosteroid injections may be given in the form of triamcinolone 2 mL and using a peppering (injecting, withdrawing, redirecting, and reinserting without emerging from the skin) technique [66].
- Retrospective studies have claimed improvement with surgery in patients who have failed to improve with conservative measures [67].

It is more common in runners who increase the distances they run, in obesity and in those who are on their feet most of the day. The condition is self-limiting in most patients and resolves within 12 months [63].

Weakness and/or sensory loss in the lower leg

FOOT DROP

A foot drop can result from:

- an L5 radiculopathy
- a lumbosacral plexus problem
- a sciatic nerve problem
- a common peroneal nerve lesion
- a peripheral neuropathy.

A careful examination to establish the pattern of weakness can help differentiate the various causes.

Figure 12.3 lists the features that help to differentiate the various causes of a foot drop. The crucial thing to note is that the tibialis posterior and tibialis anterior muscles invert the foot at the ankle. The tibialis posterior tendon can be seen and palpated behind the medial malleolus and the tibialis anterior tendon in front of the medial malleolus (see Figure 12.4).

Figure 12.4C shows both the tibialis anterior and tibialis posterior tendons contracting with inversion.

The neuroanatomy explains the signs:

- Foot drop or weakness of dorsiflexion of the foot relates to weakness of the tibialis anterior and extensor digitorum muscles. These muscles are supplied by the common peroneal nerve, the lateral branch of the sciatic nerve that arises in the popliteal fossa and traverses the neck of the fibula, a common site for compression. The 5th lumbar nerve root (L5) is the main innervation of these muscles.
- The peroneii muscles that are responsible for eversion of the foot are also innervated by the common peroneal nerve and the L5 nerve root.

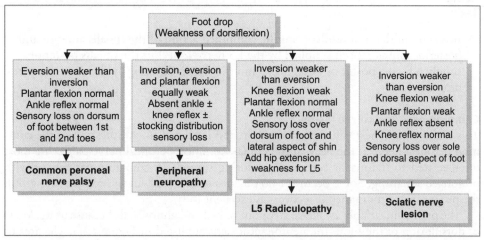

FIGURE 12.3 The patterns of weakness that help to differentiate the various causes of foot drop

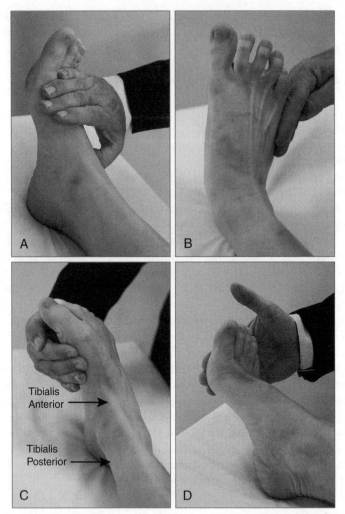

FIGURE 12.4   Testing **A** dorsiflexion, **B** eversion and **C** inversion of the foot, **D** plantar flexion

- Inversion of the foot results from the combined action of the tibialis anterior and posterior muscles, both supplied by the L5 nerve root, but the tibialis posterior is supplied by the posterior tibial nerve and the tibialis anterior by the common peroneal nerve.

Common peroneal nerve lesion

This is the commonest cause of a foot drop and is related to compression of the common peroneal nerve at the neck of the fibula. Common peroneal nerve palsies are most often related to trauma or compression during surgery, in comatose patients or with prolonged squatting. Some occur for no obvious reason [68]. In the compressive group the prognosis for spontaneous recovery is excellent [68].

The patient invariably awakens, steps out of bed and almost falls because of weakness of dorsiflexion of the foot. The neurological signs are listed in Figure 12.3. The area of sensory loss is small (between the 1st and 2nd toes on the dorsal aspect of the foot) if only the deep peroneal nerve is affected and more extensive (dorsum of foot and lateral aspect of distal half of lower leg) if the superficial peroneal nerve is also affected (see Figure 1.19).

Sciatic nerve lesion

Sciatic nerve lesions are very rare and usually result from posterior dislocation fracture of the hip or as a complication of total hip joint replacement. It has also been reported as a complication following coronary artery bypass surgery when patients were sat upright while still unconscious [69].

The neurological signs are listed in Figure 12.3. As opposed to an L5 radiculopathy, hip extension and abduction are normal and the sensory loss involves the L5 and S1 dermatomes and is over the lateral aspect of the shin, dorsum of the foot, the lateral aspect of the foot on both the dorsal and plantar surfaces and also over the calf.

L5 radiculopathy

Lumbar nerve root compression is a common cause of leg pain with or without a foot drop and occasionally patients present with a painless radiculopathy [70]. The neurological signs are listed in Figure 12.3. If sensory loss occurs, it is within the distribution of the 5th lumbar nerve root (see Figure 1.22).

Peripheral neuropathy

The list of causes of peripheral neuropathy is long and well beyond the scope of this book. Readers are referred to more definitive texts [71].

Earlier in this chapter we referred to significant hip flexion weakness related to the inflammatory demyelinating and IgA- and IgG-related peripheral neuropathies.

Other causes of peripheral neuropathy more typically present with weakness and/or sensory loss commencing in the toes and ascending up the foot and leg as the condition worsens. These neuropathies are often referred to as length dependent (because the abnormalities appear first in the longest nerves). The commonest are those related to alcohol, where weakness predominates, and diabetes, where distal symmetrical stocking distribution sensory loss is the main clinical feature.

Vitamin B_{12} deficiency is very rare, easily diagnosed and readily treatable so it should always be considered. In B_{12} deficiency the clinical picture is dominated by signs related to subacute combined degeneration of the spinal cord with marked vibration and proprioceptive loss in the limbs, resulting in significant ataxia and clumsiness exacerbated with eye closure or in the dark. Similar signs occur in paraneoplastic and Sjögren's related neuropathy as well as Friedreich's ataxia. The paraprotein related neuropathy with IgM is predominantly a length-dependent one with distal sensory loss and paraesthesia/dysaesthesia.

There are a variety of ways to classify the peripheral neuropathies:

- One way is to differentiate between single nerves being affected, referred to as mononeuropathy, multiple single nerves, the mononeuropathy multiplex, or diffuse involvement of the peripheral nervous system. In this section the peripheral neuropathies with diffuse involvement are discussed.
- A second way to characterise these neuropathies is the rapidity with which they develop, differentiating acute with onset over days to weeks, subacute with onset over months and chronic with onset over years.
- Nerve conduction studies are used to classify whether the peripheral neuropathy is axonal (affecting the axons) or whether it is demyelinating (affecting the myelin) and, in the case of demyelinating neuropathies, whether there is uniform slowing or conduction block (see additional information in Table 12.1 below).

TABLE 12.1 Features on NCS and EMG of demyelinating versus axonal neuropathies

	Demyelinating	Axonal
Amplitude of motor response	Normal or mildly reduced	Markedly reduced
Conduction velocity	Very slow	Normal or mildly reduced
Conduction block	Yes	No
Temporal dispersion[*]	Present	Absent
Distal motor latency	Prolonged	Not prolonged
Absent response	No	Possible
f-wave latencies	Prolonged	Not prolonged
EMG	No denervation	Denervation

[*]The term 'temporal dispersion' is where the proximal response (the site of stimulation is further up the arm or leg) is substantially lower in amplitude and of longer duration than the distal response.
EMG - electromyography; NCS - nerve conduction studies.

Most neuropathies are mixed axonal and demyelinating.

DIABETES AND THE PERIPHERAL NERVOUS SYSTEM

There are a number of peripheral nerve lesions that occur in the setting of diabetes.

- Acute neuropathies
  - Diabetic amyotrophy with proximal weakness and pain in the legs
  - Third nerve palsy, usually not involving the pupil
  - Truncal neuropathy with pain radiating around the lateral chest and abdominal wall toward the mid-line with sensory loss extending laterally from the mid-line anteriorly
- Chronic neuropathies
  - Distal sensory loss to pain and temperature that gradually ascends up the toes, feet and legs with increasing duration of diabetes
  - Autonomic neuropathy with postural hypotension, anhidrosis, nocturnal diarrhoea, hypothermia, dry eyes and mouth, impotence in males and bladder atony
  - Chronic proximal motor neuropathy

MANAGEMENT of PATIENTS with SUSPECTED PERIPHERAL NEUROPATHY

If a patient is suspected of having a peripheral neuropathy the initial investigation should be NCS and EMG (see Table 12.1). This will confirm the presence of peripheral neuropathy and should help characterise whether it is axonal, demyelinating or mixed axonal and demyelinating. The presence of conduction block on NCS indicates a demyelinating neuropathy in keeping with the acute and chronic inflammatory demyelinating neuropathies (AIDP, CIDP) or multifocal motor neuropathy with conduction block. If a peripheral neuropathy is confirmed, the following screening investigations would be appropriate:

- random blood glucose
- vitamin B_{12}
- immunoglobulin quantitation and protein electrophoresis
- Bence–Jones proteins.

Causes include:
- In clinical practice peripheral neuropathy most commonly relates to diabetes or alcohol in Western societies; the commonest cause worldwide is leprosy.
- The other more common causes include AIDP and CIDP, neuropathy related to mononclonal gammopathies such as IgG, IgM and IgA, drug-related neuropathy, uraemia, familial neuropathy and, although relatively rare, vitamin B12 deficiency should not be missed.
- There are many other causes including hereditary, toxic, metabolic, infectious (including HIV), inflammatory, ischaemic and paraneoplastic disorders. Occasionally, patients may present with a peripheral neuropathy in the setting of malignancy; more often the neuropathy appears after the diagnosis of the malignancy and the difficulty is to differentiate neuropathy related to drug therapy of the malignancy and a paraneoplastic neuropathy.
- In approximately 20% of patients a cause may not be established. A careful family history and examination of near relatives (including NCS) will detect a familial neuropathy in nearly half of the patients where the initial assessment fails to elucidate the cause.

Currently, peripheral neuropathies are classified as either demyelinating or axonal based largely on the results of NCS [72, 73].

The features on NCS and EMG of demyelinating versus axonal neuropathies are shown in Table 12.1 The term 'temporal dispersion' is where the proximal response (the site of stimulation is further up the arm or leg) is substantially lower in amplitude and of longer duration than the distal response and relates to differences in conduction of different fibres within the nerve. Conduction block (CB) refers to a marked reduction in the amplitude of the motor response between distal and proximal stimulation and/or prolongation of the distal motor latency, and is due to focal demyelination in the nerve. Occasionally, CB is so severe that no response can be obtained. CB cannot be diagnosed at sites where the nerve can be compressed, e.g. ulnar nerve at the elbow. The criteria for CB have varied over the years and are divided into definite or probable, based on the degree of reduction of amplitude and increase in duration of the motor response between distal versus proximal stimulation [74].

In patients with an acute onset neuropathy, e.g. AIDP, abnormalities on EMG (the study of muscle using a concentric needle electrode) are usually manifest within 7–10 days of onset of the illness but may not be evident for up to 3 weeks. When there is axonal damage, EMG demonstrates increased insertional (as the needle enters the muscle) activity, spontaneous activity in the form of fibrillation potentials and positive sharp waves (both indicative of denervation) with a reduced recruitment pattern (the diminished number of motor units recruited with voluntary contraction of the muscle is reflected in the baseline being visible between motor units). Fasciculations may be seen but are not synonymous with denervation.

Pain in the lower leg
RADICULOPATHY
Sciatica (also referred to as radiculopathy) refers to pain from compression of the nerve root, most commonly L5 or S1, less commonly L4.

Lumbar nerve root compression is a common cause of leg pain, and L5 radiculopathy accounts for 75% and L4 for 15% of these cases.

SYMPTOMS

- These patients present with pain radiating down the back of the thigh and lateral aspect of the shin to the dorsum of the foot with an L5 radiculopathy and to the medial aspect of the lower leg with an L4 radiculopathy.
- Pain related to disc herniation is exacerbated by bending forward, sitting, coughing or straining and is relieved by lying down or very rarely walking. Pain can occur in the absence of any weakness or sensory symptoms.
- If weakness does occur with an L5 radiculopathy, it affects dorsiflexion of the foot; inversion of the ankle is weaker than eversion as both the tibialis posterior and tibialis anterior muscles are affected; plantar flexion is normal.
- The area of sensory loss, if present, affects the lateral aspect of the shin and dorsal surface of the foot.
- A number of patients are seen with sciatic-like pain radiating from the buttock down to above the knee where no evidence of nerve root compression can be detected, and the aetiology of this pain is unclear.

MANAGEMENT of SCIATICA

Sciatica usually resolves without surgery within 12 months in 95% of patients [75]. If back pain is the major complaint and leg pain only a minor symptom then, in the absence of instability in the form of spondylolisthesis (one vertebra slips on another), back surgery is less likely to relieve symptoms and the patient may possibly best be treated conservatively with exercise and cognitive behaviour treatment [75, 76]. Even in patients with predominantly leg pain, the pain may settle with rest, NSAIDs, acetaminophen, skeletal muscle relaxants (for acute low back pain) or tricyclic antidepressants (for chronic low back pain). The anecdotal observation that oral corticosteroids appear to be of benefit has not been substantiated [77, 78].

Exercise-induced leg pain
LUMBAR CANAL STENOSIS (CAUDA EQUINA CLAUDICATION) VERSUS INTERMITTENT CLAUDICATION RELATED TO PERIPHERAL VASCULAR DISEASE

When a patient says they have pain in the legs, it is important to establish whether the pain is in the joints or elsewhere. This seems an obvious thing to do and yet is rarely performed. Pain in the joints exacerbated by weight bearing or by movement of the affected joint clearly indicates local pathology within the joint such as arthritis. The diagnosis of acute arthritis is not difficult when there is associated swelling, tenderness, redness and heat emanating from the joint. In long-standing arthritis there may be associated deformity of the joint; on the other hand, the joints will look normal in most patients presenting for the first time with arthritis. If the pain relates to arthritis, it should be reproduced when the joint is moved during the examination. There may also be a crackling sensation termed crepitus in the joint on movement [79].

> Localised pain and tenderness in the leg indicates local pathology and not referred pain from the back.

Pain symptoms

The pain resulting from PVD and the pain from lumbar canal stenosis (also termed cauda equina claudication) have many similarities.

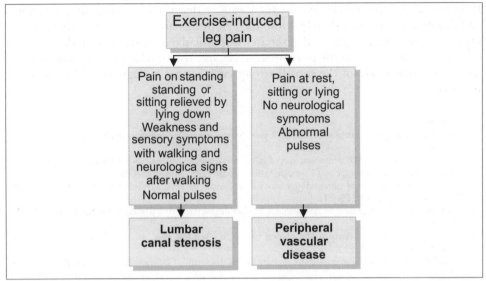

FIGURE 12.5 Organisational chart showing the different features of peripheral vascular disease versus lumbar canal stenosis

- In both, the pain is predominantly in the calves, not in the joints, and is precipitated by walking and relieved by resting for as little as a few minutes.
- The pain from lumbar canal stenosis resolves when the patient lies flat and may be precipitated by simply standing or even sitting.
- Rarely, patients with PVD and severe ischaemia may experience leg pain at rest. The rest pain is present and of the same intensity lying, sitting and standing.
- Leg pain exacerbated by an alteration in posture indicates probable lumbar canal stenosis.
- When the pain in the legs is associated with neurological symptoms, clearly the exercise-induced leg pain is related to lumbar canal stenosis. The associated neurological symptoms may consist of paraesthesia or numbness in the feet and/or the development of weakness (a foot drop).
- Much less commonly the pain may be in the genital region, resulting in priapism or vulval pain. Once again the pain is exacerbated by sitting, standing or walking and relieved by lying flat or the cessation of walking. Symptoms in the genital region indicate involvement of the sacral nerve roots.
- The pain of lumbar canal stenosis is usually but not always associated with low back pain, whereas the pain of PVD is not. In both conditions there may the associated buttock pain and in patients with PVD this relates to disease in the internal iliac vessels.

Examination
Examination of the lower limbs can differentiate between these two entities:
- In patients with PVD the peripheral pulses, particularly in the feet, are diminished or absent.
- Often, but not invariably, in patients with lumbar canal stenosis the ankle reflexes are absent, although this is not always a useful sign as many elderly patients have absent ankle reflexes as a normal finding.

It is often useful to send the patient for a walk so that the symptoms are precipitated and examine them immediately while the symptoms are still present. The development of neurological signs with exercise, in particular sensory loss in the feet, loss of reflexes that were present prior to exercise and the development of weakness, in particular dorsiflexion of the feet, is strong evidence for a diagnosis of lumbar canal stenosis.

REFERENCES

1   Chou R et al. Imaging strategies for low-back pain: Systematic review and meta-analysis. Lancet 2009; 373(9662):463–472.

2   Avrahami E et al. Early MR demonstration of spinal metastases in patients with normal radiographs and CT and radionuclide bone scans. J Comput Assist Tomogr 1989; 13(4):598–602.

3   Algra PR et al. Detection of vertebral metastases: Comparison between MR imaging and bone scintigraphy. RadioGraphics 1991; 11:219–232.

4   Madigan L et al. Management of symptomatic lumbar degenerative disk disease. J Am Acad Orthop Surg 2009; 17(2):102–111.

5   Malmivaara A et al. The treatment of acute low back pain – bed rest, exercises, or ordinary activity? N Engl J Med 1995; 332(6):351–355.

6   Assendelft WJ et al. Spinal manipulative therapy for low back pain. Cochrane Database Syst Rev 2004(1):CD000447.

7   van Tulder MW, FurlanAD, Gagnier JJ. Complementary and alternative therapies for low back pain. Best Pract Res Clin Rheumatol 2005; 19(4):639–654.

8   Waller B, Lambeck J, Daly D. Therapeutic aquatic exercise in the treatment of low back pain: A systematic review. Clin Rehabil 2009; 23(1):3–14.

9   Haim A et al. Meralgia paresthetica: A retrospective analysis of 79 patients evaluated and treated according to a standard algorithm. Acta Orthop 2006; 77(3):482–486.

10   Khalil N, Nicotra A, Rakowicz W. Treatment for meralgia paraesthetica. Cochrane Database Syst Rev 2008(3):CD004159.

11   Ducic I, Dellon AL, Taylor NS. Decompression of the lateral femoral cutaneous nerve in the treatment of meralgia paresthetica. J Reconstr Microsurg 2006; 22(2):113–118.

12   Krendel DA, Zacharias A, Younger DS. Autoimmune diabetic neuropathy. Neurol Clin 1997; 15(4): 959–971.

13   Sander HW, Chokroverty S. Diabetic amyotrophy: Current concepts. Semin Neurol 1996; 16(2):173–178.

14   Said G et al. Painful proximal diabetic neuropathy: Inflammatory nerve lesions and spontaneous favorable outcome. Ann Neurol 1997; 41(6):762–770.

15   Ogawa T et al. Intravenous immunoglobulin therapy for diabetic amyotrophy. Intern Med 2001; 40(4):349–352.

16   Courtney AE, McDonnell GV, Patterson VH. Human immunoglobulin for diabetic amyotrophy – a promising prospect? Postgrad Med J 2001; 77(907):326–328.

17   Salvarani C, Cantini F, Hunder GG. Polymyalgia rheumatica and giant-cell arteritis. Lancet 2008; 372(9634):234–245.

18   Salvarani C et al. Polymyalgia rheumatica and giant cell arteritis: A 5-year epidemiologic and clinical study in Reggio Emilia, Italy. Clin Exp Rheumatol 1987; 5(3):205–215.

19   Le Quintrec JS, Le Quintrec JL. Drug-induced myopathies. Baillieres Clin Rheumatol 1991; 5(1):21–38.

20   Kuncl RW, George EB. Toxic neuropathies and myopathies. Curr Opin Neurol 1993; 6(5):695–704.

21   Wiendl H. Idiopathic inflammatory myopathies: Current and future therapeutic options. Neurotherapeutics 2008; 5(4):548–557.

22   Walker UA. Imaging tools for the clinical assessment of idiopathic inflammatory myositis. Curr Opin Rheumatol 2008; 20(6):656–661.

23   Choy EH et al. Immunosuppressant and immunomodulatory treatment for dermatomyositis and polymyositis. Cochrane Database Syst Rev 2005(3):CD003643.

24   Tran HA. Thyrotoxic periodic paralysis. Mayo Clin Proc 2005; 80(7):960–961;author reply 961.

25   Lichtstein DM, Arteaga RB. Rhabdomyolysis associated with hyperthyroidism. Am J Med Sci 2006; 332(2):103–105.

26   Tuncel D et al. Hoffmann's syndrome: A case report. Med Princ Pract 2008; 17(4):346–348.

27   Ekbom KA. Restless legs; a report of 70 new cases. Acta Med Scand Suppl 1950; 246:64–68.

28   Satija P, Ondo WG. Restless legs syndrome: Pathophysiology, diagnosis and treatment. CNS Drugs 2008; 22(6):497–518.

29.   Benes H et al. Definition of restless legs syndrome, how to diagnose it, and how to differentiate it from RLS mimics. Mov Disord 2007; 22(Suppl18):S401–S408.

30 Oertel WH et al. State of the art in restless legs syndrome therapy: Practice recommendations for treating restless legs syndrome. Mov Disord 2007; 22(Suppl18):S466–S475.

31 Hening WA. Current guidelines and standards of practice for restless legs syndrome. Am J Med 2007; 120(1 Suppl 1):S22–S27.

32 Silber MH et al. An algorithm for the management of restless legs syndrome. Mayo Clin Proc 2004; 79(7):916–922.

33 Conti CF et al. Levodopa for idiopathic restless legs syndrome: Evidence-based review. Mov Disord 2007; 22(13):1943–1951.

34 Wagner ML et al. Randomized, double-blind, placebo-controlled study of clonidine in restless legs syndrome. Sleep 1996; 19(1):52–58.

35 Ferini-Strambi L et al. Effect of pramipexole on RLS symptoms and sleep: A randomized, double-blind, placebo-controlled trial. Sleep Med 2008; 9(8):874–881.

36 Bliwise DL et al. Randomized, double-blind, placebo-controlled, short-term trial of ropinirole in restless legs syndrome. Sleep Med 2005; 6(2):141–147.

37 Trenkwalder C et al. Efficacy of rotigotine for treatment of moderate-to-severe restless legs syndrome: A randomised, double-blind, placebo-controlled trial. Lancet Neurol 2008; 7(7):595–604.

38 Walters AS et al. Successful treatment of the idiopathic restless legs syndrome in a randomized double-blind trial of oxycodone versus placebo. Sleep 1993; 16(4):327–332.

39 Ondo WG. Methadone for refractory restless legs syndrome. Mov Disord 2005; 20(3):345–348.

40 Dressler D et al. The syndrome of painful legs and moving toes. Mov Disord 1994; 9(1):13–21.

41 Walters AS et al. Painless legs and moving toes: A syndrome related to painful legs and moving toes? Mov Disord 1993; 8(3):377–379.

42 Alvarez MV et al. Case series of painful legs and moving toes: Clinical and electrophysiologic observations. Mov Disord 2008; 23(14):2062–2066.

43 Tavee J, Zhou L. Small fiber neuropathy: A burning problem. Cleve Clin J Med 2009; 76(5):297–305.

44 Singleton JR, Smith AG, Bromberg MB. Increased prevalence of impaired glucose tolerance in patients with painful sensory neuropathy. Diabetes Care 2001; 24(8):1448–1453.

45 Penza P et al. Painful neuropathy in subclinical hypothyroidism: Clinical and neuropathological recovery after hormone replacement therapy. Neurol Sci 2009; 30(2):149–151.

46 Gonzalez-Duarte A, Robinson-Papp J, Simpson DM. Diagnosis and management of HIV-associated neuropathy. Neurol Clin 2008; 26(3):821–832.

47 Makkar RP et al. Burning feet syndrome: A clinical review. Aust Fam Physician 2003; 32(12):1006–1009.

48 Vinik AI. Diabetic neuropathy: Pathogenesis and therapy. Am J Med 1999; 107(2B):17S–26S.

49 Balakrishnan S et al. A randomized parallel trial of topical aspirin-moisturizer solution vs. oral aspirin for acute herpetic neuralgia. Int J Dermatol 2001; 40(8):535–538.

50 Buttaci CJ. Erythromelalgia: A case report and literature review. Pain Med 2006; 7(6):534–538.

51 Cohen JS. Erythromelalgia: New theories and new therapies. J Am Acad Dermatol 2000; 43(5 Pt 1):841–847.

52 Kuhnert SM, Phillips WJ, Davis MD. Lidocaine and mexiletine therapy for erythromelalgia. Arch Dermatol 1999; 135(12):1447–1449.

53 Goodgold J, Kopell HP, Spielholz NI. The tarsal-tunnel syndrome: Objective diagnostic criteria. N Engl J Med 1965; 273(14):742–745.

54 Alshami AM, Souvlis T, Coppieters MW. A review of plantar heel pain of neural origin: Differential diagnosis and management. Man Ther 2008; 13(2):103–111.

55 Sammarco GJ, Chang L. Outcome of surgical treatment of tarsal tunnel syndrome. Foot Ankle Int 2003; 24(2):125–131.

56 Patel AT et al. Usefulness of electrodiagnostic techniques in the evaluation of suspected tarsal tunnel syndrome: An evidence-based review. Muscle Nerve 2005; 32(2):236–240.

57 Erickson SJ et al. MR imaging of the tarsal tunnel and related spaces: Normal and abnormal findings with anatomic correlation. Am J Roentgenol 1990; 155(2):323–328.

58 Mullick T, Dellon AL. Results of decompression of four medial ankle tunnels in the treatment of tarsal tunnel syndrome. J Reconstr Microsurg 2008; 24(2):119–126.

59 Hassouna H, Singh D. Morton's metatarsalgia: Pathogenesis, aetiology and current management. Acta Orthop Belg 2005; 71(6):646–655.

60 Redd RA et al. Morton neuroma: Sonographic evaluation. Radiology 1989; 171(2):415–417.

61 Thomson CE, Gibson JN, Martin D. Interventions for the treatment of Morton's neuroma. Cochrane Database Syst Rev 2004(3):CD003118.

62 Prichasuk S, Subhadrabandhu T. The relationship of pes planus and calcaneal spur to plantar heel pain. Clin Orthop Relat Res 1994(306):192–196.

63 Buchbinder R. Plantar fasciitis. N Engl J Med 2004; 350:2159.

64 Batt ME, Tanji JL, Skattum N. Plantar fasciitis: A prospective randomized clinical trial of the tension night splint. Clin J Sport Med 1996; 6(3):158–162.

65   Kudo P et al. Randomized, placebo-controlled, double-blind clinical trial evaluating the treatment of plantar fasciitis with an extracorporeal shockwave therapy (ESWT) device: A North American confirmatory study. J Orthop Res 2006; 24(2):115–123.

66   Kalaci A et al. Treatment of plantar fasciitis using four different local injection modalities: A randomized prospective clinical trial. J Am Podiatr Med Assoc 2009; 99(2):108–113.

67   Cole C, Seto C, Gazewood J. Plantar fasciitis: Evidence-based review of diagnosis and therapy. Am Fam Physician 2005; 72(11):2237–2242.

68   Berry H, Richardson PM. Common peroneal nerve palsy: A clinical and electrophysiological review. J Neurol Neurosurg Psychiatry 1976; 39(12):1162–1171.

69   Kempster P et al. Painful sciatic neuropathy following cardiac surgery. Aust N Z J Med 1991; 21(5): 732–735.

70   Lipetz JS, Misra N, Silber JS. Resolution of pronounced painless weakness arising from radiculopathy and disk extrusion. Am J Phys Med Rehabil 2005; 84(7):528–537.

71   Dyck PJ, Thomas PK. Peripheral neuropathy, 4th edn. Philadelphia: Saunders; 2005.

72   Donofrio PD, Albers JW. AAEM minimonograph No. 34: Polyneuropathy: Classification by nerve conduction studies and electromyography. Muscle Nerve 1990; 13(10):889–903.

73   Tankisi H et al. Pathophysiology inferred from electrodiagnostic nerve tests and classification of polyneuropathies: Suggested guidelines. Clin Neurophysiol 2005; 116(7):1571–1580.

74   Olney RK. Guidelines in electrodiagnostic medicine: Consensus criteria for the diagnosis of partial conduction block. Muscle Nerve Suppl 1999; 8:S225–S229.

75   Legrand E et al. Sciatica from disk herniation: Medical treatment or surgery? Joint Bone Spine 2007; 74(6):530–535.

76   Mirza SK, Deyo RA. Systematic review of randomized trials comparing lumbar fusion surgery to nonoperative care for treatment of chronic back pain. Spine 2007; 32(7):816–823.

77   Chou R et al. Correction: Diagnosis and treatment of low back pain. Ann Intern Med 2008; 148(3): 247–248.

78   Chou R, Huffman LH. Medications for acute and chronic low back pain: A review of the evidence for an American Pain Society/American College of Physicians clinical practice guideline. Ann Intern Med 2007; 147(7):505–514.

79   Apley AG, Solomon L. Osteoarthritis and related disorders. In: Concise system of orthopaedics and fractures. Oxford: Butterworth–Heinemann; 1994:36–41.

chapter 13

Abnormal Movements and Difficulty Walking Due to Central Nervous System Problems

In the previous chapter difficulty walking that is related to peripheral nervous system problems was discussed. The first half of this chapter deals with the more common central nervous system problems that result in difficulty walking; the second half discusses abnormal movements affecting the face, head and limbs, some of which lead to difficulty walking.

Difficulty walking related to weakness and/or sensory disturbances in one or both lower limbs occurs with spinal cord, brainstem or cerebral hemisphere problems affecting the motor and/or sensory pathways. Unsteadiness in the legs in the absence of weakness can occur with vertigo or with problems in the cerebellar pathways including the cerebellar connections in the brainstem, in the extrapyramidal system such as Parkinson's syndrome or a frontal lobe disorder referred to as an apraxic gait. Patients with severe visual impairment due to either ocular or occipital lobe problems will have difficulty walking but this is not discussed in this chapter.

'My legs are weak, Doc.' When a patient states that their legs are weak, ask them to clarify exactly what they mean. Patients often use the term weakness as a non-specific way to say that something is wrong with their legs, and they do not necessarily mean that there is an actual loss of strength in their legs. Often, in fact, the legs are strong and the difficulty relates to other neurological and non-neurological problems.

DIFFICULTY WALKING

When a patient complains that they are have difficulty walking, simply ask if the difficulty relates to a sense of instability in the head or something wrong with their legs or if they are uncertain why they are having problems. Figure 13.1 shows the diagnostic possibilities in each of these three scenarios.

Difficulty walking related to weakness
The presence of weakness in the legs infers a problem involving the motor pathway, which extends from the motor cortex to the muscle.

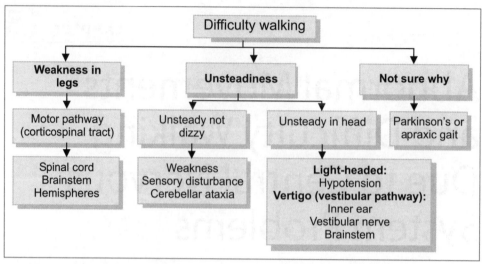

FIGURE 13.1   The clinical approach to difficulty walking related to central nervous system problems

One needs to determine if the weakness is related to spinal cord, brain stem or cerebral hemisphere pathology. This can be very difficult if weakness is the only symptom. Although bilateral leg weakness is more common in patients with spinal cord problems, it can occur in conditions that affect the brainstem and very rarely the parafalcine region of the cerebral hemispheres. Unilateral leg weakness is more in keeping with a cerebral hemisphere problem but, once again, can occur with brainstem or spinal cord involvement. Some potential clues that may help determine the site of the pathology are listed below.

Clues that the *spinal cord is the site of the problem*:
- Back or neck pain that coincides with the development of neurological symptoms in the lower limbs
- Alteration in sphincter function with constipation and/or urinary retention
- Altered sensation with a sensory level on the trunk (a strong indicator)

Clues that the *brainstem is the site of the problem*:
- Vertigo
- Diplopia
- Dysphagia (to a lesser extent)
- Ipsilateral facial sensory loss and contralateral loss to pain and temperature affecting the limbs (lateral brainstem involvement)
- A 12th, 6th or 3rd nerve palsy on the side opposite to the weakness points to the medulla, pons and midbrain, respectively (see Chapter 4, 'The cranial nerves and understanding the brainstem')

Clues that the *cerebral hemisphere is the site of the problem*:
- When there is upper motor neuron facial weakness in addition to the weakness in the arm and leg, the lesion must be above the mid pons on the contralateral side and, therefore, cannot be any lower in the brainstem or in the spinal cord. If areas in the hemispheres other than the motor pathway are affected, it may be possible to localise the lesion to the hemispheres, in particular the cerebral cortex.

- Dysphasia (dominant hemisphere lesions affecting the cortex)
- Gerstmann's syndrome
- Visual field loss (hemianopia or quadrantanopia) if the visual pathways are affected
- Visual inattention if the parietal cortex is affected
- Cortical sensory signs (2-point discrimination, graphaesthesia, stereognosis or sensory inattention) (Other cortical phenomena are described in Chapter 5, 'The cerebral hemispheres and cerebellum'.)

SPINAL CORD PROBLEMS

The three common spinal cord problems that result in leg weakness are cervical spondylitic myelopathy, thoracic cord compression, most often due to malignancy, and transverse myelitis.

There are many other rarer conditions that can affect the spinal cord and are traditionally divided into:

1 lesions external to the dura (traumatic spinal cord compression, prolapsed intervertebral discs, epidural abscess)
2 lesions beneath the dura but external to the spinal cord (neurofibroma, Chiari malformation)
3 intrinsic spinal cord problems (glioma, ependymoma, sarcoidosis, vasculitis, syphilis, arteriovenous malformation, spinal cord infarction and adrenomyeloneuropathy). These *are very rare conditions and are beyond the scope of this book.*

The features that point to intrinsic cord pathology are:

- early development urinary or anal sphincter dysfunction
- early involvement of the spinothalamic tract
- suspended sensory loss, which is a classical feature of an intrinsic spinal cord problem where there is altered pain and temperature sensation in a pattern that resembles a cape with impaired sensation on the upper trunk but sparing the lower trunk and lower limbs.
- early sacral sensory loss occurs with extrinsic compression and sacral sparing is seen with intrinsic spinal cord lesions; the presence of radicular pain indicates lesions extrinsic to the dura.

No neurology textbook would be complete without mentioning the Brown–Sequard hemicord syndrome that consists of ipsilateral weakness and ipsilateral impairment of vibration and proprioception with contralateral impairment of pain and temperature sensation indicative of involvement of one half of the spinal cord. The explanation for this clinical syndrome is that the motor fibres and dorsal columns cross the midline at the level of the foramen magnum while the spinothalamic tract crosses in the spinal cord close to the entry into the spinal cord of the dorsal nerve root conveying sensation.

Cervical spondylotic myelopathy (CSM)

Cervical spondylotic myelopathy (CSM) is the commonest cause of spinal cord dysfunction in elderly patients. It is also the commonest cause of paraparesis or quadriparesis not related to trauma. Repeated occupational trauma, such as carrying axial loads, genetic predisposition and Down syndrome all predispose to an increased risk of cervical spondylosis.

Cervical spondylosis relates to degenerative changes initially in the cervical discs with subsequent subperiosteal bone formation, referred to as osteophytes. Cervical disc protrusion or extrusion, osteophytes and hypertrophy of the ligamentum flavum

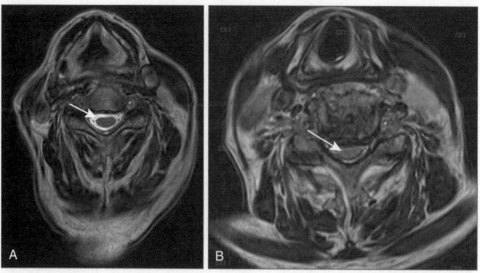

FIGURE 13.2 MRI scan of **A** normal cervical spine and **B** spinal cord compression due to cervical spondylosis

together result in spinal cord compression, and secondary spinal cord ischaemia can occur with severe compression. Rarely spondylolisthesis may occur and cause cord compression.

Cervical cord compression (see Figure 13.2) can be seen in younger patients with congenitally narrow spinal canals (10–13 mm). The spinal cord is stretched during flexion of the cervical spine and buckling of the ligamentum flavum occurs during extension of the cervical spine. Thus, repeated flexion and extension in the patient with significant canal narrowing may cause intermittent acute compression of the spinal cord, and it is thought that this may also account for the clinical deterioration seen in many cases of CSM [1].

The natural course of CSM for any given individual is variable and precise prognostication is not possible. Once moderate signs and symptoms develop, however, patients are less likely to spontaneously improve. Worsening occurs more commonly in older patients whereas patients with mild disability are less likely to worsen [1].

CSM can present in a variety of ways.

1 The commonest presentation is with the insidious onset of difficulty walking related to weakness and/or stiffness (due to spasticity). Some patients will have neck pain from the cervical spondylosis; pain in the arm related to nerve root compression is less common.

2 Older patients in particular may present with weakness and wasting of the small muscles of the hands related to nerve root compression, and the signs of spinal cord compression are noted when they are examined.

3 A presentation that is much less common is the central cord syndrome resulting from a hyperextension injury in the setting of cervical canal stenosis where the weakness is greater in the upper than the lower limbs with or without a suspended sensory loss (affecting the shoulders and upper torso like a cape) and urinary retention.

4 Patients with cervical cord compression may experience an electric shock-like ensation radiating down their back or into their limbs with neck flexion, the so-called L'Hermitte phenomena commonly seen in patients with multiple sclerosis (MS).

The examination will reveal someone who may walk with a stiff-legged gait if there is associated spasticity, the tone will be increased with or without sustained ankle clonus, the knee reflexes will be abnormally brisk; ankle reflexes are often absent in the elderly and this should not exclude consideration of cervical cord compression. The plantar should be up-going but this is not universal.

> Some elderly patients assume that the gradual onset of difficulty walking is simply the result of advancing age and tend not to seek medical attention until the cord compression and limb weakness are severe.

MANAGEMENT of CERVICAL SPONDYLOTIC MYELOPATHY

Investigations

- A plain X-ray of the cervical spine may demonstrate degenerative disease, but this is common in elderly patients in the absence of cervical cord compression.
- Similarly, a CT scan of the cervical spine may demonstrate degenerative disease but currently is not sensitive enough to adequately evaluate the presence of cervical nerve root or cervical spinal cord compression.
- Magnetic resonance imaging (MRI) is currently the imaging modality of choice in patients suspected of having cervical cord compression.

Treatment

There are no prospective randomised controlled trials comparing medical management with surgery for CSM. The choice of therapy will be dictated by the patient's attitude to surgery, the severity of the cervical cord compression and the fitness from the medical point of view of the patient to undergo surgery. Patients are advised that the goal of surgery is to prevent worsening and that improvement cannot be guaranteed, although many patients do in fact improve following appropriate surgery. Many neurosurgeons would recommend a period of observation in patients with mild symptoms and signs, but it would seem reasonable to recommend surgery for patients with moderate disability. Once moderate signs and symptoms develop, however, patients are less likely to spontaneously improve and such patients should consider surgical decompression.

Thoracic cord compression

Thoracic spinal cord compression most commonly occurs with metastatic malignancy, less commonly with a thoracic disc, epidural abscess or extrinsic spinal cord tumour such as a meningioma or a neurofibroma. There is an aphorism that 'a thoracic cord lesion in a middle-aged to elderly female is a meningioma (benign tumour arising from the meninges) until proven otherwise'. Back pain is rare with a meningioma, more common but not a universal feature of thoracic discs, but *increasingly severe* back pain occurs for on average 8 weeks or longer in 80–95% of patients who subsequently develop malignant cord compression [2]. Patients who are not known to suffer from malignancy, but who develop increasingly severe midline (especially thoracic) back pain, should be investigated promptly in the hope of preventing malignant cord compression.

Although initially the pain is localised to the vertebra, subsequent nerve root compression can result in radicular pain. The back pain is often worse after lying down and this can be *a vital clue*. Rapidly developing weakness in the legs is the initial and dominant neurological symptom once malignant spinal cord compression occurs; sensory symptoms are less common and sphincter disturbance occurs late. A delay in the diagnosis of malignant cord compression is common with many patients only diagnosed after they lose their ability to walk [2, 3] and, unfortunately, once significant cord compression related to malignancy occurs the prognosis for recovery is poor.

In patients with preexisting malignancy, particularly breast and prostate, the development of back pain should raise the suspicion of possible secondary malignancy in the spinal column and prompt investigation (see Figure 13.3).

The following suggest spinal metastases:
- pain in the thoracic or cervical spine
- severe unremitting or progressive lumbar spinal pain
- spinal pain aggravated by straining
- nocturnal spinal pain preventing sleep
- localised spinal tenderness [4].

It has been recommended that patients with known malignancy should be advised to return urgently within 24 hours for review should they develop back pain in the midline [4].

Severe thoracic back pain followed by the rapid development of spinal cord compression can be the initial manifestation of malignancy in as many as one-third of patients with cancer of unknown primary origin, non-Hodgkin lymphoma, myeloma and lung cancer [2]. Metastatic disease less commonly affects the cervical or lumbar spine. Although almost any systemic cancer can metastasise to the spinal column, prostate, breast and lung are the most common [2].

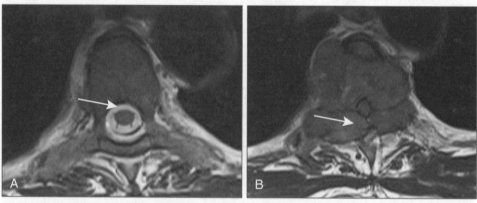

FIGURE 13.3 MRI scan of **A** thoracic spinal cord normal (the arrow shows normal CSF around the spinal cord) and **B** malignant thoracic spinal cord compression (the arrow points to the malignancy; the CSF space is obliterated)

MANAGEMENT of MALIGNANT CORD COMPRESSION

Investigations
- Plain X-rays and nuclear bone scans may detect metastases in the vertebrae but will not detect cord compression [5].
- MRI is currently the modality of choice in the detection of malignant cord compression [6, 7].

Treatment
- Corticosteroids result in a significantly better outcome in terms of ambulation in patients undergoing radiotherapy for malignant cord compression [8]. Dexamethasone at a dose in the range of 16–100 mg/day is probably appropriate [2].
- Surgical decompression combined with postoperative radiotherapy result in more patients able to walk than radiotherapy alone [9].

Intrinsic spinal cord problems

Transverse myelitis is the commonest intrinsic cord lesion resulting in dysfunction in the lower limbs and difficulty walking in the younger patient while spinal cord ischaemia is seen in the elderly. Spinal cord ischaemia can develope abruptly or insidiously. *Other intrinsic spinal cord problems such as tumours and the cavitating lesion referred to as syringomyelia are very rare* and are beyond the scope of this book.

TRANSVERSE MYELITIS

Acute transverse myelitis (ATM) is a focal inflammatory disorder of the spinal cord, resulting in motor, sensory and autonomic dysfunction with many infectious and non-infectious causes [10].

The Transverse Myelitis Consortium Working Group [11] has established diagnostic criteria that require:

- bilateral signs and/or symptoms of spinal cord dysfunction affecting the motor, sensory and autonomic systems
- a clearly defined sensory level
- the exclusion of cord compression
- the demonstration of inflammation within the cerebrospinal fluid (CSF). If none of the inflammatory criteria is met at symptom onset, repeat MRI and lumbar puncture evaluation should be performed between 2 and 7 days following symptom onset.

The development of neurological symptoms and signs is often preceded by a febrile illness up to 4 weeks prior to onset [12], typically an upper respiratory tract infection. Patients present with an ascending sensory loss, with the development of a sensory level in the majority of patients with or without a paraparesis, paraplegia, quadriplegia and urinary retention [12, 13]. The *symptoms may develop rapidly over as little as 4 hours or more slowly over several weeks.*

In one study of acute transverse myelitis, a parainfectious cause was diagnosed in 38% of patients but the underlying infectious agent was identified in a minority of patients. In 36% of patients the aetiology remained uncertain and in 22% it was the first manifestation of possible MS. The MRI scan (see Figure 13.4) was abnormal in 96% of cases (i.e. a normal MRI is rare but does not exclude a diagnosis) [12].

> Patients whose spinal cord symptoms reach maximal severity in < 4 hours from onset should be presumed to have an ischaemic aetiology [1].

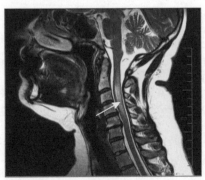

FIGURE 13.4   MRI scan of transverse myelitis

Acute non-compressive myelopathies can also be classified according to their aetiology [14]:

1 multiple sclerosis
2 systemic disease (e.g. systemic lupus erythematosus [SLE], antiphospholipid syndrome, Sjögren's syndrome
3 parainfectious
4 delayed radiation myelopathy
5 spinal cord infarct
6 idiopathic myelopathy.

MANAGEMENT of TRANSVERSE MYELITIS

Patients suspected of having transverse myelitis should have an MRI scan and a lumbar puncture.
 The CSF is abnormal [14] with:

• mildly elevated protein (except in post-infectious myelopathy where it may exceed 1 g/L)
• lymphocytic pleocytosis (as low as 1 cell/mm^3 in delayed radiation myelopathy to as high as 320 cells/mm^3 in post-infectious myelopathy)
• a normal CSF glucose
• negative CSF cytology for malignant cells.

 MRI scanning usually but not invariably reveals abnormalities that may be restricted to one or many spinal segments [13]. Typically the MRI signal changes extend at least three segments above the sensory level.

 In western countries transverse myelitis may be the presenting feature of MS or it may manifest during the course of this disease. Patients who are ultimately diagnosed with MS are more likely to have asymmetric clinical findings, predominant sensory symptoms with relative sparing of motor systems, MRI lesions extending over fewer than two spinal segments, abnormal brain MRI and oligoclonal bands in the CSF [11]. It is important to test for oligoclonal bands in the CSF and serum to detect intrathecal synthesis seen with MS.

CONUS MEDULLARIS LESION

This chapter has discussed central nervous system causes of difficulty walking whereas the previous chapter discussed peripheral nervous system problems. There is one very rare syndrome that produces both upper and lower motor neuron signs in the lower limbs and this is a lesion at the level of the conus medullaris (the lower end of the spinal cord at the level of the 2nd lumbar vertebra) with or without the involvement of the cauda equina (the sheath of lumbosacral nerve that extends from the lower end of the spinal cord through the spinal canal exiting at the appropriate level and that looks like a horse's tail, hence the name).

The clinical signs in a pure conus medullaris lesion consist of impaired sensation affecting the lower sacral nerve roots (S3–S5) with urinary retention and urinary or faecal incontinence. If the cauda equina is also involved there will be low back pain, weakness and sensory loss in the lower limbs that is asymmetrical, but it usually affects the lower lumbar and upper sacral nerve roots (L5–S1), resulting in foot drop and absent ankle reflexes.

BRAINSTEM PROBLEMS CAUSING WEAKNESS IN THE LEG(S)

Weakness caused by brainstem problems is usually unilateral or bilateral weakness affecting the lower limbs with or without involvement of the upper limbs and, if above the mid pons, the face. It is the presence of symptoms and signs pointing to the brainstem (see Chapter 4, 'The cranial nerves and understanding the brainstem') that is the clue to the site of the pathology.

As brainstem tumours are very rare, the most likely causes of motor weakness related to brainstem pathology are cerebral ischaemia in older patients, where the onset will be sudden, and demyelinating disease in younger patients, where the onset will be over hours to days.

CEREBRAL HEMISPHERE PROBLEMS CAUSING WEAKNESS IN THE LEG(S)

Weakness related to cerebral hemisphere problems is almost invariably unilateral, although bilateral lower limb weakness can occur with involvement of the parafalcine region, typically with cerebral infarction in the distribution of the anterior cerebral artery. The presence of abulia (see Chapter 5, 'The cerebral hemispheres and cerebellum') is the clue that the lesion is affecting the distribution of the anterior cerebral artery.

Cerebrovascular disease is the most likely cause of motor weakness related to the motor pathways in the cerebral hemispheres, either ischaemia or haemorrhage. Demyelinating diseases and both benign and malignant (primary or secondary) tumours are the other more common causes although both of these are rare. CT scanning, but in particular MRI scanning, can readily establish the pathology.

Difficulty walking due to unsteadiness

When patients complain that they are unsteady on their feet, it is important to clarify whether this sense of instability relates to a feeling of dizziness or instability in the head or whether it relates to something wrong in the legs suggesting a problem in either the spinal cord or peripheral nervous system.

UNSTEADINESS RELATED TO DIZZINESS IN THE HEAD

Vertigo is 'an illusion of movement', often rotary, with the sensation as if the room or head is spinning and it renders the patient unable to walk. The presence of vertigo with the head or room spinning clearly indicates the problem is either in the peripheral vestibular system, where there may be associated tinnitus and/or deafness, or in the brainstem where the presence of diplopia, weakness and sensory symptoms may accompany the vertigo.

A less marked vertigo includes a sensation of instability, a feeling of disequilibrium like being on a ship, but can also include sensations of tipping, tilting, falling etc. The more one strays from the sense of rotation, the less one can be sure that the problem causing instability is within the vestibular system. This sense of dizziness in the head could also relate to hypotension.

UNSTEADINESS IN THE ABSENCE OF WEAKNESS OR DIZZINESS

Patients with bilateral vestibular hypofunction (e.g. due to aminoglycoside toxicity) do not present with vertigo but with a sense of disequilibrium.

Patients with marked impairment of proprioception in the lower limbs will be very unsteady on their feet, particularly in the dark and when they close their eyes, e.g. while having a shower or washing their hair. This is often referred to as a sensory ataxia. Vitamin B_{12} deficiency with subacute combined degeneration of the cord is probably the commonest cause now that syphilis has largely been eradicated. *Very rarely, impairment of proprioception results from a dorsal root ganglionopathy or sensory neuronopathy.* This occurs as a paraneoplastic phenomenon [15, 16], in patients with Sjögren's syndrome [17] or pyridoxine abuse [18]. The sensory ganglionopathies are extremely rare and are mentioned here because the neurological problem may antedate the diagnosis of malignancy or indicate recurrence in a patient with known malignancy and should prompt a search for malignancy [16].

Another cause of difficulty walking from unsteadiness in the absence of dizziness in the head or weakness in the legs is the ataxia related to cerebellar disease. Ataxia in the limbs reflects problems in the cerebellar hemispheres whereas ataxia affecting the trunk (truncal ataxia) is seen in patients with problems related to the midline vermis of the cerebellum.

Truncal ataxia occurs with hypothyroidism [19] and alcoholism [20]. Patients with isolated truncal ataxia walk with a wide-based gait with little in the way of nystagmus or ataxia in the limbs.

The commonest cause of ataxia related to cerebellar disease would be cerebellar infarction. Two less common causes of cerebellar ataxia affecting the cerebellar hemispheres are the paraneoplastic cerebellar syndrome [21] and the hereditary spinocerebellar atrophies (SCA) [22]. The paraneoplastic cerebellar syndrome may be the initial presenting symptom of malignancy or develop after the diagnosis of malignancy is established. The clinical picture is one of very disabling ataxia affecting the limbs and trunk, together with dysarthria and nystagmus evolving rapidly over days to weeks. On the other hand, the hereditary spinocerebellar atrophies present with the insidious onset of ataxia affecting the limbs with or without nystagmus and dysarthria.

Difficulty walking not sure why

There are two conditions, Parkinson's and the apraxia of gait, where patients have increasing difficulty walking in the absence of any obvious weakness or sensory disturbance in the lower limbs or any sensation of instability in the head, and the patients are uncertain why they are having difficulty. In both conditions the patient will appear to walk with short steps: in Parkinson's the patients shuffle while they walk whereas with the apraxia of gait the steps are short but the patient does not shuffle. It can be very difficult at times to differentiate Parkinson's disease from the apraxic gait.

PARKINSON'S SYNDROME

Parkinson's syndrome is a term used to describe patients with clinical features that include one or more of:
- a resting tremor
- stooped posture
- slowness of movement referred to as bradykinesia
- cogwheel rigidity (increased tone that has a sensation of the muscle giving way in little jerks).

The commonest cause of Parkinson's syndrome is Parkinson's disease, but drugs (such as phenothiazines, butyrophenones, metoclopramide, reserpine and tetrabenazine) may cause a reversible Parkinson's syndrome, and toxins (such as manganese dust or carbon disulfide) and the recreational drug N-methyl-4-phenyl-1,2,3,6-tetrahydropyridine (MPTP) cause an irreversible Parkinson's syndrome [23] by destroying the dopamine neurons in the midbrain. The term 'Parkinson's disease' is reserved for patients with the above clinical features who have the characteristic neuropathology of loss of pigmentation in the substantia nigra and the presence of the Lewy bodies.

Parkinson's is largely a disease of the elderly, although in up to 10% of patients the onset is before the age of 50. The patient with Parkinson's disease affecting both lower limbs walks with small shuffling steps where the sole of the shoe is often heard scraping along the ground. As the patient walks there is a lack of arm swing. They may also develop an involuntary sensation where they cannot stop themselves from walking with short accelerating steps, the so-called festinating gait. Occasionally, patients present with unilateral involvement mimicking a hemiparesis and are thought to have had a 'stroke'. The insidious onset and the presence of tremor and cogwheel rigidity on examination should alert the clinician to the correct diagnosis.

As the Parkinson's disease becomes more severe, patients will have difficulty getting out of bed and low chairs and will walk with a stooped posture. Patients may have a fixed expression on their face, blink infrequently and lose the ability to smile. Curiously, many patients with Parkinson's can still dance. The other characteristic feature of Parkinson's is the resting tremor, and this is discussed in the next section together with the principles of management of Parkinson's.

APRAXIA OF GAIT

Apraxia of gait is an inability to walk in the absence of weakness, sensory deficit, instability or incoordination. It is a perseveration of posture and an inability to perform the serial movements necessary for ambulation. In the initial stage there is difficulty in starting to walk or changing direction. Patients walk with small steps referred to as the 'marche a petit pas' (walks with little steps); unlike in Parkinson's they do not shuffle but lift their feet off the ground. The features that help differentiate apraxia of gait from Parkinson's disease are listed in Table 13.1.

To the inexperienced clinician these patients appear to have cogwheel rigidity but it is in fact Gegenhalten or 'an involuntary, voluntary resistance to passive movement'. The way to differentiate between the cogwheel rigidity of Parkinson's and the apparent cogwheel rigidity in frontal lobe disorders is that, in patients with Parkinson's, the cogwheel rigidity is evident from the moment testing begins whereas, in patients with Gegenhalten, the increased tone that has the sensation of cogwheel rigidity is not present initially but, the more the clinician tests for increased tone, the greater the degree of resistance creating the impression of a cogwheel rigidity. If testing is momentarily interrupted by simply lowering the hand and wrist and then started again, the increased tone is not present initially but once again increases with further testing.

TABLE 13.1   The clinical features that help differentiate Parkinson's from frontal lobe apraxia, two commonly confused conditions

Clinical feature	Parkinson's	Frontal lobe apraxia
Resting tremor	Yes	No
Shuffles when walks	Yes	No
Lifts feet when walks with small steps	No	Yes
Swings arms when walking	No	Yes
Smiles spontaneously	No	Yes
Bradykinesia	Yes	Yes
Difficulty arising from chair	Yes	Yes
Grasp and palmo-mental reflexes	No*	Yes
Cogwheel rigidity (rigidity constant during testing)	Yes	No
Gegenhalten rigidity (rigidity increases with testing)	No	Yes

*May occur late in the course when cognitive decline is present.

The method of testing tone in patients with suspected extrapyramidal or frontal lobe apraxia of gait is different from the method when one suspects altered tone due to a problem affecting the motor pathway. One passively extends and then flexes the wrist repeatedly while compressing the wrist as if you are trying to push or compact the hand into the distal aspect of the radius and ulnar. Subtle degrees of increased tone can be detected by using a technique referred to as Jendrassik's manoeuvre, a distracting technique in which the patient simultaneously clenches the opposite fist, lifts the arm with the clenched fist in the air and shakes their head from side to side. This is a particularly useful technique when looking for alteration in tone in patients with early suspected Parkinson's.

Note: Jendrassik's manoeuvre is also used to overcome the voluntary suppression of reflexes or to elicit reflexes that initially appeared to be absent without reinforcement. While the attention is being diverted, the lower extremity reflexes are tested while the patient hooks the flexed fingers of the two hands together forming a 'monkey grip' and forcibly tries to pull them apart.

The apraxic gait, although not confined to frontal lobe pathology, is characteristic of patients with disorders of the frontal lobe, most frequently on the basis of degenerative or vascular diseases of the brain. There are several treatable causes that should always be excluded:
- communicating ('normal pressure') hydrocephalus [24]
- bilateral subdural haematomas
- sub-frontal meningioma.

Communicating or 'normal pressure' hydrocephalus
Communicating hydrocephalus is relatively rare but important because it is treatable. The diagnosis is a largely a clinical one and is based on the triad of:
- gait impairment
- mild cognitive dysfunction
- unwitting urinary incontinence.

The lateral, 3rd and 4th ventricles are enlarged with little or no atrophy of the cerebral hemispheres. It presents with a fairly rapid onset over weeks or months of gait apraxia associated with unwitting urinary incontinence and *mild* cognitive impairment. Patients with significant cognitive impairment who subsequently develop apraxia of gait and patients in whom the decline is very slow over years are less likely to have communicating hydrocephalus.

The term 'normal pressure' is a misnomer as continuous intracranial pressure monitoring has demonstrated intermittent elevation of the intracranial pressure. One theory is that there is decreased arterial blood flow into the head because of closing down of the arterioles with advancing age, resulting in less venous blood flow out and consequently less CSF resorption via the transparenchymal/transvenous route. Patients with 'normal pressure' hydrocephalus may already have enlarged ventricles due to decreased CSF resorption via the arachnoid granulations and villi. When the decreased absorption via the transparenchymal/transvenous route is added, this leads to increased CSF pressure, expansion of the lateral ventricles and increased shearing forces on the local white matter tracts, particularly the corticospinal tracts to the legs that are adjacent to the ventricles.

If there is an alteration in the rapidity with which a patient with Parkinson's worsens, it is important to consider another cause. A common and readily reversible cause of a rapid deterioration in patients with Parkinson's disease is a urinary tract infection. Worsening has also been described in patients with subdural haematoma [30]. Other

MANAGEMENT of 'NORMAL PRESSURE' HYDROCEPHALUS

The aetiology of normal pressure hydrocephalus is unknown. Imaging such as a CT scan of the brain demonstrates enlargement of all the ventricles.

A number of diagnostic tests designed at predicting response to ventricular shunting have been described. These include various MRI abnormalities [25], external continuous lumbar drainage [26], continuous intraventricular pressure monitoring [27] and the CSF tap test [28], where a lumbar puncture is performed and CSF is removed to see if the patient temporarily improves. None has been validated in terms of ruling out a response to surgery. The problem with ventricular-peritoneal CSF drainage is the risk of reducing the intracranial pressure too much, resulting in subdural haematomas or hygromas. This risk has been reduced in recent years with the use of adjustable pressure shunts [29].

In patients with chronic neurological diseases such as Parkinson's, the rate of worsening tends to be fairly constant in the individual patient and, therefore, a rapid deterioration should alert the clinician to an alternative diagnosis.

examples of this principle seen by this author include spinal cord compression and dermatomyositis, which lead to a more rapid decline in the patient's ability to walk than had occurred with their Parkinson's disease.[1]

ABNORMAL MOVEMENTS

Abnormal movements of the head, face and neck

Abnormal movements that affect the head, face and neck are:

- essential/familial tremor
- tardive dyskinesia
- Tourette syndrome
- oculogyric crisis.

Two uncommon causes of abnormal movements of the face and head, hemifacial spasm and spasmodic torticollis; the latter has been discussed in the section 'Neck pain' in Chapter 11, 'Common neck, arm and upper back problems'.

HEAD TREMOR

Head tremor is usually a manifestation of benign essential/familial tremor or cerebellar disease; it is very rare in Parkinson's disease [31]. Essential/familial tremor may also affect the mouth and at times the voice. Benign essential/familial tremor is discussed in more detail in the section on abnormal movements of the upper limbs where this form of tremor is more common.

TARDIVE DYSKINESIA

Tardive dyskinesia is a neurological syndrome first recognised in the 1950s [32] that consists of repetitive, involuntary, purposeless movements affecting the mouth, lips and tongue with tongue protrusion; lip smacking, puckering and pursing; facial grimacing and rapid eye blinking. The involuntary movements occur during most of the waking hours. Typically it relates to side effects from certain drugs with an increased incidence in the elderly, although it may occur in the absence of any drug therapy, particularly

---

1 Personal observation.

in elderly edentulous patients. Tardive dyskinesia may also affect the limbs and trunk where the abnormal movements are more athetoid (repetitive involuntary, slow, sinuous, writhing movements) in nature.

MANAGEMENT of TARDIVE DYSKINESIA

This is one of the extrapyramidal syndrome side effects of central dopamine-blocking drugs such as the antipsychotics. It also occurs as a side effect of drugs used to treat Parkinson's disease and some of the antiemetics such as prochlorperazine. The higher the dose and the longer the duration of treatment, the more likely is this condition to develop. It is less common with the new generation antipsychotic drugs [33]. Sometimes withdrawing the drug may lead to a resolution of the problem, particularly if the condition is identified very early, although improvement may take some time and the condition may persist for years after withdrawal of the offending drug. Tetrabenazine [34] and deep brain stimulation have been reported to be of benefit [35].

The other extrapyramidal side effects that can occur with the antipsychotic and antidepressant drugs include akathisia (unpleasant sensations of 'inner' restlessness that manifests itself as an inability to sit still or remain motionless), the neuroleptic malignant syndrome [36] and the serotonin syndrome. These entities are discussed below in the section, 'Rare but life-threatening movement disorders'.

TOURETTE SYNDROME

Tourette syndrome is a condition predominantly seen in school-aged children [37]. The syndrome consists of tics that are sudden, brief, intermittent, involuntary or semi-voluntary movements (motor tics), such as blinking, nose twitching, head and limb jerking, mouth opening, torticollis, shoulder rotation and sustained eye closure (blepharospasm). More complex motor tics may occur, such as making obscene gestures (copropraxia) and imitating others' gestures (echopraxia). Burping, retching, vomiting, fist shaking, trunk bending, jumping or kicking are also seen. Phonic or vocal tics can also occur and these may include simply sniffing, grunting, coughing, clearing the throat, barking, screaming, shouting obscenities (coprolalia) and repeating one's own utterances (echolalia). *One of the diagnostic characteristics is the ability of the patient to suppress their tics.* The motor and phonic tics may persist during sleep. It is much more common in males and is often associated with attention-deficit/hyperactivity disorder or obsessive–compulsive disorder.

MANAGEMENT of TOURETTE SYNDROME

The Tourette Syndrome Classification Study Group has created diagnostic criteria [38]. The aetiology is uncertain and treatment consists of behaviour therapy, particularly informing people who come into contact with the patient. Alpha-2 adrenergic agonists (clonidine) or dopamine receptor-blocking drugs (neuroleptics such as haloperidol and pimozide) are used to control the motor tics [37]. In severe and disabling motor tics, botulinum toxin (Botox) or deep brain stimulation may useful. Vocal cord injections can help phonic tics.

OCULOGYRIC CRISIS

This refers to the sudden involuntary contractions of some of the eye muscles that result in repetitive, conjugate ocular deviations usually, although not always, in an upward direction. The attack or crisis may last from seconds to minutes. Oculogyric crisis is most commonly seen following exposure to neuroleptic drugs. The incidence of oculogyric crises in patients treated with chronic neuroleptic therapy may be as high as 10%.

AETIOLOGY and MANAGEMENT of OCULOGYRIC CRISIS

Tetrabenazine, gabapentin, domperidone, carbamazepine and lithium carbonate have all been reported to trigger oculogyric crises. Oculogyric crisis may occur in patients with dopa-responsive dystonia, bilateral paramedian thalamic infarction, herpes encephalitis, cystic glioma of the posterior 3rd ventricle and Wilson's disease.

The acute oculogyric crises can be terminated with an injection of intravenous anticholinergics or diphenhydramine. Diphenhydramine, 25 or 50 mg IV, is probably the treatment of choice for this condition. Oral clonazepam may be effective for patients with chronic neuroleptic-induced oculogyric crises that are resistant to anticholinergics [39].

HEMIFACIAL SPASM

Hemifacial spasm consists of brief clonic movements of the facial muscles on one side. Involvement of the orbicularis oculi results in repetitive blinking whereas involvement of the orbicularis oris causes repetitive twitching of the side of the mouth. It is believed to be due to a blood vessel irritating the proximal facial nerve near where it emerges from the brainstem.

Abnormal movements of the limbs

There are a large number of abnormal movements in the limbs. The more common seen in clinical practice are:

- benign essential or familial tremor
- the tremor of Parkinson's disease
- cerebellar or intention tremor
- myoclonus
- hemiballismus
- chorea and athetosis
- orthostatic tremor
- paroxysmal kinesogenic choreoathetosis.

Some abnormal movements occur only with activity, others occur at rest and the patient is unable to keep still (see Figure 13.5). Most are abolished by sleep, but myoclonus and hemiballismus can occur while the patient is asleep.

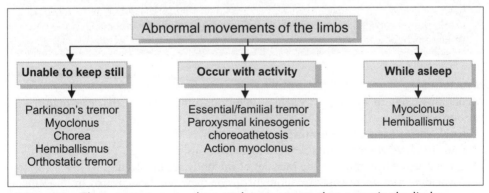

FIGURE 13.5   The more common abnormal movements that occur in the limbs

ABNORMAL MOVEMENTS WHERE THE PATIENT CANNOT KEEP STILL

Parkinson's disease

Parkinson's disease was first described by James Parkinson in 1817 [40]. Resting tremor abolished by movement is often the initial symptom although occasional patients with Parkinson's disease may have a non-resting tremor. The associated features of rigidity and bradykinesia that are characteristic of Parkinson's may be minimal or absent in the very early stages. Patients do not complain that their limbs are rigid or stiff; they tend to say that the muscles in the arms and legs ache and they do not work as well. With advanced disease there is increasing inability to undertake activities of daily living that results from the bradykinesia, although patients often assume it is simply the ageing process! Patients with Parkinson's disease walk with a slightly stooped posture and do not swing their arms when they are walking.

AETIOLOGY and MANAGEMENT of PARKINSON'S DISEASE

The aetiology of Parkinson's disease is unknown, although in some patients there is a genetic predisposition and mutations in the parkin gene are linked to autosomal recessive juvenile parkinsonism [41].

At the time of writing there is no effective treatment to arrest the progression of the disease. Management is largely directed towards alleviation of the symptoms of Parkinson's while trying to minimise the short- and long-term side effects of the drugs. In essence, the initial response to levodopa is very gratifying, and the first few years of treatment consist of gradually increasing drug therapy as the condition becomes more severe. This is replaced in later years by the progressive reduction in the doses of drugs to manage the side effects.

When reviewing patients with Parkinson's disease, it is important to clarify the exact time of day that they take each of their medications and how long the benefit persists after taking the individual dose. This will help differentiate between the motor fluctuations that represent end-of-dose failure (the beneficial effect of the drug wearing off after a period of time) and the motor fluctuations referred to as the 'on–off phenomena' that can be likened to someone pushing a button on and pushing a button off, where the patient develops increasingly severe symptoms of Parkinson's unrelated to the timing of medication. The former may respond to more frequent doses of levodopa and drugs that prolong the duration of benefit of levodopa; the latter is very difficult to treat but may respond to dopamine agonists.

Although levodopa is the recognised 'gold standard' drug for the symptomatic relief of Parkinson's disease, the efficacy diminishes after 4–5 years and is supplanted by significant motor fluctuations [42]. Initially the duration of benefit from a single dose may last several hours; after many years the duration of benefit is significantly shorter. The combination of pramipexole and levodopa is superior to levodopa alone [43]. Stereotactic surgery and deep brain stimulation are other treatment modalities in drug-resistant cases. Patients have significant depression, dementia, psychosis and psychosocial issues that need considerable attention in addition to control of the tremor and the other motor manifestations of Parkinson's disease [44].

Myoclonus

Myoclonus refers to sudden, shock-like, involuntary movements that can manifest in various patterns:

- focal, where a few adjacent muscles are involved
- multifocal, where many muscles jerk asynchronously
- generalised, where most of the muscles of the body are involved.

Myoclonic movements may be spontaneous or they may be activated by movement. Myoclonus is most commonly related to epilepsy and this has been discussed in Chapter 8,

'Seizures and epilepsy'. Myoclonus might also occur after hypoxic brain damage either acutely, within 24 hours and while the patient is still comatose, or as a late complication. The myoclonus related to hypoxia is usually movement-induced, but it can be triggered by noise, touching the patient or tracheal suctioning. The acute form is associated with a poor prognosis. The chronic form develops days or weeks after the hypoxic insult and predominantly consists of an action myoclonus affecting the limbs. Violent flexion movements of the body, head and neck are precipitated by movement.

Propriospinal myoclonus (PSM) is a rare movement disorder characterised by myoclonic jerks arising in muscles corresponding to a single myotome and spreading rostrally and caudally to the other myotomes. PSM can be idiopathic, related to spinal cord lesions, drug use, malignancy or infection [45]. Patients present with myoclonic jerks involving abdominal wall muscles which worsen when lying down.

MANAGEMENT OF **MYOCLONUS**

MRI with diffusion tensor imaging detects abnormalities in patients with PSM [45]. Clonazepam, piracetam and valproic acid are the first-line treatments for post-hypoxic action myoclonus or PSM. Propofol and midazolam may be needed in the acute hypoxic form [46]. Zonisamide has been recommended for PSM [45].

Chorea and athetosis

Chorea is the ceaseless irregular, rapid, uncontrolled complex body movements that look well coordinated and purposeful but are in fact involuntary. The term 'chorea' is derived from the Greek word 'choreia' or 'khoreia' for dancing. Chorea was thought to be suggestive of a grotesque dance. Chorea can affect the face, arms or legs. The abnormal movements are almost continuous.

Athetosis consists of repetitive involuntary, slow, sinuous, writhing movements, especially severe in the hands.

Choreoathetosis is a movement of intermediate speed, between the quick, flitting movements of chorea and the slower, writhing movements of athetosis.

Chorea is very uncommon; Huntington's disease is now the main cause with Sydenham's chorea largely disappearing along with rheumatic fever. A very rare but treatable cause of chorea is Wilson's disease [47]. There are a number of even rarer inherited movement disorders that could result in dystonia, chorea or ataxia [48, 49], but are beyond the scope of this book.

HUNTINGTON'S DISEASE

Huntington's disease [50] is a hereditary disorder with the genetic defect on the short arm of chromosome 4. The genetic defect leads to altered function of the ubiquitous protein, huntingtin, that culminates in neuronal loss in the caudate nucleus. The number of tri-nucleotide repeats (cysteine-adenine-guanidine; CAG) influences whether the disease shows incomplete or complete penetrance and also influences the age of onset, with juvenile-onset Huntington's patients typically having more than 55 tri-nucleotide repeats.

Huntington's disease is characterised by the insidious onset in middle age (35–44 years of age) of progressive cognitive decline associated with abnormal movements and psychiatric disturbances. The chorea may not be present at onset; often the initial symptoms are unsteadiness and a lack of coordination with the cognitive decline and psychiatric disturbances appearing later. Chorea is the typical movement disorder but often rigidity, bradykinesia and dystonia may predominate and be more disabling. Rarely does it develop before the age of 20 where it is referred to as juvenile Huntington's disease. In juvenile

Huntington's disease, the symptoms are quite different – the patient often presents rigid and akinetic (absence or poverty of movement) – and the progression to disability is more rapid. The inheritance pattern of Huntington's disease is autosomal dominant.

SYDENHAM'S CHOREA

Sydenham's chorea was first described in 1686 by Thomas Sydenham in a work entitled 'Schedula monitoria de novae febris ingress', but it was not until 180 years later (in 1866) that the association with rheumatic fever was appreciated by Roger. It is a complication of rheumatic fever following infection with particular strains of streptococci (i.e. group A beta-hemolytic streptococci). It predominantly affects children although it can be seen in adults. It is much rarer these days since the virtual abolition of rheumatic fever.

The antecedent sore throat, polyarthritis and subcutaneous nodules the size of peas at joints such as the elbows and knees, together with the characteristic pink-red macular rash referred to as erythema marginatum, are the clues to the diagnosis. Sydenham's chorea is a self-limiting illness that initially worsens over 2–4 weeks and then subsequently resolves spontaneously over 3–6 months, although some patients may have waxing and waning symptoms for up to 12 months [51].

WILSON'S DISEASE

Wilson's disease is an autosomal recessive disease caused by mutations in the ATP7B gene. The mutated gene prevents the transport protein from functioning properly, allowing copper to accumulate in the liver, brain, kidneys and skeletal system [47].

The neurological manifestations are the most common presentation; patients with liver disease present with jaundice. Although chorea occurs in Wilson's disease, it is not the commonest manifestation; the majority present with features of parkinsonism, dystonia, ataxia, pyramidal signs, seizures, myoclonus and athetosis.

MANAGEMENT OF **WILSON'S DISEASE**

The diagnosis of Wilson's disease is established by the presence of Kayser–Fleischer rings on the cornea, decreased serum ceruloplasmin, elevated 24-hour urine copper or increased hepatic copper content. Unfortunately, none of these findings is entirely sensitive or specific [48]. Characteristic MRI abnormalities in patients with Wilson's disease consist of axial T_2WI bilateral basal ganglionic and thalamic hyperintensity in addition to mild to moderate diffuse atrophy [47]

Treatment is usually with drugs that reduce copper absorption (zinc acetate or zinc sulfate) or chelating agents such as penicillamine. Liver transplantation is an option in patients who fail to respond or cannot tolerate medical therapy [52]

Symptomatic treatment for chorea can be achieved with dopamine-depleting agents such as tetrabenazine or reserpine, benzodiazepines such as clonazepam or diazepam and dopamine antagonists such as the neuroleptic drug haloperidol.

ABNORMAL MOVEMENTS THAT OCCUR WITH ACTIVITY
Benign essential or familial tremor

Essential and familial essential tremor [53, 54] are the most common movement disorders in the elderly and the most common cause of an action tremor [55]. It can occur in patients in their teens.

Typically, the benign essential/familial tremor occurs when patients are either moving their arms or holding an object such as a book or a cup of tea where the cup rattles in the saucer and patients have to resort to half-filling their cup in order not to spill the tea. Eating becomes more difficult as the patient repeatedly spills food off the fork or soup out of the spoon. Although the tremor is bilateral, one side may be more severely affected than the other. The tremor sometimes leads to physical disability but progression to disability is usually very slow. Many patients are socially disabled as they are 'too embarrassed' to go out. Familial tremor is usually inherited as an autosomal dominant trait but with variable penetrance. Apart from the tremor, neurological examination is otherwise normal, in particular there is no rigidity or bradykinesia.

Differentiating Parkinson's from essential/familial tremor

Table 13.2 shows the differences between the tremor of Parkinson's and that of familial essential tremor.

INVESTIGATION and TREATMENT of ESSENTIAL TREMOR

It is important to exclude hyperthyroidism in patients with 'essential tremor'. Genetic susceptibility loci have been identified in the FET1 (also known as ETM1) gene located on chromosome 3q1 [56] and ETM mapped to chromosome 2p22–25 [57].

There is no cure and many patients simply require reassurance about the benign nature of the tremor. Small doses of alcohol can be used to reduce the severity of mild tremor. In patients with more severe tremor, low-dose primidone (commencing with ¼ of a tablet or 62.5 mg and increasing to the minimum required or maximally tolerated dose, as much as 250 mg/day) or moderate dose propranolol (commencing with 10 mg and increasing slowly up to 120 mg/day) has been shown to reduce the severity of the tremor [58]. Osteoporosis commonly coexists in the elderly and primidone can exacerbate osteoporosis. Other medications include alprazolam, gabapentin, topiramate, nimodipine, clozapine and clonidine. In patients who are resistant to pharmacological therapy, either thalamotomy or deep brain stimulation may be of benefit [58].

Cerebellar or intention tremor

Cerebellar tremor is also referred to as intention tremor. These patients present with tremor when using their arms. There is no tremor at rest, little or no tremor with the hands outstretched but obvious tremor when the patient is asked to perform finger-to-nose or heel-to-shin testing where instability is noticed as the patient stretches to reach the distant target. The oscillations of intention tremor are perpendicular to the direction of movement and usually of low frequency, less than 5 Hz.

Intention tremor occurs in patients with MS, Friedreich's ataxia, cerebellar infarction and degeneration.

TREATMENT for INTENTION TREMOR

There is no specific treatment for intention tremor; drugs such as clonazepam, carbamazepine, odansetron, isoniazid and physostigmine have all been tried with variable success [59]. In refractory cases, brain stimulation may be of benefit [60, 61].

ORTHOSTATIC TREMOR

Orthostatic tremor is a condition where the patient finds it impossible to stand still for any length of time without developing an increasingly severe sensation of instability (not dizziness) with their body developing a tremulous sensation. Patients rarely fall and usually hang on to something, sit or commence walking. Many patients avoid stopping while walking in order to avoid this sensation. The neurological examination is otherwise normal. Most cases are idiopathic [62], but it has been described in progressive supranuclear palsy [63] and following head injury [64].

TABLE 13.2   The different features of the tremor of Parkinson's disease and essential/familial tremor

Clinical feature	Parkinson's	Essential/familial
Affects the head and voice	No	Yes
Present at rest	Yes	No
Present when holding objects	No	Yes
Worse with walking	Yes	No
Influenced by alcohol	No	Yes
Frequency	3–6 Hz	5–12 Hz
Family history	Occasional	Often (familial)

TREATMENT of ORTHOSTATIC TREMOR

Clonazepam and primidone, particularly a combination of both drugs [65], and pramipexole [66] have been reported to reduce the severity of orthostatic tremor although none has been subjected to randomised controlled trials. Benefit from deep brain stimulation has also been described [67].

Action myoclonus

Myoclonus is the one abnormal movement that occurs at rest and also persists in sleep. Action myoclonus refers to sudden arrhythmic muscular jerking induced by voluntary movement. The condition is usually associated with diffuse neuronal disease, such as post-hypoxic encephalopathy [68], uraemia and various forms of progressive myoclonic epilepsy such as the Ramsay–Hunt syndrome [69].

Paroxysmal kinesogenic choreoathetosis

Paroxysmal kinesogenic choreoathetosis (PKC) has its onset in childhood or early adulthood. The characteristic feature is discrete episodes of *abnormal movements precipitated by sudden movement* such as standing up from sitting or being startled. Chorea occurs as does hyperkinesias, dystonia, athetosis and ballism. The neurological exam is normal between the events. The attacks are brief (< 5 minutes) and may occur several times a day.

MANAGEMENT of PAROXYSMAL KINESOGENIC CHOREOATHETOSIS

Linkage has been established in eight Japanese families to chromosome 16p11.2-q12.1 [70]. The condition responds very well to low-dose anticonvulsant therapy such as carbamazepine or phenytoin [71].

ABNORMAL MOVEMENTS THAT OCCUR DURING SLEEP

Myoclonus has already been discussed; the other abnormal movement that occurs during sleep is hemiballismus.

Hemiballismus

Hemiballismus (derived from the Greek word 'ballismos' that means jumping about or dancing) is considered a rare form of chorea and is almost continuous, violent, coordinated involuntary motor restlessness of half (very rarely bilateral, referred to as paraballism) of the body. The movements are usually continuous contorting movements and often rotatory in nature. It is most marked in the upper extremities and usually caused by a lesion involving the subthalamic nucleus of the opposite side of the brain, but it can arise from contralateral lesions in the cortex, basal ganglia and thalamus [72]. The commonest cause is an infarct, but it has been reported with demyelinating disease.

Although spontaneous remission is common, hemiballismus is a potentially life-threatening disorder and therapy is essential.

MANAGEMENT of HEMIBALLISMUS

An MRI scan, in particular a diffusion-weighted MRI scan, may define the site of the pathology in patients with hemiballismus. Pharmacological agents include haloperidol, risperadone, clonazepam and baclofen. Pallidotomy or thalamotomy may be necessary in intractable cases.

Rare but life-threatening movement disorders

These have also been referred to as movement disorder emergencies and are defined as any movement disorder that evolves over hours to days and include acute parkinsonism, dystonia, chorea, tics and myoclonus. The commonest is drug-induced (neuroleptics and antiemetics) parkinsonism, and cyanide, methanol, carbon monoxide, carbon disulfide, organophosphate pesticides and the designer drug MPTP are some of the toxins that may produce a severe encephalopathy with clinical features of parkinsonism. Only neuroleptic malignant syndrome and serotonin syndrome will be discussed here. For an excellent review of movement disorder emergencies see the review by Poston [39].

NEUROLEPTIC MALIGNANT SYNDROME

Neuroleptic malignant syndrome is a very rare potentially life-threatening but treatable idiosyncratic response to D_2-dopamine receptor agonists such as antiemetics, droperidol, anaesthetic agents and antipsychotic drugs. A rapid increase in the dose may increase the risk of neuroleptic malignant syndrome. It can also occur if treatment for Parkinson's is suddenly withdrawn.

The clinical features consist of rigidity, fever, sweating, severe hypertension and altered conscious state. Creatinine kinase is elevated and liver function abnormalities occur. Dehydration leads to renal impairment. Features of parkinsonism and the presence of fever should alert the clinician to the possibility of this condition. It can occur at any age and in either sex.

TREATMENT of NEUROLEPTIC MALIGNANT SYNDROME

Dopamine agonists, levodopa, lisuride and dantrolene are the pharmacological agents used to treat neuroleptic malignant syndrome.

SEROTONIN SYNDROME

Serotonin syndrome [73] is caused mainly by the serotonin-specific reuptake inhibitors (sertraline, fluoxetine, paroxetine and fluvoxamine), clomipramine, ecstasy and the combination of monoamine oxidase inhibitors and meperidine that result in an increase in the biological activity of serotonin.

Serotonin syndrome consists of fever with confusion, hypomania, agitation, tachycardia, fever, sweating, shivering, tremor, diarrhoea, hypertension, incoordination, myoclonus, rigidity and hyperreflexia. The clinical features of serotonin syndrome and neuroleptic malignant syndrome overlap; it is the presence of myoclonus that distinguishes serotonin syndrome from neuroleptic malignant syndrome.

TREATMENT of SEROTONIN SYNDROME

Propranolol, chlorpromazine, diazepam, methysergide and, in particular, cyproheptadine are recommended for the treatment of serotonin syndrome [74, 75].

REFERENCES

1 Baron EM, Young WF. Cervical spondylotic myelopathy: A brief review of its pathophysiology, clinical course, and diagnosis. Neurosurgery 2007; 60(Suppl 1):S35–S41.
2 Prasad D, Schiff D. Malignant spinal-cord compression. Lancet Oncol 2005; 6(1):15–24.
3 Husband DJ. Malignant spinal cord compression: Prospective study of delays in referral and treatment. BMJ 1998; 317(7150):18–21.
4 White BD et al. Diagnosis and management of patients at risk of or with metastatic spinal cord compression: Summary of NICE guidance. BMJ 2008; 337:a2538.
5 Portenoy RK et al. Identification of epidural neoplasm. Radiography and bone scintigraphy in the symptomatic and asymptomatic spine. Cancer 1989; 64(11):2207–2213.
6 Hyman RA et al. 0.6 T MR imaging of the cervical spine: Multislice and multiecho techniques. Am J Neuroradiol 1985; 6(2):229–236.
7 Loblaw DA et al. Systematic review of the diagnosis and management of malignant extradural spinal cord compression: The Cancer Care Ontario Practice Guidelines Initiative's Neuro-Oncology Disease Site Group. J Clin Oncol 2005; 23(9):2028–2037.
8 Sorensen S et al. Effect of high-dose dexamethasone in carcinomatous metastatic spinal cord compression treated with radiotherapy: A randomised trial. Eur J Cancer 1994; 30A(1):22–27.
9 Patchell RA et al. Direct decompressive surgical resection in the treatment of spinal cord compression caused by metastatic cancer: A randomised trial. Lancet 2005; 366(9486):643–648.
10 al Deeb SM et al. Acute transverse myelitis: A localized form of postinfectious encephalomyelitis. Brain 1997; 120(Pt 7):1115–1122.
11 Transverse Myelitis Consortium Working Group. Proposed diagnostic criteria and nosology of acute transverse myelitis. Neurology 2002; 59(4):499–505.
12 Harzheim M et al. Discriminatory features of acute transverse myelitis: A retrospective analysis of 45 patients. J Neurol Sci 2004; 217(2):217–223.
13 Misra UK, Kalita J, Kumar S. A clinical, MRI and neurophysiological study of acute transverse myelitis. J Neurol Sci 1996; 138(1–2):150–156.
14 de Seze J et al. Acute myelopathies: Clinical, laboratory and outcome profiles in 79 cases. Brain 2001; 124(Pt 8):1509–1521.
15 Croft P. Neuromuscular syndromes associated with malignant disease. Br J Hosp Med 1977; 17(4):356, 360–362.
16 Rudnicki SA, Dalmau J. Paraneoplastic syndromes of the peripheral nerves. Curr Opin Neurol 2005; 18(5):598–603.
17 Malinow K et al. Subacute sensory neuronopathy secondary to dorsal root ganglionitis in primary Sjögren's syndrome. Ann Neurol 1986; 20(4):535–537.
18 Schaumburg H et al. Sensory neuropathy from pyridoxine abuse: A new megavitamin syndrome. N Engl J Med 1983; 309(8):445–448.
19 Jellinek EH, Kelly RE. Cerebellar syndrome in myxoedema. Lancet 1960; 2(7144):225–227.
20 Skillicorn SA. Presenile cerebellar ataxia in chronic alcoholics. Neurology 1955; 5(8):527–534.
21 Bariety M et al. ["Paraneoplastic" psychic and cerebellar syndrome reversible by radiotherapeutic treatment of its cause: "Anaplastic bronchial epithelioma".] Bull Mem Soc Med Hop Paris 1960; 76:650–661.
22 Richter R. The hereditary nature of late cortical cerebellar atrophy. Trans Am Neurol Assoc 1948; 73(73 Annual Meet):85–78.
23 Davis GC et al. Chronic parkinsonism secondary to intravenous injection of meperidine analogues. Psychiatry Res 1979; 1(3):249–254.
24 Messert B, Baker NH. Syndrome of progressive spastic ataxia and apraxia associated with occult hydrocephalus. Neurology 1966; 16(5):440–452.
25 Dixon GR et al. Use of cerebrospinal fluid flow rates measured by phase-contrast MR to predict outcome of ventriculoperitoneal shunting for idiopathic normal-pressure hydrocephalus. Mayo Clin Proc 2002; 77(6):509–514.

26 Panagiotopoulos V et al. The predictive value of external continuous lumbar drainage, with cerebrospinal fluid outflow controlled by medium pressure valve, in normal pressure hydrocephalus. Acta Neurochir (Wien) 2005; 147(9):953–958;discussion 958.

27 Pfisterer WK et al. Continuous intraventricular pressure monitoring for diagnosis of normal-pressure hydrocephalus. Acta Neurochir (Wien) 2007; 149(10):983–990:discussion 990.

28 Wikkelso C et al. Normal pressure hydrocephalus. Predictive value of the cerebrospinal fluid tap-test. Acta Neurol Scand 1986; 73(6):566–573.

29 Bret P et al. [Clinical experience with the Sp[hy adjustable valve in the treatment of adult hydrocephalus: A series of 147 cases.] Neurochirurgie 1999; 45(2):98–108:discussion 108–109.

30 Wiest RG, Burgunder JM, Krauss JK. Chronic subdural haematomas and Parkinsonian syndromes. Acta Neurochir (Wien) 1999; 141(7):753–757:discussion 757–758.

31 Gan J et al. Possible Parkinson's disease revealed by a pure head resting tremor. J Neurol Sci 2009; 279(1–2): 121–123.

32 Schonecker VM. Ein eigentumliches syndrom in oralen Bereich bei Negaphenapplikation. Nervenarzt 1957; 28:35.

33 Tarsy D, Baldessarini RJ. Epidemiology of tardive dyskinesia: Is risk declining with modern antipsychotics? Mov Disord 2006; 21(5):589–598.

34 Kenney C, Jankovic J. Tetrabenazine in the treatment of hyperkinetic movement disorders. Expert Rev Neurother 2006; 6(1):7–17.

35 Sun B et al. Subthalamic nucleus stimulation for primary dystonia and tardive dystonia. Acta Neurochir Suppl 2007; 97(Pt 2):207–214.

36 Nisijima K, Shioda K, Iwamura T. Neuroleptic malignant syndrome and serotonin syndrome. Prog Brain Res 2007; 162:81–104.

37 Jankovic J. Tourette's syndrome. N Engl J Med 2001; 345(16):1184–1192.

38 The Tourette Syndrome Classification Study Group. Definitions and classification of tic disorders. Arch Neurol 1993; 50(10):1013–1016.

39 Poston KL, Frucht SJ. Movement disorder emergencies. J Neurol 2008; 255(Suppl 4):2–13.

40 Parkinson J. An essay on the shaking palsy. London: Whittingham and Roland; 1817.

41 Polymeropoulos MH et al. Mutation in the alpha-synuclein gene identified in families with Parkinson's disease. Science 1997; 276(5321):2045–2047.

42 Miyasaki JM et al. Practice parameter: Initiation of treatment for Parkinson's disease: An evidence-based review: Report of the Quality Standards Subcommittee of the American Academy of Neurology. Neurology 2002; 58(1):11–17.

43 Parkinson Study Group. Pramipexole vs levodopa as initial treatment for Parkinson disease: A randomized controlled trial. JAMA 2000; 284(15):1931–1938.

44 Miyasaki JM et al. Practice parameter: Evaluation and treatment of depression, psychosis, and dementia in Parkinson disease (an evidence-based review): Report of the Quality Standards Subcommittee of the American Academy of Neurology. Neurology 2006; 66(7):996–1002.

45 Roze E et al. Propriospinal myoclonus revisited: Clinical, neurophysiologic, and neuroradiologic findings. Neurology 2009; 72(15):1301–1309.

46 Venkatesan A, Frucht S. Movement disorders after resuscitation from cardiac arrest. Neurol Clin 2006; 24(1):123–132.

47 Taly AB et al. Wilson disease: Description of 282 patients evaluated over 3 decades. Medicine (Baltimore) 2007; 86(2):112–121.

48 Sharma N, Standaert DG. Inherited movement disorders. Neurol Clin 2002; 20(3):759–778,vii.

49 Jen JC et al. Primary episodic ataxias: Diagnosis, pathogenesis and treatment. Brain 2007; 130(Pt 10):2484–2493.

50 Huntington G. On chorea. The Medical and Surgical Reporter: A Weekly Journal 1872; 26(15):317–321.

51 Gordon N. Sydenham's chorea, and its complications affecting the nervous system. Brain Dev 2009; 31(1):11–14.

52 Cox DW, Roberts E. Wilson's disease. 2006. Gene Tests website. Available: http://www.ncbi.nlm.nih.gov/bookshelf/br.fcgi?book=gene&part=wilson#wilson (14 Dec 2009).

53 Critchley M. Observations on essential (heredofamial) tremor. Brain 1949; 72(Pt 2):113–139.

54 Davis CH, Kunkle EC. Benign essential (heredofamilial) tremor. Trans Am Neurol Assoc 1951; 56:87–89.

55 Thanvi B, Lo N, Robinson T. Essential tremor – the most common movement disorder in older people. Age Ageing 2006; 35(4):344–349.

56 Gulcher JR et al. Mapping of a familial essential tremor gene, FET1, to chromosome 3q13. Nat Genet 1997; 17(1):84–87.

57 Higgins JJ, Pho LT, Nee LE. A gene (ETM) for essential tremor maps to chromosome 2p22-p25. Mov Disord 1997; 12(6):859–864.

58 Zesiewicz TA et al. Practice parameter: Therapies for essential tremor: Report of the Quality Standards Subcommittee of the American Academy of Neurology. Neurology 2005; 64(12):2008–2020.

59 Bhidayasiri R. Differential diagnosis of common tremor syndromes. Postgrad Med J 2005; 81(962): 756–762.

60 Nandi D, Aziz TZ. Deep brain stimulation in the management of neuropathic pain and multiple sclerosis tremor. J Clin Neurophysiol 2004; 21(1):31–39.

61 Wishart HA et al. Chronic deep brain stimulation for the treatment of tremor in multiple sclerosis: Review and case reports. J Neurol Neurosurg Psychiatry 2003; 74(10):1392–1397.

62 Gates PC. Orthostatic tremor (shaky legs syndrome). Clin Exp Neurol 1993; 30:66–71.

63 de Bie RM, Chen R, Lang AE. Orthostatic tremor in progressive supranuclear palsy. Mov Disord 2007; 22(8):1192–1194.

64 Sanitate SS, Meerschaert JR. Orthostatic tremor: Delayed onset following head trauma. Arch Phys Med Rehabil 1993; 74(8):886–889.

65 Poersch M. Orthostatic tremor: Combined treatment with primidone and clonazepam. Mov Disord 1994; 9(4):467.

66 Finkel MF. Pramipexole is a possible effective treatment for primary orthostatic tremor (shaky leg syndrome). Arch Neurol 2000; 57(10):1519–1520.

67 Guridi J et al. Successful thalamic deep brain stimulation for orthostatic tremor. Mov Disord 2008; 23(13):1808–1811.

68 Fahn S. Posthypoxic action myoclonus: Literature review update. Adv Neurol 1986; 43:157–169.

69 Lance JW. Action myoclonus, Ramsay Hunt syndrome, and other cerebellar myoclonic syndromes. Adv Neurol 1986; 43:33–55.

70 Tomita H et al. Paroxysmal kinesigenic choreoathetosis locus maps to chromosome 16p11.2-q12.1. Am J Hum Genet 1999; 65(6):1688–1697.

71 Wein T et al. Exquisite sensitivity of paroxysmal kinesigenic choreoathetosis to carbamazepine. Neurology 1996; 47(4):1104–1106.

72 Dewey RB, Jr, Jankovic J. Hemiballism-hemichorea: Clinical and pharmacologic findings in 21 patients. Arch Neurol 1989; 46(8):862–867.

73 Sternbach H. The serotonin syndrome. Am J Psychiatry 1991; 148(6):705–713.

74 Lappin RI, Auchincloss EL. Treatment of the serotonin syndrome with cyproheptadine. N Engl J Med 1994; 331(15):1021–1022.

75 Graudins A, Stearman A, Chan B. Treatment of the serotonin syndrome with cyproheptadine. J Emerg Med 1998; 16(4):615–619.

chapter **14**

Miscellaneous Neurological Disorders

The principal aim of this textbook has been to introduce simple concepts to help the 'student of neurology' understand the diagnostic process and to discuss the more common neurological problems encountered in everyday clinical practice. There are a number of conditions that are not common in everyday clinical practice, and yet no neurology textbook would be complete without at least some discussion of those entities. This chapter will discuss:
* assessment of patients with a depressed conscious state
* assessment of the confused or demented patient
* disorders of muscle and the neuromuscular junction
* multiple sclerosis
* malignancy and the nervous system
* infections of the nervous system.

ASSESSMENT OF PATIENTS WITH A DEPRESSED CONSCIOUS STATE

The definitive text on this subject has been written by Fred Plum and Jeremy Posner in a superb text, entitled *The Diagnosis of Stupor and Coma* [1], that is required reading for every neurologist in training.

Essentially there are three patterns of a depressed conscious state:
1 Diffuse – consciousness is depressed in the absence of neurological signs. The main causes include:
  * drugs (alcohol, opiates and sedatives)
  * hypothermia (may cause coma if the temperature is less than 31°C), meningitis, encephalitis
  * subarachnoid haemorrhage, acute hydrocephalus
  * severe hypotension from any cause
  * metabolic disturbances such as hypoxaemia, hepatic coma, hyponatraemia or hypernatraemia, hypercapnia
  * most importantly, hypoglycaemia.
  Note: The presence of fever indicates the possibility of meningitis, encephalitis or subarachnoid haemorrhage. Examination of the fundi may reveal papilloedema to indicate raised intracranial pressure or the tell-tale **subhyaloid haemorrhages** that are pathognomonic for subarachnoid haemorrhage, but these are only present with haemorrhage in the anterior aspect of the cerebral hemisphere.

2 Cerebral hemisphere problems – the conscious state is depressed in the setting of a hemiparesis or hemiplegia. Conditions that produce a mass effect cause downward herniation of the brain through the tentorium and secondary compression of the brainstem. Such conditions include:
- extradural, subdural and intracerebral haemorrhage
- tumours
- brain abscess
- herpes simplex encephalitis.

3 Diseases in the brainstem – the conscious state is depressed and there are abnormalities in the brainstem reflexes. These include:
- brainstem haemorrhage
- brainstem infarction.

In a comatose patient, even before a neurological examination is performed and while a second person checks the blood glucose to exclude hypoglycaemia or hyperglycaemia, it is important to check the following:
- The *airway* is not obstructed.
- The patient is *breathing* adequately; if not, intubate them.
- The *circulation*, pulse and blood pressure and, if the patient is hypotensive, treat with appropriate fluids and if necessary pharmacological agents.

Currently, pressor drugs are used to treat severe hypotension and these are sympathomimetic agents, vasoconstrictor drugs or cardiostimulatory drugs.

Hypotension suggests possible drug overdose, severe internal haemorrhage in a body cavity such as the chest or abdomen, sepsis, severe hypothyroidism or an Addisonian crisis.

1 *Look at the pupils.* If they are pinpoint, administer naloxone. (Pontine haemorrhage and narcotic or barbiturate overdose result in pinpoint pupils.)
2 *Smell the breath* for alcohol or ketones.
3 *Check the blood alcohol.*
4 *Look for IV needle puncture marks.*

Neurological examination of patients in a depressed conscious state
Having ensured that the patient is stable from the cardiac and respiratory point of view and having excluded hypothermia, hypoglycaemia and hyponatraemia, the next step is to obtain as much information as possible and to perform a neurological examination.

Often patients are found unconscious and a detailed history is not possible.
- As much information as possible should be obtained from an eyewitness, if there is one, or from the person who found the patient.
- Attempt to establish when the patient was last seen well, as this helps to narrow down the time the patient may have been unconscious for.
- Have people check for empty bottles or a suicide note near where the patient was found, which indicate the possibility of a drug overdose.
- Question ambulance officers rather than rely on the ambulance report.
- Telephone relatives, neighbours or anybody who might be able to provide clues to the diagnosis.
- Ask about evidence to suggest trauma, e.g. overturned furniture, blood on the floor, syringes to suggest possible drug overdose from medications (e.g. insulin or hypoglycaemics) the patient takes.
- See if there is anything in the past medical history that may provide a clue.

The neurological examination in patients with a depressed conscious state is completely different to the standard neurological examination. It is designed to detect:

1 the level of arousal
2 the response to pain
3 abnormalities within the cranial nerves that indicate involvement of the brainstem.

Initially the patient should be *observed for spontaneous movements* of the limbs or lack thereof, the latter suggesting possible paralysis. Observe whether they spontaneously open their eyes and look around, indicating a lesser degree of depression of the conscious state. It is important to *look for focal seizure activity* in the face or limbs.

The next step is to *attempt to arouse the patient with verbal stimuli* and, if it fails, *painful stimuli* (Figure 14.1). One of the most useful techniques is to pinch the skin on the medial aspect of the elbows and knees between your fingernails. A normal response is abduction of the limbs away from the painful stimulus; an abnormal response is adduction of the limbs towards the painful stimulus or extension of the limbs. Before testing the response to painful stimuli in front of the family, explain to them that it is the way to test when someone is unconscious. The family should also be warned that this technique may leave bruises.

The *brainstem reflexes* are then examined. The region tested is shown in brackets.
- The *pupil responses* – the afferent pathway is the 2nd nerve; the efferent pathway is the parasympathetic pathway on the surface of the 3rd nerve (midbrain and 3rd nerve)
- *Doll's eye reflexes* – spontaneous and head movement-evoked eye movements (vertical eye movements = midbrain, horizontal eye movements = pons) (Figure 14.1)
- The *corneal and nasal tickle reflexes* – the afferent pathway is the 5th cranial nerve; the efferent pathway is the 7th nerve (pons) (Figure 14.1)
- The *gag reflex* – the afferent pathway is the 9th cranial nerve; the efferent pathway is the 10th cranial nerve (medulla)
  Note: This reflex is not as useful as the others because many healthy people may not have a gag reflex.

Normal pupil responses, doll's eye testing and corneal or nasal tickle reflexes indicate that the brainstem is intact and that the cause of the coma is either in the cerebral hemispheres or due to a diffuse problem. A 3rd or 6th nerve palsy does not necessarily indicate brainstem involvement. A 3rd can occur with a hemisphere lesion with downward herniation, and a 6th can occure with raised intracranial pressure as a false localising sign.

Response to pain

If the patient abducts or withdraws the limb away from the painful stimulus applied to the medial aspect of the elbow or knee, this implies that the motor pathway is intact. On the other hand, if the patient does not withdraw the limb, but the arm or leg moves towards the painful stimulus or it straightens, this indicates that the motor pathway is damaged.

Decorticate and decerebrate rigidity are two terms used to describe certain postures that may occur in the comatose patient and were formerly thought to provide localising value, although this is now in question. Decorticate rigidity refers to flexion of the elbows and wrists and supination of the arms and was said to indicate bilateral damage above (rostral) to the midbrain; decerebrate rigidity consists of extension of the elbows and wrists with pronation of the forearms indicating damage to the motor pathways in the midbrain or lower part (caudal) of the diencephalon (thalamus and hypothalamus). Similarly, the pattern of respiration is not of great localising value. For example, the cyclic breathing with periods of apnoea referred to as Cheyne–Stokes respiration can occur with bilateral hemisphere damage or metabolic suppression of the conscious state.

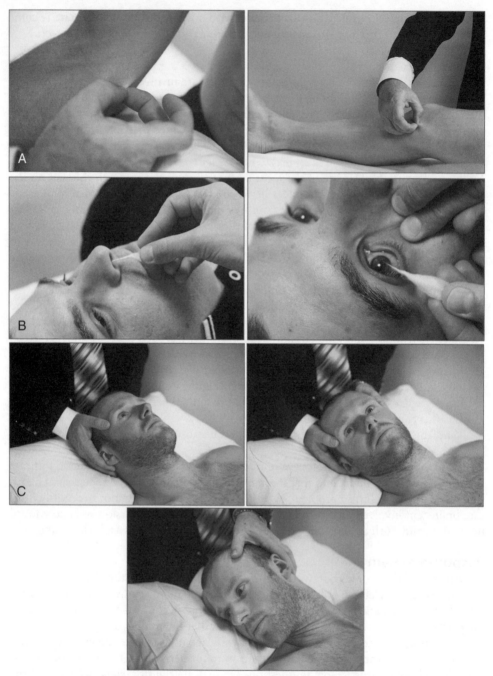

FIGURE 14.1 Methods of **A** applying painful stimuli to the limbs, **B** testing the nasal and corneal reflexes and **C** testing eye movements using the doll's eye procedure

The pupil responses

The response of the pupils to a *bright* light is one of the most important aspects of the examination (see Figure 14.2). It may be necessary to use a magnifying glass to see slight reactions. The size of the pupil and the reaction to light are used to exclude or localise pathology in or affecting the midbrain and pons of the brainstem.

- Bilateral normal size (2.5–5mm) and reactive pupils:
  - Essentially excludes midbrain damage
- Unilateral dilated (> 6 mm) and non-reactive pupil + contralateral weakness:
  - Compression of the ipsilateral 3rd cranial nerve with herniation due a mass lesion (tumour, haemorrhage, oedema related to a cerebral infarct) in the cerebral hemisphere
- Bilateral dilated and non-reactive pupils:
  - Bilateral midbrain pathology
- Bilateral small (1–2.5 mm) and reactive pupils:
  - Metabolic encephalopathy or bilateral deep hemisphere lesions
- Bilateral pinpoint pupils that react to light:
  - Pontine haemorrhage, narcotic or barbiturate overdose

The eye movements

In normal patients the eyes may be divergent in sleep.

- Spontaneous movements of the eyes, referred to as 'roving eyes', *exclude damage to the midbrain and pons.*
- If the eyes are *deviated to one side,* this is either due to an ipsilateral hemisphere lesion, where the eyes look to the side of the lesion and away from the side of the paralysis, or alternatively may indicate pontine pathology, where the eyes look away from the side of the lesion and towards the side of the paralysis or hemiparesis.

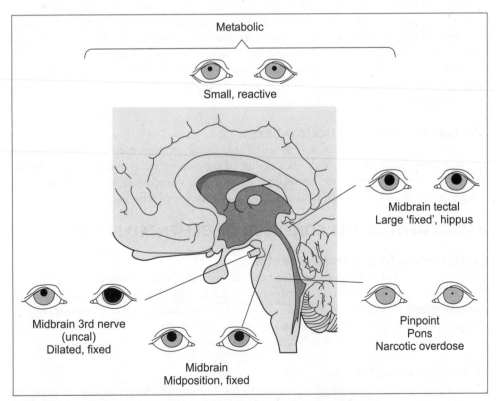

FIGURE 14.2 Abnormal pupil responses in the comatose patient

Reproduced from *Diagnosis of Stupor and Coma.* 2nd edn, by F Plum, JB Posner, 1972, FA Davis.

One exception to this rule is that with irritating hemisphere lesions the eyes may be deviated away from the side of the lesion and towards the side of the paralysis.
* *Ocular bobbing* indicates bilateral pontine damage, most often seen with basilar artery thrombosis. It consists of the absence of horizontal eye movements and a characteristic brisk downward movement of both eyes and then a slow upward movement to return to the normal position.

In the absence of these spontaneous ocular signs, the brainstem can be tested using the technique referred to as the *oculocephalic reflex* or doll's eye test (see Figure 14.1C).

> Eyes that spontaneously deviate away from the side of the paralysis indicate a hemisphere lesion on the side opposite to the paralysis; eyes that deviate to the side of the paralysis indicate a brainstem lesion on the side opposite the paralysis.

* The head is moved rapidly horizontally and then vertically while the movement of the eyes in the opposite direction to the movement of the head is observed.
* When the head is turned to the right, the eyes deviate fully left and vice versa.
    * If the eye movement is full, i.e. the eyes move in the orbits to their full extent so that no sclera can be seen, this indicates that the brainstem is intact and therefore not the site of the pathology causing the impaired consciousness.
    * If the eyes fail to move, this suggests damage to the ipsilateral brain stem nuclei.
* In patients with severe depression of the conscious state due to drug overdose, the oculocephalic reflexes may be abnormal and not indicate any structural damage to the brainstem. In this latter setting the pupils would usually be of normal size and react to light, something that would not occur in destructive brainstem lesions.

More intense stimulation of the oculocephalic reflex can be produced with caloric stimulation, where either warm or cold water is used to irrigate the external ear canal (ensure that the external ear canal is not occluded by wax before performing this test). Tonic deviation of the eyes with nystagmus to the opposite side with cold water and to the same side with warm water indicates that the brainstem is intact. If the eyes fail to deviate this indicates brainstem damage.

The corneal and nasal tickle reflexes

The cornea of the eye or the nostril is stimulated using cotton wool (not tissue paper as this may damage the cornea), and reflex closure of the eyes indicates that the pons is intact. Absent reflexes may occur with hemisphere lesions, drug overdose or structural brainstem lesions and, thus, absent corneal reflexes are not particularly useful for localising the problem.

ASSESSMENT OF THE CONFUSED OR DEMENTED PATIENT

Confusion, delirium and dementia

Students often have difficulty understanding the difference between delirium and dementia because of the similar symptoms. Patients with delirium develop it quickly, become agitated, and can go in and out of consciousness over time. Delirium is usually reversible and memory problems are usually short-term. Dementia develops more gradually, and the effects on memory are more permanent.

CONFUSION AND DELIRIUM

Delirium is an acute and relatively sudden (developing over hours to days) decline in attention–focus, perception and cognition. The patient appears out of touch with their surroundings and is spontaneously producing evidence of this confusion, such as a lack of clear and orderly thought and behaviour, disorientation with muttering, restlessness, rambling and shouting (often offensively and continuously) with evidence of delusion and hallucinations. *It is not synonymous with drowsiness* and may occur without it. Other features of delirium can include: depression, memory problems, difficulty writing or finding words and disturbances of the sleep–wake cycle.

The *International Classification of Diseases*, 10th edition [2], defines delirium as:

* impairment of consciousness and attention;
* global disturbance of cognition (including illusions, hallucinations, delusions and disorientation);
* psychomotor disturbances;
* disturbance of the sleep–wake cycle;
* emotional disturbances.

There are many causes of delirium and often it is multifactorial in origin. Even after extensive investigation it is not always possible to define the particular aetiology in all patients and in such patients the delirium usually resolves spontaneously. Delirium in the absence of any clearly definable alternative explanation is not uncommon in hospital in the postoperative period following prolonged anaesthesia. Delirium occurs more commonly in patients with mild cognitive impairment and it can be precipitated by a chest or urinary tract infection, electrolyte disturbances, cardiac, liver or renal failure, drug toxicity and drug withdrawal.

It is important to review all medications, particularly those that have recently been commenced or ceased. Clinical signs of chronic liver disease and the characteristic odour on the breath referred to as 'fetor hepaticus' (the breath of the dead where the breath has a sweet or fecal smell related to mercaptans, ammonia and ketones) identifies patients with portal hypertension and hepatic encephalopathy. Patients with a metabolic encephalopathy due to any cause may also have an abnormality referred to as asterixis: a short, flapping tremor elicited by having the patient hold their arms out in front of them with their wrists extended. Asterixis is also seen in patients with hypercapnia (elevated carbon dioxide) and anticonvulsant overdose. A tremor together with myoclonic jerks may be seen in patients with renal failure or patients exposed to antipsychotic drugs. Delirium may also be a manifestation of hypoxia in the setting of cardiac or respiratory failure or a chest infection.

Patients with delirium should have a full workup for sepsis, including looking for fever and tachycardia, examining the chest for evidence of infection, palpating the abdomen to look for tenderness that might suggest abdominal pathology and checking for neck rigidity by flexing the neck. Check the urine with a dip stick to look for evidence of infection (protein, blood and nitrites) and request a full blood examination, ESR, CRP and urine, blood and, if appropriate, sputum cultures. In the absence of obvious infection, assessments of hepatic and renal function, blood gases and electrolytes (in particular sodium, calcium and magnesium) should be undertaken. Very rarely, delirium may be the presenting feature of meningitis or encephalitis and a lumbar puncture may be necessary.

One clue is that patients with confusion and delirium are usually restless and agitated, whereas patients with symptoms related to parietal lobe pathology are not as a rule agitated.

This is particularly so for problems in the dominant parieto-temporal lobe with fluent dysphasia, word salad, literal and verbal paraphasic errors and

It is not uncommon for patients with hemisphere lesions affecting the parietal lobes to be diagnosed with confusion or delirium.

neologisms (see Chapter 5, 'The cerebral hemispheres and cerebellum') or non-dominant parietal lobe lesions with patients 'lost in space'. A quick screening examination (if the patient can cooperate) with double simultaneous stimuli in the visual fields and asking the patient to hold their arms out could detect the visual inattention and parietal drift that would alert one to focal rather than diffuse brain pathology.

MANAGEMENT of DELIRIUM

The main goal in managing delirium is keeping each patient comfortable and safe. Place the patient in a quiet, well-lit room with familiar people and objects, a visible clock and wall calendar.

Alcohol withdrawal or delirium tremens, 'the DT's', is a common cause of delirium. Benzodiazepines are the treatment of choice. A meta-analysis of nine prospective controlled trials [3] concluded that sedative-hypnotic agents (diazepam, chlordiazepoxide, pentobarbital paraldehyde and barbital) are more effective than neuroleptic agents (chlorpromazine, promazine and thioridazine) in reducing duration of delirium and mortality. Adequate doses should be used to maintain light somnolence for the duration of delirium. Coupled with comprehensive supportive medical care, this approach is highly effective in preventing morbidity and mortality. In general it is best to use one drug at a time, using the minimal effective dose, increasing the dose as required and reviewing the treatment on a regular basis [4]. The atypical antipsychotics such as risperidone and olanzapine have the advantage of producing less sedation and are less likely to be associated with extrapyramidal side effects.

For patients with delirium unrelated to alcohol withdrawal, there are no randomised trials but most clinicians would follow the same principles of management used in treating patients with delirium tremens [5]. Imaging in the form of a CT or MRI scan is often performed but rarely rewarding.

DEMENTIA

Dementia is derived from the Latin 'de-', meaning apart or away, + 'mens' (genitive mentis), meaning mind. It consists of a progressive global deterioration of intellectual and cognitive function with defects in orientation, memory, intellect, judgement and affect. Dementia is often associated with depression and apathy. As cognitive function declines the patient loses the ability to be independent with regard to all activities of daily living.

There are many causes of dementia; the more common include Alzheimer's disease (AD), vascular dementia, alcoholism and Parkinson's disease.

Potentially treatable causes of dementia include:
- hypothyroidism
- vitamin B_1 or vitamin B_{12} deficiency
- normal pressure hydrocephalus
- subdural haematoma
- drug intoxication
- cerebral vasculitis
- heavy metal intoxication
- brain tumours
- chronic infections or inflammation such as syphilis, meningitis related to tuberculosis, cryptococcus, sarcoidosis and *the extremely rare entity of Whipple's disease*. It is anticipated that future discoveries will lead to even more cases of treatable dementia.

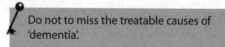
Do not to miss the treatable causes of 'dementia'.

Alzheimer's disease

Alzheimer's disease is the commonest cause of dementia and, at the time of writing this textbook, the definitive diagnosis still requires histopathological demonstration of sufficient numbers of amyloid plaques and neurofibrillary tangles and is therefore not usually possible in life. The risk of Alzheimer's increases with advancing age and 20–40% of patients over the age of 85 will have Alzheimer's disease. A positive family history is not uncommon. Patients with Down syndrome (trisomy 21) have an increased risk of Alzheimer's disease after the age of 40.

Most patients with Alzheimer's disease will present with the insidious onset over many years of memory impairment, particularly short-term memory. As cognitive function declines the patient develops increasing difficulties with daily activities and it is this difficulty that differentiates mild cognitive impairment from true dementia. A reversal of the sleep cycle with patients sleeping during the day and wandering at night is not uncommon. Some patients with Alzheimer's disease are unaware of their cognitive impairment and it is concerned relatives that urge them to seek medical attention. Patients may cope well in their home environment, but often the dementia is unmasked when they are admitted to hospital or when they travel and are placed in an unfamiliar environment. As the disease relentlessly progresses, patients become lost when they go for walks or when they are driving, and they have difficulty with finances, housekeeping, shopping and following instructions. Leaving the stove on is a common complaint. Walking becomes difficult and patients may develop a characteristic disorder of gait referred to as the apraxic gait (see Chapter 13, 'Abnormal movements and difficulty walking due to central nervous system problems'). Language function deteriorates with difficulty naming objects, comprehension and then subsequently the development of aphasia. In advanced Alzheimer's patients are no longer able to care for themselves in terms of dressing, bathing and feeding and eventually lose control of bladder and bowels.

Depression can present with many of the clinical features of dementia that resolve with treatment of the depression and this is referred to as 'pseudodementia'. It is the intellectual impairment in patients with a primary psychiatric disorder, in which the features of intellectual abnormality resemble, at least in part, those of a neuropathologically induced cognitive deficit. These patients often complain of memory disturbance and yet are often able to recant the history of their 'cognitive decline' without much difficulty. The correct diagnosis may only reveal itself when the patient improves with treatment for depression. Reynolds et al [6] in a small study found that significantly greater pretreatment early morning awakening, higher ratings of psychological anxiety and more severe impairment of libido were features of pseudodementia whereas patients with dementia showed significantly more disorientation to time, greater difficulty finding their way about familiar streets or indoors and more impairment with dressing.

In very rare instances dementia may begin with focal neurological deficits [7–10] and a number of syndromes have been identified, such as posterior cortical atrophy (PCA), corticobasal syndrome (CBS), behavioural variant frontotemporal dementia (bvFTD), progressive non-fluent aphasia (PNFA) (or a mixed aphasia) and semantic dementia (SD). In some instances these patients will have the pathological features of Alzheimer's disease. These focal syndromes may remain pure for many years before the subsequent appearance of other signs of dementia. The underlying neuropathology does not uniquely associate the clinical syndromes with distinctive patterns of pathological markers. A detailed discussion of these entities is beyond the scope of this textbook [7, 9, 10].

Rapidly progressive dementia (RPD)

Rapidly progressive dementias can develop subacutely over months, weeks or even days and be quickly fatal. Prion disease (Creutzfeldt–Jakob disease) is the commonest cause, but some cases of frontotemporal dementia (FTD), corticobasal degeneration (CBD), Alzheimer's disease, dementia with Lewy bodies (DLB) and progressive supranuclear palsy may sometimes present in a fulminant form with death occurring in less than 3 years [11].

Antibody-mediated limbic encephalitis (LE) associated with cancer (paraneo-plastic) or occurring without cancer (non-paraneoplastic) and Hashimoto's encepha-lopathy (HE) with associated antineuronal antibodies are potentially treatable causes of RPD. Multiple sclerosis and neurosarcoidosis may also cause rapidly progressive dementia.

Limbic encephalitis presents with rapid memory loss, depression, anxiety and changes in personality followed by impaired cognitive function and seizures. Anti-neuronal antibodies may be found in the serum or cerebrospinal fluid and hyponatraemia due to the syndrome of inappropriate anti-diuretic hormone secretion may also be present.

Creutzfeldt–Jakob disease (CJD) presents with cerebellar ataxia and behavioural disturbances in addition to the rapid dementia. There is a variant form of vCJD, 'mad-cow disease', where the initial manifestations are major psychiatric symptoms with the ataxia and dementia associated with chorea and myoclonus occurring later in the course.

Forgetfulness or early dementia

Forgetfulness or absent-mindedness is a feature of the ageing process. Most patients over the age of 70 complain of problems with memory and many patients seek medical attention concerned about the possibility of dementia. It can be very difficult in the early stages to differentiate between these two processes [12]. Episodic memory loss precedes widespread cognitive decline in early AD [13].

DIAGNOSIS and MANAGEMENT of ALZHEIMER'S DISEASE

Magnetic resonance imaging including volumetric studies can detect specific changes in patients with minimal cognitive disturbance that may predict progression to dementia [14].

Apo E was the first gene demonstrated to increase the risk of Alzheimer's disease and a point mutation in APP results in the early onset of Alzheimer's disease that is inherited in an autosomal dominant pattern. Presenelin-1 on chromosome 14 and presenelin-2 on chromosome 1 have been associated with extremely rare instances of familial Alzheimer's disease of early onset.

There are a number of cholinesterase inhibitors that provide symptomatic benefit and may decrease the rate of cognitive decline in the first few years. The management of patients with Alzheimer's disease is predominantly providing support for the family and the patient, treatment of depression and treatment of seizures if they occur. In the early stages patients can be instructed to write lists or put up little reminders where they will see them of what they need to do that day. It is also helpful if patients with Alzheimer's develop a daily routine including physical exercise. Caring for patients with Alzheimer's disease is very demanding day in and day out, and organising a period of family relief where the patient is admitted to an interim care facility while the supportive family member has a break will often enable the patient to remain at home for a longer period of time.

DISORDERS OF MUSCLE AND THE NEUROMUSCULAR JUNCTION

Diseases of muscle and conditions affecting the neuromuscular junction are very rare. For example, the prevalence of inflammatory muscle disease is estimated to be 1 in 100,000 and of myasthenia gravis is 8 in 100,000. A complete discussion of all disorders of muscle is well beyond the scope of this text and interested readers will find many excellent reviews, textbooks and websites [15–18].

Although symptoms such as myalgia (muscle pain), muscle cramps, muscle stiffness, fatigue and exercise intolerance occur in patients with muscle disease, many of these are somewhat non-specific. Patients should be suspected of suffering from muscle disease when they complain of weakness with or without wasting of muscles in the absence of other neurological symptoms. The weakness will develop very slowly over years in most of the disorders, of muscle other than the inflammatory myopathies although, even in the inflammatory myopathies where the weakness usually evolves over weeks to months, occasionally the onset may also be more gradual. As many muscle diseases are hereditary, there will often be a positive family history.

- *Muscle pain* or *myalgia,* apart from (therapeutic) drug-induced muscle pain, is rare in muscle diseases and more often relates to rheumatological, psychiatric or orthopaedic disorders, although it may occur in patients with congenital or endocrine myopathies and myositis. It is important to question about the use of prescription and non-prescription medications when a patient presents with muscle pain. For a recent review on drug-induced myopathies, refer to Klopstock [19].
- *Fatigue* is also a very non-specific symptom. Patients with depression, for example, often complain of fatigue; however, fatigue in the form of exercise intolerance may point to involvement of the neuromuscular junction with conditions such as myasthenia gravis and the Lambert–Eaton syndrome. Fatigue is also a prominent symptom in patients with motor neuron disease.
- *Muscle cramps* are seen with hyponatraemia, renal failure, hypothyroidism and many other conditions that affect peripheral nerves.
- *Myotonia* is the inability to relax a muscle after forced voluntary contraction, for example gripping an object with the hands. It is seen in some of the hereditary disorders of muscle such as myotonic dystrophy and Thompson's disease as well as acquired disorders such as neuromyotonia (Isaac's syndrome).

There are many approaches to patients with suspected muscle disease; one is shown in Figure 14.3.

1 The initial step is to establish if there is a *family history*, as many diseases of muscle, such as the muscular dystrophies and the congenital, metabolic and mitochondrial myopathies, are inherited disorders of muscle and there will be another member of the family affected. It is important to remember that a negative family history does not exclude hereditary disorders of muscle. Some patients are so mildly affected that they are not aware of the problem or have not sought medical attention. This is not uncommon in patients with muscular dystrophy.

2 The *age of onset* can provide another clue, e.g. congenital myopathies may be present at birth, the muscular dystrophies often develop in the first few years of life and inclusion body myositis is predominantly seen in elderly patients.

3 Consider the *rapidity of onset of the weakness*. Many disorders of muscle, particularly the inherited disorders of muscle, develop gradually over many, many years; most of the acquired disorders of muscle, for example the inflammatory myopathies, on the other hand progress rapidly over months. Patients with congenital myopathies

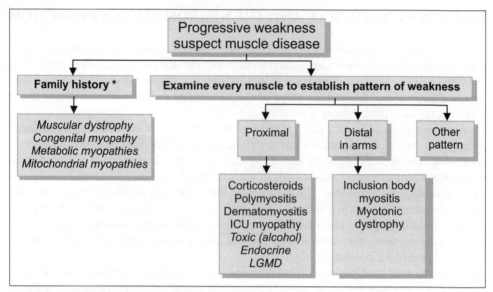

FIGURE 14.3   An approach to patients with suspected muscle disease

Note: The uncommon diseases are in italics.

*A 'negative' family history does not exclude inherited disorders of muscle. 'Other' pattern refers to patterns of weakness other than proximal or distal, for example fascioscapulohumeral.

ICU = intensive care unit; LGMD = limb-girdle muscular dystrophy

may not progress at all. *Fluctuating weakness* suggests disorders of the neuromuscular junction, such as myasthenia gravis and the Lambert–Eaton syndrome. Recurrent attacks of weakness are a feature of the periodic paralyses and certain glycolytic pathway disorders.

4 *Define the pattern of weakness.* Many conditions of muscle have been labelled according to the pattern of weakness, for example limb-girdle muscular dystrophy or fascioscapulohumeral dystrophy. This may be less important in the future. As the underlying genetic bases for the muscle diseases are defined, it is increasingly apparent that there is great variability in the phenotypic expression (the pattern of weakness), reflecting the severity of the underlying the genetic defect. For example, with mutations in the dysferlin gene, patients can present with the pattern of a limb-girdle muscular dystrophy, a distal anterior compartment myopathy or the classic Miyoshi myopathy with multifocal weakness and wasting [20]. The term 'dysferlin deficient muscular dystrophy' has replaced the term 'Miyoshi myopathy'. The classification of the limb-girdle dystrophies continues to be revised on the basis of the elucidation of the underlying protein and genetic abnormalities [21]. In everyday clinical practice, other than a proximal muscle weakness, the 'proximal myopathy' that is probably the most common pattern and distal weakness in the forearms, most of the other disorders of muscle are extremely rare.

5 *Look for associated phenomena* that may help differentiate one condition from another.
  • Muscle hypertrophy
    • Duchenne and Becker muscular dystrophy
    • Hypothyroidism
  • Respiratory failure:
    • Myotonic dystrophy
    • Centronuclear myopathy

- Nemaline myopathy
- Acid maltase deficiency
- Cardiac disease:
  - Myotonic dystrophy
  - Duchenne or Becker muscular dystrophies
  - Limb-girdle muscular dystrophies 1B, 2I, 2C–F, 2G
  - Emery–Dreifuss muscular dystrophy
- Hepatomegaly: metabolic or alcoholic myopathies
- Central nervous system involvement may occur in patients with mitochondrial myopathies [15]

6 Blood tests
  - *Measure the creatinine kinase (CK).* CK is elevated in most but not all disorders of muscle and in itself is not a particularly useful test to differentiate one disorder of muscle from another; however, a markedly elevated CK is seen with Duchenne muscular dystrophy and the dysferlinopathies.
  - Thyroid function tests and electrolytes should be routine and parathyroid hormone and human immuno-deficiency virus (HIV) in selected cases.
  - Inflammatory myopathies can be associated with connective tissue diseases such as systemic lupus erythematosus and rheumatoid arthritis; thus an antinuclear factor (ANF), double-stranded DNA and rheumatoid factor tests should be performed in these patients.

7 The urine should be examined for myoglobinuria in patients with exercise-induced muscle pain.

8 A *forearm ischaemic lactate test* is performed in patients suspected of having a metabolic myopathy; a less than threefold increase in the lactate is abnormal.

9 *Perform nerve conduction studies and in particular electromyography.* Nerve conduction studies are normal in patients with muscle disease (exceptions include mitochondrial disorders, myotonic dystrophy and inclusion body myositis). Electromyography (EMG) can confirm the presence of a myopathy with the demonstration of brief small amplitude polyphasic potentials (BSAPPs) and a full recruitment pattern with minimal effort; exclude other conditions such as motor neuron disease, peripheral neuropathy and disorders of the neuromuscular junction. Occasionally the nerve conduction studies and EMG can be completely normal in patients with muscle disease. The presence of fibrillation potentials and positive sharp waves with the myopathic changes described above indicate a likely inflammatory myositis such as polymyositis, dermatomyositis or inclusion body myositis. The sound of a motorbike or dive bomber on EMG is seen with myotonia in myotonic and congenital muscular dystrophies.

10 *Biopsy an affected muscle.* This can be performed using an open biopsy procedure or a needle biopsy; the latter is less invasive and multiple samples can be taken but the size of the individual samples is small. It is important to remember that pathological changes may be focal and thus a normal biopsy does not exclude muscle disease. It is more rewarding to biopsy an affected muscle, but not one that is so severely affected that the likely pathology will be non-diagnostic end-stage muscle. It is also important not to biopsy a muscle at the site of EMG as the EMG needle will cause abnormal pathology. Increasingly sophisticated pathological methods, such as immunohistochemical staining with a panel of antibodies, quantitative analysis of proteins by western blotting and DNA analysis, are now a routine part of the pathological examination of muscle and help to determine the cause of muscle weakness in most patients.

Note: The unravelling of the genome is in some instances already replacing muscle biopsy with non-invasive molecular genetics studies in the hereditary muscle diseases [15, 22]. DNA analysis is becoming the gold standard for the diagnosis.

In everyday clinical practice there are two common clinical presentations of patients with muscle disease: proximal weakness (referred to as the proximal myopathy) and distal weakness.

Proximal limb weakness, 'the proximal myopathy'

Patients with proximal muscle weakness complain of difficulty sitting in and getting out of chairs, getting up off the floor, climbing up and down stairs, lifting objects above their head or brushing their hair. The term 'proximal myopathy' is very non-specific and both hereditary and acquired conditions will result in weakness of the proximal muscles (shoulder abduction and hip flexion). The list is very extensive and includes limb-girdle muscular dystrophy, endocrine and metabolic disturbances, drugs and infections, osteo-malacia and hyperparathyroidism, polymyositis and dermatomyositis, corticosteroids, HIV, Cushing's disease and hyperthyroidism. The commonest causes would be iatrogenic corticosteroid use, critical illness or ICU myopathy, the inflammatory myopathies and thyroid disease, although with early detection of thyroid disease weakness is increasingly uncommon.

Muscle diseases causing distal weakness in the arms

Patients with distal weakness will complain of difficulty opening jars, turning the key in the lock or doing up buttons. Distal weakness in the legs related to muscle disease is extremely rare and is more common in patients with peripheral neuropathies. If present, distal weakness in the legs causes patients to complain of difficulty walking on uneven ground often associated with tripping due to catching their toe due to a foot drop.

Although there are many causes of distal weakness in the arms [16], myotonic dystrophy and inclusion body myositis are the two commonest conditions that result in distal weakness in the forearms. Some of the limb-girdle muscular dystrophies may involve distal as well as proximal weakness [21].

> **TREATMENT of MUSCULAR DYSTROPHIES**
>
> At present there is no established therapy that can cure muscular dystrophy. Corticosteroids have a defined role in patients with Duchenne muscular dystrophy, but not in other muscular dystrophies [23].

The inflammatory myopathies
POLYMYOSITIS AND DERMATOMYOSITIS

Polymyositis and dermatomyositis should be suspected in patients who develop weakness over a period of months. The weakness is symmetrical and affects proximal muscles in the limbs with weakness of shoulder abduction and hip flexion; associated neck flexion weakness is a clue to the diagnosis. Rarely, the bulbar (muscles innervated by the 9th, 10th and 12th cranial nerves) and respiratory muscles may be affected. Patients with dermatomyositis have characteristic skin changes such as the heliotrope rash resulting in violaceous discoloration of the eyelids, scaly erythema over the joints on the dorsal aspect of the hands, macular erythema on the posterior neck and shoulders or on the anterior neck and chest or a violaceous erythema associated with increased pigment and telangiectasia on the anterior neck, chest, posterior shoulders, back and buttocks.

TREATMENT of POLYMYOSITIS and DERMATOMYOSITIS

Treatment of polymyositis and dermatomyositis is largely empirical. Corticosteroids remain the agent of first choice, despite the lack of randomised controlled data [24]. Other immunosuppressive agents are recommended for patients who fail to respond to corticosteroids or are used in combination with corticosteroids to reduce the incidence of side effects from the steroids.

- The initial dose of prednisolone is 1–2 mg/kg body weight for 2–4 weeks, slowly reducing the dose over a period of 6 months and changing to an alternate day regimen as maintenance therapy.
- If the response to corticosteroids is suboptimal at 3 months, other immunosuppression is recommended [25]. Azathioprine (it may take 3–6 months before seeing any benefit), cyclophosphamide [26], cyclosporine and methotrexate [27] have all been advocated in corticosteroid-resistant cases.
- Plasmapheresis was not shown to be of any benefit in a randomised controlled trial [28].
- A randomised controlled trial has confirmed the efficacy of intravenous immunoglobulin in corticosteroid-resistant polymyositis [29] and is currently recommended by the European Federation of Neurological Societies [30]. Treatment may need to continue for 1–3 years to prevent relapse.

INCLUSION BODY MYOSITIS

Inclusion body myositis (IBM) is a sporadic condition seen predominantly in patients over the age of 50. IBM has a pathognomonic pattern of weakness affecting the quadriceps muscle with severe weakness of knee extension resulting in frequent falls as the knees give way in addition to the distal weakness in the forearms and hands with weakness of flexion of the fingers. Hip flexion weakness is much less severe than the knee extension weakness. Dysphagia is common but involvement of the respiratory muscles is rare [31]. The muscle biopsy demonstrates inflammatory cells and vacuoles in muscle fibres.

TREATMENT OF INCLUSION BODY MYOSITIS

Many immunosuppressive drugs have been tried in IBM, including corticosteroids, azathioprine, cyclosporine, methotrexate and intravenous immunoglobulin and interferon-beta-1a, all to no avail. Current recommendations encourage exercise for patients with IMB [32].

Drug-induced myopathies

Side effects from the use of drugs are rare and occur in less than 0.5% of patients. They include muscle pain that can be mild and not require cessation of the drug or severe and associated with fatigue and elevation of the CK to more than 10 times the upper limit of normal (ULN). Other complications include a proximal muscle weakness or rhabdomyolysis which at times is fatal. Myopathy is more common in patients on multiple therapeutic agents and may relate to drug–drug interactions. Although the CK is usually elevated, a normal value does not exclude a drug-induced myopathy [33]. The myopathy may take months or even years to develop, and symptoms may persist for some time after cessation of the drug [34].

Statins, fibrates, antidepressants, antipsychotic drugs, benzodiazepines, calcium channel blockers, corticosteroids, alcohol, cocaine, amphetamines, colchicines and heroin are some of the drugs that can produce myopathy including rhabdomyolysis.

Weakness and fatigue
MYASTHENIA GRAVIS AND LAMBERT–EATON SYNDROME

The term 'myasthenia' literally means muscle weakness and is derived from the Latin 'myos', meaning muscle, and the Greek 'asthenes', meaning a- (without) + sthenos (strength).

The two currently recognised disorders that affect the neuromuscular junction (NMJ) are myasthenia gravis [35] and the Lambert–Eaton syndrome, also referred to as the Lambert–Eaton myasthenic syndrome [36]. Patients with myasthenia gravis observe that their weakness is exacerbated by exercise, whereas patients with the Lambert–Eaton syndrome complain of weakness and fatigue unrelated to exercise. Patients with amyotrophic lateral sclerosis (motor neuron disease) may also complain of a significant exacerbation of weakness with exercise, but the severe fixed weakness, wasting and fasciculations seen in motor neuron disease are not seen in the disorders of the NMJ [37].

> Disorders of the neuromuscular junction should be suspected in patients who have weakness that is associated with fatiguability.

Both are immune-mediated disorders.[1] Lambert–Eaton syndrome is often associated with malignancy, particularly small cell carcinoma of the lung [40], but may also occur as an autoimmune disease in the absence of malignancy [41]. Myasthenia gravis may be associated with a tumour of the thymus [42], either benign or malignant; this is more common in elderly patients and younger patients tend to have thymic hyperplasia or aplasia of the thymus.

Myasthenia gravis is classified as either ocular if it just affects the ocular muscles (including the eyelids) or generalised if it affects the facial, bulbar and limb muscles. The characteristic feature is the exacerbation of the weakness with exercise or prolonged use of the muscles. Variable ptosis (drooping of the eyelid) and variable diplopia with a mixture of horizontal and vertical diplopia at different times occur with ocular myasthenia gravis, although the occasional patient does not observe variable diplopia leading to the incorrect diagnosis of a 3rd, 4th or 6th nerve palsy or an internuclear ophthalmoplegia (a lesion of the median longitudinal fasciculus in the brainstem).[2] The ocular muscles may also be affected in patients with generalised myasthenia gravis. Patients with generalised myasthenia may complain of difficulty holding their head up while watching television due to weakness of the extensor muscles of the neck, increasing dysarthria the more they speak; problems with chewing or swallowing food, again worse with prolonged chewing; increasing weakness leading to difficulty holding the arms up above the head when washing the hair or putting clothes on the clothes line. Patients have to rest momentarily before they can continue this activity. During the examination increasing degrees of ptosis and diplopia can be elicited by asking the patient to look up for a prolonged period of time; fatiguable weakness in the limbs can be elicited with repetitive exercise. A quick test in patients with suspected ocular myasthenia is to place ice on the eyelid and see the temporary resolution of the ptosis [43]. Changes in the degree of diplopia with the ice test should be interpreted with caution [44].

The reflexes are normal and are not influenced by exercise. There are a number of diagnostic tests for myasthenia gravis with variable sensitivity but high specificity (see Table 14.1).

---

1 In the majority of patients with myasthenia gravis, antibodies are directed against the acetylcholine receptor, although in recent years other antibodies have been identified [38, 39]. The Lambert–Eaton syndrome is due to antibodies directed against the P/Q-type calcium channels at the motor nerve terminals.
2 Personal observation.

TABLE 14.1 Sensitivity and specificity of diagnostic tests in myasthenia gravis

Test	Sensitivity (%) (95% CI)	Specificity (%) (95% CI)
Tensilon test [45]	92 (83–100%)	97 (91–100)
Ice test [43]	95 (87–100)	97 (90–100)
ACHR antibody* [46]	54 (44–63)	98 (96–100)
Repetitive nerve stimulation [47]	26 (15–44)	95 (94–100)
SFEMG [48]	89 (83–95)	88 (78–96)

Note: These figures were calculated from the table in the article entitled 'A systematic review of diagnostic studies in myasthenia gravis' [49]. Benatar assessed the quality of the studies as well as the reported results of sensitivity and specificity. The individual figures from each of the studies quoted were summed and divided by the number of studies to obtain the sensitivity, specificity and 95% confidence intervals quoted in this table.
*The figures for the ACHR antibody assay are at variance with the accepted figure of approximately 85% sensitivity [50] and the explanation for this is unclear.

Diagnostic tests
THE TENSILON TEST
The tensilon (edrophonium hydrochloride) test demonstrates transient improvement lasting 30–60 seconds.

1 The patient should be pre-treated with atropine 600 µg to reduce the gastrointestinal side effects of the edrophonium hydrochloride.
2 10 mg of edrophonium is mixed with 9 mL of normal saline (1 mg of edrophonium per mL).
3 Initially 2 mg is injected; if the patient fails to respond to 2 mg, the other 8 mg is injected.
4 Observe the patient for at least 3 minutes after the injection (longer in older patients due to a slower circulation time).

In some patients 2 mg is too much and in other patents 8 mg may be insufficient [51]. In normal patients the tensilon test does not produce any change in strength.

ACETYLCHOLINE RECEPTOR ANTIBODIES
Acetylcholine receptor (ACHR) antibodies are positive in 85% of patients with myasthenia gravis [50]. ACHR antibodies may be detected with repeat testing in some patients with myasthenia gravis in whom they are initially negative [52]. It is likely that further antibodies will be discovered in the sero-negative (the ACHR antibody negative) patients with myasthenia gravis.

Musk antibodies are an IgG antibody against the muscle-specific kinase (MuSK). The presence of antibodies against MuSK appears to define a subgroup of patients with sero-negative myasthenia gravis who have predominantly localised, in many cases bulbar, muscle weaknesses (face, tongue, pharynx etc) and reduced response to conventional immunosuppressive treatments [53].

Anti-titin antibodies may identify patients with a thymoma [39].

NERVE CONDUCTION STUDIES
Nerve conduction studies can differentiate between myasthenia gravis and Lambert–Eaton syndrome.

A repetitive stimulation study is where the nerve is stimulated at 3 per second for 8 impulses immediately before exercise, 20 seconds after sustained exercise and then at intervals of 1 minute for several minutes. The test may demonstrate a decremental response (the 5th response is of lower amplitude compared to the 1st response) in patients with myasthenia gravis and an incremental response in patients with the Lambert–Eaton syndrome.

Single fibre electromyography (SFEMG) can demonstrate instability at the neuromuscular junction (referred to as increased jitter) but cannot differentiate between Lambert–Eaton syndrome and myasthenia gravis. Increased jitter is also seen in motor neuron disease.

TREATMENT of MYASTHENIA GRAVIS

Treatment of myasthenia gravis is influenced by the presence or absence of a thymic tumour. Most authorities would recommend thymectomy [54] in patients with thymic tumours as it is difficult to differentiate between benign and malignant tumours prior to surgery. Thymic tumours are locally malignant, invading the lung and/or pericardium; they do not metastasise.

In patients with isolated *ocular myasthenia gravis,* the treatment options include nothing, pyridostigmine or other anticholinesterase drugs to provide symptomatic relief or full immunosuppressive treatment. In patients with generalised myasthenia gravis the options include immunosuppression or thymectomy in the presence of thymic hyperplasia.

In *generalised myasthenia gravis* corticosteroids are often the first drug of choice and limited evidence from randomised controlled trials has demonstrated short-term benefit [56]. Small randomised controlled trials suggest that cyclosporine, as monotherapy or with corticosteroids, or cyclophosphamide with corticosteroids significantly improve myasthenia gravis. Azathioprine, either as monotherapy or with steroids, has not been shown to be of benefit in randomised controlled trials. Mycophenolate mofetil (as monotherapy or with either corticosteroids or cyclosporine) or tacrolimus (with corticosteroids or plasma exchange) has also been advocated in resistant cases [57]. Although intravenous immunoglobulin has been shown to be superior to placebo but no different to plasma exchange, the ease of use means that intravenous immunoglobulin is regarded by most as the treatment of choice for a myasthenic crisis or preoperatively in patients undergoing thymectomy or other surgery if the myasthenia is unstable at the time. Pyridostigmine may provide some symptomatic benefit, but gastrointestinal upset and the fact that an excess dose can cause similar symptoms to worsening myasthenia gravis makes this a difficult drug to use. Excess salivation and abdominal discomfort with diarrhoea are the two clues that there may be an excess of pyridostigmine.

Currently corticosteroids, azathioprine, plasmapheresis, intravenous immunoglobulins and 3,4-diaminopyridine are used in treatment of Lambert–Eaton myasthenic syndrome with limited success. Some evidence from randomised controlled trials shows that either 3, 4-diaminopyridine or intravenous immunoglobulin improves muscle strength scores and compound muscle action potential amplitudes in patients with Lambert–Eaton myasthenic syndrome [58]. 3,4 diaminopyridine works by blocking K^+ channel efflux in nerve terminals so that action potential duration is increased. Ca^{2+} channels thus remain open for a longer period of time, which allows greater acetylcholine release to stimulate the muscle at the end plate.

CHRONIC FATIGUE OR POST-VIRAL FATIGUE SYNDROME

The post-viral fatigue syndrome is very common. It was initially described at the Royal Free Hospital [59] and was referred to as benign myalgic encephalomyelitis [60]. The aetiology remains obscure, although a similar syndrome of fatigue and depression is common following infectious mononucleosis [61], suggesting a possible viral aetiology and thus the term post-viral fatigue syndrome.

---

3   First described by Mary Walker who administered prostigmin [neostigmine] and performed the 'miracle of St Alfeges' [55]; until then myasthenia gravis was regarded as an incurable progressive neurological disease.

Although post-viral fatigue can occur in epidemics, it is usually sporadic. It occurs at any age but is more common in young and middle-aged females. The overwhelming complaint is one of severe fatigue with muscle aches and pains developing after a flu-like illness. Depression and excessive sleep are common, as are complaints of poor memory and difficulty concentrating [62].

> **MANAGEMENT of POST-VIRAL FATIGUE**
>
> There is at this stage no specific test. The diagnosis is a clinical one and requires the presence of a definite viral infection followed by severe fatigue. There is no specific treatment but fortunately it is a self-limiting illness in most patients, although some may be troubled for months or even years.

MULTIPLE SCLEROSIS

After more than a century of study (multiple sclerosis was first described by the French pathologist Charcot in 1868), the aetiology of multiple sclerosis (MS) remains unknown. There is no gold standard test to confirm the diagnosis and there is no curative treatment. It is highly likely that everything written in this section will very rapidly be out of date.

Currently the diagnosis is based on the clinical features, the results of MRI, analysis of the cerebral spinal fluid and visual evoked potentials [63] (see Tables 14.2–14.4). These criteria have been modified on several occasions and are likely to change in the future. The diagnosis of MS can be very difficult as there are a number of conditions that can result in multifocal involvement of the central nervous system and thus mimic MS. These include central nervous system or systemic vasculitis including systemic lupus erythematosus, acute disseminated encephalomyelitis, antiphospholipid antibody syndrome, sarcoidosis, Wilson's disease, paraneoplastic syndromes and central nervous system lymphoma.

MS as it is currently defined is more common in women and in younger patients between the ages of 15 and 50, with a mean age of onset of 29–33 years. It can occur in children or in adults over the age of 50. There is probably a genetic predisposition [64]. The natural history is highly variable from the very benign, where it is accidentally discovered at autopsy in old age, to the very malignant with death within the first few years of onset. This variability makes it very difficult to assess therapeutic interventions. In general, at 10 years 50% of patients with MS will have a neurological deficit requiring the use of a cane to walk while 15% will be in a wheelchair [65].

MS may present as a clinically isolated syndrome, a relapsing/remitting course with or without secondary progressive MS or primary progressive MS where progression to disability occurs without remission.

Presentations of multiple sclerosis
CLINICALLY ISOLATED SYNDROME

Younger patients with the disease may present with a *clinically isolated syndrome* affecting the optic nerve, such as optic or retrobulbar neuritis, the spinal cord with transverse myelitis or involvement of the brainstem with vertigo and/or diplopia. The latter relates to involvement of the median longitudinal fasciculus resulting in an internuclear ophthalmoplegia. These episodes are usually self-limiting with resolving over several weeks. The presence of gadolinium-enhancing abnormalities or juxtacortical lesions on an MRI scan increases the risk of progression to clinically definite MS in patients with clinically isolated syndromes.

RELAPSING AND REMITTING MULTIPLE SCLEROSIS

The course in the great majority of patients is relapsing and remitting with initially complete resolution of symptoms and signs. Some patients may be left with a residual deficit that accumulates with subsequent relapses.

SECONDARY PROGRESSIVE MULTIPLE SCLEROSIS

Many patients with the relapsing/remitting form of MS will subsequently develop a *secondary progressive* course with increasing disability in the absence of any obvious relapses or develop a cumulative neurological deficit when the relapses do not completely resolve.

PRIMARY PROGRESSIVE MULTIPLE SCLEROSIS

There is a primary progressive form of MS where increasing disability occurs in the absence of any obvious relapses or attacks. This typically occurs in patients of middle age who develop progressive cervical spinal cord involvement.

When to suspect multiple sclerosis

MS should be suspected in patients who present with the gradual onset of focal neurological symptoms associated with impaired function that evolves over a period of hours to days.

OPTIC OR RETROBULBAR NEURITIS

Unilateral blurring of vision associated with pain on movement of the eye evolving over hours to days is a very typical initial

> Not all patients with optic neuritis will subsequently develop MS.

presentation and represents *optic or retrobulbar neuritis*. As described in Chapter 4, 'The cranial nerves and understanding the brainstem', patients with optic neuritis will have markedly impaired visual acuity with a swollen optic disc and an afferent pupillary defect with or without impairment of colour vision, whereas patients with retrobulbar neuritis will have the same features but without the optic disc swelling.

TRANSVERSE MYELITIS

Weakness commencing in the lower limbs that may spread to affect the

> Not all patients with transverse myelitis will develop MS.

upper limbs or an ascending sensory disturbance once again commencing in the lower limbs and spreading up onto the trunk and sometimes into the arms represents involvement of the spinal cord and is referred to as *transverse myelitis*. Sphincter disturbance is common in patients with spinal cord involvement. This may manifest as either acute urinary retention or incontinence of either urine or faeces.

It is important to remember that transverse myelitis is a syndrome and not a diagnosis. Although MS is a common cause of transverse myelitis, transverse myelitis also occurs with infectious and post-infectious diseases, as a paraneoplastic phenomenon and in collagen vascular diseases. Patients with transverse myelitis and a normal MRI scan of the brain have a low risk of developing clinically definite MS [66].

NEUROMYELITIS OPTICA

The term *neuromyelitis optica* (NMO) is used to describe an entity where severe attacks of optic neuritis and transverse myelitis occur either simultaneously or in succession. Although a monophasic form exists, the tendency is for recurrent optic neuritis and transverse myelitis. The original description was of transverse myelitis with bilateral optic neuritis or bilateral retrobulbar neuritis. MS, systemic lupus erythematosus, acute disseminated encephalomyelitis and Behçet's can present with clinical features resembling NMO. Some authorities regard NMO as a distinct disorder separate from MS [67]. On MRI there are extensive longitudinal *central* spinal cord T2 lesions over several segments. Oligoclonal bands are usually negative in the cerebral spinal fluid and 70% will have a unique bio-marker in the serum, the NMO-IgG or aquaporin [67]. In contrast, in patients with MS the spinal cord abnormality on MRI usually involves fewer than two segments, is asymmetrical and in the peripheral aspect of the spinal cord. Patients with NMO often succumb to respiratory failure. The pathogenesis of NMO is likely to be different to that of MS.

BILATERAL INTERNUCLEAR OPHTHALMOPLEGIA

Another classical presentation is with horizontal diplopia with or without vertigo due to involvement of the brainstem. The diplopia results from involvement of the median longitudinal fasciculus and this causes ipsilateral failure of adduction (looking towards the nose) and leading eye nystagmus in the opposite eye, the so-called internuclear ophthalmoplegia. *Bilateral internuclear ophthalmoplegia* is regarded as almost pathognomonic of MS. Pseudo-internuclear ophthalmoplegia can occur with the Miller Fisher variant of acute inflammatory demyelinating peripheral neuropathy, myasthenia gravis and thyroid eye disease, although in these conditions other signs are the clue to the diagnosis.

SPHINCTER DISTURBANCE

Neurologists are often asked to see young patients with disturbances of micturition and, although this can be a presenting symptom in a very small number of patients with MS, most of these patients do not have MS.

UHTHOFF'S PHENOMENON

Transient worsening of symptoms in patients with MS is not uncommon in the setting of excessive heat or an infection that causes fever. This is referred to as Uhthoff's phenomenon. Patients with established MS will often confuse this with a relapse of their MS; the clue is that it is a transient worsening of preexisting symptoms and signs rather than the appearance of new symptoms or signs that would indicate involvement of a different part of the nervous system. Uhthoff's phenomenon may be the only symptom of, for example, a urinary tract infection in patients with MS.

L'HERMITTE'S PHENOMENON

Electric shock-like sensations that radiate from the neck down the body and into the limbs with neck flexion is referred to as the L'Hermitte's phenomenon. Although characteristic of MS it is not pathognomonic and can occur with severe cervical cord compression.

TRIGEMINAL NEURALGIA IN YOUNG PATIENTS

Although trigeminal neuralgia (see Chapter 4, 'The cranial nerves and understanding the brainstem') can occur in patients with MS, MS is rarely the cause.

Investigation in suspected multiple sclerosis

MRI has revolutionised the management of patients with MS, both in terms of diagnosis and also as a surrogate end-

> The MRI scan must not be used in isolation to diagnose MS; the findings must be carefully correlated with the clinical presentation.

point in therapeutic trials. The current McDonald criteria [63] used for the diagnosis of MS rely heavily on the MRI scan findings. The criteria are given in Appendix I.

MALIGNANCY AND THE NERVOUS SYSTEM

Direct effects of malignancy
PRIMARY TUMOURS OF THE NERVOUS SYSTEM

Primary tumours of the nervous system can affect the brain, spinal cord or rarely the peripheral nervous system and they are named according to their cell of origin (see Table 14.2). Tumours can develop from:

- Glial cells
  - Astrocytes
  - Ependyma (inner lining of the brain)
  - Oligodendrocytes
- Neuroectoderm (external lining of the brain)
  - Meninges
  - Schwann cell
- Pituitary gland

Neurological problems are very common in patients with malignancy. The symptoms may relate to:

1. direct effects of the malignancy on the central nervous system – patients present with focal neurological deficits, seizures or headache
2. remote effects of the malignancy, the paraneoplastic syndrome – patients present with diffuse neurological problems
3. complications of therapy (chemotherapy or radiotherapy) for the malignancy
4. an entirely separate problem and unrelated to either the malignancy or its treatment.

Just because a patient has malignancy it does not mean they cannot develop an unrelated neurological problem.

Classifications of tumours of the nervous system, such as that of the World Health Organization [68, 69], will continue to evolve with new discoveries [70].

Primary central nervous system tumours declare themselves with seizures, headache or the development of a progressive focal neurological deficit. Gliomas can affect any part of the nervous system but are less common in the brainstem or spinal cord. They can infiltrate the corpus collosum, spreading to both hemispheres and forming a butterfly glioma, or they can infiltrate throughout the entire brain rather than forming a discrete mass and this is referred to as gliomatosis cerebri.

TABLE 14.2   Primary tumours of the nervous system named according to their cell of origin

Central nervous system	Cell of origin	Name of tumour
	Astrocytes	Astrocytoma*
	Ependyma	Ependymoma*
	Oligodendrocytes	Oligodendrogliomas*
	Neuroectoderm	Medulloblastoma, pinealoblastoma
	Meninges	Meningioma
	Schwann cell	Neurofibroma
Peripheral nervous system		
	Schwann cell	Neurofibroma
	Neuroectoderm	Ewing's sarcoma

*Astrocytomas, ependymomas and oligodendrogliomas are referred to as gliomas.
Note: All these tumours can be either malignant or benign.

Tumours of the pituitary gland represent about 10% of primary central nervous system tumours. Symptoms arise from pituitary tumours in three ways:

1 a direct result of the tumour (visual loss due to compression of the optic chiasm or optic nerves and headache)
2 destruction of the pituitary gland and loss of hormone function, in particular hypo-thyroidism and amenorrhoea
3 excess hormone secretion, e.g. growth hormone causing either gigantism or acro-megaly or prolactin causing galactorrhoea.

Most pituitary tumours are macroadenomas whereas hormone-secreting tumours such as prolactinomas can be microadenomas.

Secondary tumours of the nervous system

In non-central nervous system malignancy the neurological manifestations may be the presenting symptom of that malignancy or they may develop in a patient with an estab-lished diagnosis. Any tumour can potentially metastasise to the brain, but the com-mon ones are lung and breast, while the paired organs (thyroid, lung, breast, kidney and prostate) metastasise to the spinal column. Secondaries tend to occur in patients between the ages of 40 and 60. Spinal cord compression due to malignancy is discussed in Chapter 13, 'Abnormal movements and difficulty walking due to central nervous system problems'.

Paraneoplastic syndromes

Paraneoplastic syndromes are rare except for myasthenia gravis (thymoma), Lambert–Eaton syndrome (small cell carcinoma of the lung) and the demyelinating peripheral neuropathy associated with the osteosclerotic plasmacytoma.

Paraneoplastic syndromes refer to neurological symptoms and signs in a patient with malignancy that are not the direct result of the tumour but rather an immune-mediated remote effect. Paraneoplastic syndromes are seen in both the central and peripheral nervous systems (see Tables 14.3 and 14.4). Similar clinical syndromes mediated by antibodies may also be seen in the absence of malignancy. Anti-neuronal antibodies that react with the underlying tumour and the target cells within the central nervous system can be detected [71–74].

These neurological syndromes are very severe, often disabling and sometimes fatal. They can develop rapidly over days but more commonly weeks to a few months. The neurological symptoms and signs often but not invariably precede the diagnosis of malignancy for months and sometimes years; in other patients they may herald a recur-rence of the tumour. The malignancy may initially elude detection, despite extensive investigations and be diagnosed some time later. It is thought that effective antitumour immunity is associated with autoimmune brain disease [71, 75–81]. Increasing num-bers of antibodies are being recognised and the type of malignancy can vary consider-ably; the ones listed in the tables are the more common (see Tables 14.3 and 14.4). It is now recognised that pure presentations of these syndromes are the exception rather than the rule and it is not uncommon for a patient with malignancy and paraneoplastic phenomena to have multifocal symptoms and signs.

Positron emission tomography (PET) scanning is able to detect malignancy even in patients where a CT scan is negative. In patients with paraneoplastic syndromes, PET scanning has a sensitivity and specificity of 80% and 67%, respectively [82].

Self-examination, mammography, ultrasound, MRI and a new modality termed elas-ticity imaging are all used to detect breast cancer [83].

INVESTIGATION and MANAGEMENT of PARANEOPLASTIC SYNDROMES

The exact pathogenesis of most paraneoplastic syndromes is currently unknown, and it is possible that both humoral and cell-mediated immunity are involved. In patients suspected of having paraneoplastic syndrome, anti-neuronal antibodies, a whole body PET scan and in females mammography and ultrasound or CT scan of the ovaries are recommended. New anti-neuronal antibodies are being increasingly identified; the particular antibody is often a guide to the site of the underlying malignancy (see Tables 14.3 and 14.4).

TABLE 14.3   Central nervous system paraneoplastic syndromes

Clinical syndrome	Antibodies	Underlying malignancy
Carcinoma-associated retinopathy	Antirational	SCLC, melanoma, gynaecologic
Limbic encephalitis	Anti-Hu, anti-Ma2	SCLC, testicular
Brainstem encephalitis	Anti-Ma1, anti-Ma2	Lung, testicular
Encephalomyelitis	Anti-amphiphysin, anti-PCA-2, anti-CRMP5, ANNA-3, anti-NMDA-receptor	SCLC, breast, thymoma, ovarian
Cerebellar degeneration	Anti-Yo, anti-Hu, anti-Tr anti-Ma1, anti-mGluR1, anti-PCA-2, anti-CRMP5	SCLC, ovarian, breast, bladder, Hodgkin's lymphoma
Opsoclonus–myoclonus	Anti-Ri	Ovarian, breast, bladder, lung
Chorea	Anti-CRMP5 (anti-CV2)	SCLC, breast, thymoma
Necrotising myelopathy	None identified	Not specific
Stiff-person syndrome	Anti-amphiphysin	SCLC, breast

SCLC = small cell lung cancer
Compiled from Darnell and Posner [71], Dalmau [72] and Anderson and Barber [73]

TABLE 14.4   Peripheral nervous system paraneoplastic syndromes

Clinical syndrome	Antibodies	Underlying malignancy
Dorsal root ganglionopathy	Anti-Hu, anti-CRMP5 (anti-CV2), ANNA-3	Lung, SCLC, thymoma
Peripheral neuropathy	Anti-MAG	Waldenstrom's
Autonomic neuropathy	Anti-Hu, anti-nicotinic AchR	SCLC, bladder, thyroid
Myasthenia gravis	AchR, anti-titin	Thymoma
Lambert–Eaton syndrome	Anti-VGCC, anti-PCA-2	SCLC
Dermatomyositis	None identified	Ovarian, breast, lung
Necrotising myopathy	None identified	No specific neoplasm
Neuromyotonia	Anti-VGKC	SCLC, thymoma
Stiff-person syndrome	Anti-amphiphysin	SCLC, breast

SCLC = small cell lung cancer
Compiled from Darnell and Posner [71], Dalmau [72], Rudnicki [74] and Anderson and Barber [73]

The most effective treatment is removal of the antigen by treatment of the underlying malignancy but, as already stated, the tumour may not be detectable at the time of the initial presentation. Unfortunately, many patients are severely disabled at the time of presentation. Myasthenia gravis, the Lambert–Eaton syndrome, peripheral neuropathy associated with osteosclerotic plasmacytoma and opsoclonus–myoclonus may respond to treatment of the underlying malignancy, immunosuppression or both. In most patients treatment consists of immunosuppression.

Complications of therapy

When neurological symptoms develop in a patient undergoing therapy for malignancy it is important to consider the possibility of side effects due to the therapy. There are many recognised complications of radiotherapy and chemotherapy and, with the emergence of newer chemotherapeutic agents including monoclonal antibodies and proteasome inhibitors in recent years, the list of neurological complications is expanding.

COMPLICATIONS OF CHEMOTHERAPY

The most common side effect of chemotherapeutic agents is *peripheral neuropathy* [84, 85]. The neuropathy is dose-dependent, develops gradually and increases in severity with subsequent doses. It is almost invariably a length-dependent peripheral neuropathy in which patients develop a distal sensory loss in the lower limbs with or without distal weakness. Very rarely the autonomic nervous system may be affected, for example with vincristine. Oxaliplatin has been reported to cause an acute reversible peripheral neuropathy developing within hours of commencing intravenous therapy [86]. Improvement often but not invariably occurs if no further doses are given, although this may be unavoidable in order to treat the malignancy. Peripheral neuropathy is seen with many of the currently employed chemotherapeutic agents, including thalidomide and an analogue of thalidomide, lenalidomide, the vinca alkaloids (vincristine and vinblastine), platinum compounds (cisplatin, carboplatin and oxaliplatin), the taxanes (paclitaxel and docetaxel) and cytarabine.

Cognitive decline may occur with chemotherapy and is referred to as 'chemobrain' [85].

COMPLICATIONS OF INTRATHECAL THERAPY

Occasionally drugs, for example methotrexate and cytarabine, are administered via the intrathecal route (into the cerebral spinal fluid via a lumbar puncture). This route of administration can be complicated by *chemical meningitis, myelopathy* (spinal cord involvement) or *seizures. Multifocal leucoencephalopathy* has been reported with capecitabine [87]. The inadvertent intrathecal administration of vincristine causes a severe myelopathy with tetraplegia that is often fatal [88].

COMPLICATIONS OF RADIOTHERAPY

The neurological complications of radiotherapy can be divided into early and delayed [89]. The early complications are usually mild and transient whereas the delayed complications are often progressive and disabling. Complications occur when central nervous system tumours are irradiated or as a result of incidental damage when the radiation is applied to soft tissue tumours adjacent to the nervous system. The site of the neurological complications will relate directly to the site of radiotherapy. Necrosis resulting in swelling and a mass effect may occur with radiation to the brain. The onset of symptoms usually commences 1–3 years after therapy but may begin as early as 3 months or be delayed for as long as 12 years. The symptoms and signs relate to the mass. At times it can be difficult to differentiate between recurrent tumour and radiation necrosis. Radiation necrosis-induced masses may also, like tumours, enhance with contrast on a CT scan of the brain. Careful correlation with the sight of maximum irradiation may sometimes help to differentiate recurrent tumour from radiation necrosis. MR spectroscopy or computer-assisted stereotactic biopsy is used to differentiate tumour recurrence from radiation necrosis [90, 91].

Immediate radiation damage to the spinal cord is usually transient. A transient myelopathy develops within weeks of radiation with numbness and paraesthesia without weakness or objective neurological signs. These sensory symptoms spread from the site of radiation down into the limbs and are often associated with L'Hermitte phenomena. Symptoms usually resolve within months.

Non-reversible radiation myelopathy can occur acutely, with paraplegia or quadriplegia evolving over days and is thought to relate to arterial occlusion [92]. This acute form of myelopathy is very rare and more common is the chronic progressive myelopathy developing within 1 year, although it may occur as early as 4 months or as late as 13 years after radiation. The patient develops ascending sensory loss and weakness often associated with sphincter disturbance. The symptoms and signs are usually bilateral but may be unilateral. The myelopathy progresses over months, often to severe disability. An MRI scan demonstrates swelling of the spinal cord, focal contrast enhancement, low signal over several segments on T1-weighted images and high signal on T2-weighted images [93, 94].

Radiation injury may also occur to cranial nerves, either single or multiple cranial nerves may be affected. The brachial plexus is another site where radiation damage can occur. It can be difficult to differentiate between radiation injury to the brachial plexus and malignant infiltration; perhaps the only clue is that pain is much more common with the latter.

There is little effective treatment for radiation damage to the nervous system. Treatment with corticosteroids, surgery or antioxidants is often ineffective and the role of anticoagulation remains unclear [95, 96].

INFECTIONS OF THE NERVOUS SYSTEM

Meningitis, which is one of the more common infections of the nervous system, has already been discussed in Chapter 9, 'Headache and facial pain'. Central nervous system infections, particularly opportunistic infections, are more common in immunocompromised patients such as patients with HIV or those on immunosuppressive therapy. A complete discussion of central nervous system infections is beyond the scope of this book.

Encephalitis

Encephalitis literally means inflammation of the brain. Many patients also have associated meningitis and often the term meningo-encephalitis is used. A complete review is beyond the scope of this book. It can occur in HIV, related to malignancy, as a paraneoplastic a phenomena (Bickerstaff brainstem encephalitis) or secondary to viral infection. Viral encephalitis can occur either in epidemics (e.g. Murray–Valley or Japanese encephalitis) or it can be sporadic with the commonest cause being herpes simplex encephalitis (HSE). The essential clinical features are fever, confusion, focal or generalised seizures, focal neurological signs, signs of meningism and often impairment of consciousness.

HERPES SIMPLEX ENCEPHALITIS

Herpes simplex encephalitis (HSE) is seen sporadically and is probably the commonest form of encephalitis encountered in clinical practice. Left untreated it can either be fatal or result in a devastating neurological deficit, in particular with regards to memory. Untreated the mortality approaches 70% and only 10% of patients can return to a normal life [97]. The advent of effective therapy (see below) has reduced mortality to approximately 20% [97], although rates as low as 7% have been reported [98]. A poor outcome still occurs in 30–40% of patients [98].

Herpes simplex encephalitis should be suspected in patients presenting with *fever, focal deficit and a fit* (seizure). Dysphasia or hemiparesis and either focal or generalised seizures are seen. An altered mental state is common, coma may ensue, but headache, nausea and vomiting are uncommon. *Treatment should be initiated immediately the diagnosis is considered, while investigations are performed to confirm or exclude the diagnosis.*

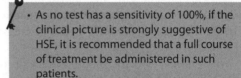

- As no test has a sensitivity of 100%, if the clinical picture is strongly suggestive of HSE, it is recommended that a full course of treatment be administered in such patients.

- Imaging should be performed immediately prior to a lumbar puncture as swelling of the temporal lobe can occur in patients with HSE without obvious deterioration, and this could result in transtentorial herniation.

MANAGEMENT of HERPES SIMPLEX ENCEPHALITIS

Periodic lateralised epileptiform discharges and/or focal temporal slowing can be present on the electroencephalogram of patients with HSE in the first 24–48 hours; the sensitivity is decreased after 48 hours. While low density abnormalities may be seen on the CT scan, the findings are not always present in the early stages [99]. MRI scanning enables the early diagnosis of HSE [100] and is abnormal in more than 80% of patients in the first 24–48 hours [101]. A repeat MRI scan is indicated in suspected cases if the initial scan is normal. Increased signal is seen on T2-weighted images in one or both temporal lobes. The diagnosis can be confirmed by polymerase chain reaction (PCR) of the herpes simplex type 1 or 2 viral genome in the CSF [102].

Treatment consists of supportive measures, but specifically the antiviral agent acyclovir 10–15 mg/kg 8-hourly for 10 days is the treatment of choice for HSE [97, 103]. Although combination with corticosteroids has been recommended based on a retrospective study [104], uncertainty remains with regards to their use in HSE [105].

Approach to immunocompromised patients with disorders of the central nervous system

Human (HIV) or acquired immune deficiency (AIDS) virus results in severe immune deficiency, but immune deficiency is more commonly seen in patients with malignancy on chemotherapy and with immune-mediated disorders such as vasculitis treated with immunosuppressants. In addition to the typical complications seen in patients who are immunocompromised, HIV also results in a variety of peripheral nervous system complications, in particular a painful peripheral neuropathy, a vacuolar myelopathy and an inflammatory myopathy [106]. Direct invasion of the virus into the central nervous system results in the AIDS dementia complex [107]. These are beyond the scope of this book; please refer to the book entitled *AIDS and the Nervous System* by Rosenblum, Levy and Bredesen (New York: Raven Press; 1998). In particular Chapter 19 of that book contains excellent algorithms to aid in the management of patients with AIDS and neurological symptoms.

Immunosuppressed patients develop opportunistic infections of the central nervous system, such as toxoplasmosis, cytomegalovirus, tuberculous and cryptococcal meningitis, primary central nervous system lymphoma and progressive multifocal encephalopathy (PML). *Note*: Toxoplasmosis, primary central nervous system lymphoma and progressive multifocal encephalopathy are the commonest causes of focal disease in patients with AIDS.

Patients present with meningitis, intracerebral or brainstem symptoms or with focal mass lesions. In patients with malignancy it can at times be very difficult to establish whether the mass represents recurrent malignancy, primary lymphoma, toxoplasmosis or PML.

MRI and stereotactic biopsy is the approach to patients with mass lesions who are alert, while open biopsy and decompression is necessary if there is imminent herniation. Analysis of CSF, MRI and empirical treatment for toxoplasmosis is the approach if there are multiple lesions and the patient is alert and stable.

REFERENCES

1 Plum F, Posner JB. Diagnosis of stupor and coma, 2nd edn. Philadelphia: FA Davis; 1972:286.
2 World Health Organization. International Statistical Classification of Diseases and Related Health Problems 2003, 10th Revision. 2007. Available: http://apps.who.int/classifications/apps/icd/icd10online/ (14 Dec 2009).
3 Mayo-Smith MF et al. Management of alcohol withdrawal delirium: An evidence-based practice guideline. Arch Intern Med 2004; 164(13):1405–1412.
4 Attard A, Ranjith G, aylor D. Delirium and its treatment. CNS Drugs 2008; 22(8):631–644.
5 Lonergan E et al. Benzodiazepines for delirium: Cochrane Database Syst Rev 2009(1):CD006379.
6 Reynolds CF, 3rd et al. Bedside differentiation of depressive pseudodementia from dementia. Am J Psychiatry 1988; 145(9):1099–1103.
7 Kertesz A. Clinical features and diagnosis of frontotemporal dementia. Front Neurol Neurosci 2009; 24:140–148.
8 Alladi S et al. Focal cortical presentations of Alzheimer's disease. Brain 2007; 130(Pt 10):2636–2645.
9 Mesulam MM. Primary progressive aphasia. Ann Neurol 2001; 49(4):425–432.
10 Petersen RC. Focal dementia syndromes: In search of the gold standard. Ann Neurol 2001; 49(4):421–423.
11 Geschwind MD et al. Rapidly progressive dementia. Ann Neurol 2008; 64(1):97–108.
12 Pokorski RJ. Differentiating age-related memory loss from early dementia. J Insur Med 2002; 34(2): 100–113.
13 Linn RT et al. The 'preclinical phase' of probable Alzheimer's disease: A 13-year prospective study of the Framingham cohort. Arch Neurol 1995; 52(5):485–490.
14 Meyer JS, Huang J, Chowdhury MH. MRI confirms mild cognitive impairments prodromal for Alzheimer's, vascular and Parkinson–Lewy body dementias. J Neurol Sci 2007; 257(1–2):97–104.
15 Jackson CE. A clinical approach to muscle diseases. Semin Neurol 2008 Apr. Available: http://www.medscape.com/viewarticle/572269 (28 Feb 2009).
16 Washington University. Myopathy and neuromuscular junction disorders: Differential diagnosis. Available: http://neuromuscular.wustl.edu/maltbrain.html (3 Jul 2009).
17 Karpati G, Hilton-Jones D, Griggs RD. Disorders of voluntary muscle, 7th edn. New York: Cambridge University Press; 2001.
18 Mendell JR. Approach to the patient with muscle disease. In: Hauser SL (ed). Harrison's neurology in clinical medicine. San Francisco: McGraw–Hill; 2006.
19 Klopstock T. Drug-induced myopathies. Curr Opin Neurol 2008; 21(5):590–595.
20 Klinge L et al. New aspects on patients affected by dysferlin deficient muscular dystrophy. J Neurol Neurosurg Psychiatry 14 Jun 2009 [Epub ahead of print].
21 Norwood F et al. EFNS guideline on diagnosis and management of limb girdle muscular dystrophies. Eur J Neurol 2007; 14(12):1305–1312.
22 Hilton-Jones D, Kissel JT. The examination and investigation of the patient with muscle disease. In: Karpati G, Hilton-Jones D, Griggs R (eds). Disorders of voluntary muscle. New York: Cambridge University Press; 2001:349–373.

23 Moxley RT, 3rd et al. Practice parameter: Corticosteroid treatment of Duchenne dystrophy: Report of the Quality Standards Subcommittee of the American Academy of Neurology and the Practice Committee of the Child Neurology Society. Neurology 2005; 64(1):13–20.

24 Choy EH et al. Immunosuppressant and immunomodulatory treatment for dermatomyositis and polymyositis. Cochrane Database Syst Rev 2005(3):CD003643.

25 Wiendl H. Idiopathic inflammatory myopathies: Current and future therapeutic options. Neurotherapeutics 2008; 5(4):548–557.

26 Fries JF et al. Cyclophosphamide therapy in systemic lupus erythematosus and polymyositis. Arthritis Rheum 1973; 16(2):154–162.

27 Vencovsky J et al. Cyclosporine A versus methotrexate in the treatment of polymyositis and dermatomyositis. Scand J Rheumatol 2000; 29(2):95–102.

28 Miller FW et al. Controlled trial of plasma exchange and leukapheresis in polymyositis and dermatomyositis. N Engl J Med 1992; 326(21):1380–1384.

29 Dalakas MC et al. A controlled trial of high-dose intravenous immune globulin infusions as treatment for dermatomyositis. N Engl J Med 1993; 329(27):1993–2000.

30 Elovaara I et al. EFNS guidelines for the use of intravenous immunoglobulin in treatment of neurological diseases: EFNS task force on the use of intravenous immunoglobulin in treatment of neurological diseases. Eur J Neurol 2008; 15(9):893–908.

31 Oldfors A, Lindberg C. Diagnosis, pathogenesis and treatment of inclusion body myositis. Curr Opin Neurol 2005; 18(5):497–503.

32 Greenberg SA. Inclusion body myositis: Review of recent literature. Curr Neurol Neurosci Rep 2009; 9(1):83–89.

33 Phillips PS et al. Statin-associated myopathy with normal creatine kinase levels. Ann Intern Med 2002; 137(7):581–585.

34 Sailler L et al. Increased exposure to statins in patients developing chronic muscle diseases: A 2-year retrospective study. Ann Rheum Dis 2008; 67(5):614–619.

35 Willis T. De anima brutorum. Oxford: Oxonii Theatro Sheldoniano; 1672:404–407.

36 Eaton LM, Lambert EH. Electromyography and electric stimulation of nerves in diseases of motor unit: Observations on myasthenic syndrome associated with malignant tumors. J Am Med Assoc 1957; 163(13):1117–1124.

37 Mulder DW, Lambert EH, Eaton LM. Myasthenic syndrome in patients with amyotrophic lateral sclerosis. Neurology 1959; 9:627–631.

38 Hoch W et al. Auto-antibodies to the receptor tyrosine kinase MuSK in patients with myasthenia gravis without acetylcholine receptor antibodies. Nat Med 2001; 7(3):365–368.

39 Aarli JA et al. Patients with myasthenia gravis and thymoma have in their sera IgG autoantibodies against titin. Clin Exp Immunol 1990; 82(2):284–288.

40 Kennedy WR, Jimenez-Pabon E. The myasthenic syndrome associated with small cell carcinoma of the lung (Eaton–Lambert syndrome). Neurology 1968; 18(8):757–766.

41 Gutmann L et al. The Eaton–Lambert syndrome and autoimmune disorders. Am J Med 1972; 53(3): 354–356.

42 Ackerman LV et al. Thymoma in a case of myasthenia gravis. Mo Med 1949; 46(4):270–272.

43 Sethi KD, Rivner MH, Swift TR. Ice pack test for myasthenia gravis. Neurology 1987; 37(8):1383–1385.

44 Larner AJ, Thomas DJ. Can myasthenia gravis be diagnosed with the 'ice pack test'? A cautionary note. Postgrad Med J 2000; 76(893):162–163.

45 Osserman KE, Kaplan LI. Rapid diagnostic test for myasthenia gravis: Increased muscle strength, without fasciculations, after intravenous administration of edrophonium (tensilon) chloride. JAMA 1952; 150(4):265–268.

46 Aharonov A et al. Humoral antibodies to acetylcholine receptor in patients with myasthenia gravis. Lancet 1975; 2(7930):340–342.

47 Schwartz MS, Stalberg E. Single fibre electromyographic studies in myasthenia gravis with repetitive nerve stimulation. J Neurol Neurosurg Psychiatry 1975; 38(7):678–682.

48 Stalberg E, Ekstedt J, Broman A. Neuromuscular transmission in myasthenia gravis studied with single fibre electromyography. J Neurol Neurosurg Psychiatry 1974; 37(5):540–547.

49 Benatar M. A systematic review of diagnostic studies in myasthenia gravis. Neuromuscul Disord 2006; 16(7):459–467.

50 Vincent A et al. Antibodies in myasthenia gravis and related disorders. Ann N Y Acad Sci 2003; 998: 324–335.

51 Osserman KE, Genkins G. Critical reappraisal of the use of edrophonium (tensilon) chloride tests in myasthenia gravis and significance of clinical classification. Ann N Y Acad Sci 1966; 135(1):312–334.

52 Vincent A, Newsom-Davis J. Acetylcholine receptor antibody as a diagnostic test for myasthenia gravis: Results in 153 validated cases and 2967 diagnostic assays. J Neurol Neurosurg Psychiatry 1985; 48(12):1246–1252.

53 Vincent A et al. Seronegative generalised myasthenia gravis: Clinical features, antibodies, and their targets. Lancet Neurol 2003; 2(2):99–106.

54 Sonett JR, Jaretzki A, 3rd. Thymectomy for nonthymomatous myasthenia gravis: A critical analysis. Ann N Y Acad Sci 2008; 1132:315–328.

55 Walker MB. Treatment of myasthenia gravis with physostigmine. Lancet 1934; 1:1200–1201.

56 Schneider-Gold C et al. Corticosteroids for myasthenia gravis. Cochrane Database Syst Rev 2005(2):CD002828.

57 Hart IK, Sathasivam S, Sharshar T. Immunosuppressive agents for myasthenia gravis. Cochrane Database Syst Rev 2007(4):CD005224.

58 Maddison P, Newsom-Davis J. Treatment for Lambert–Eaton myasthenic syndrome. Cochrane Database Syst Rev 2003(2):CD003279.

59 Ramsay AM, O'Sullivan E. Encephalomyelitis simulating poliomyelitis. Lancet 1956; 270(6926): 761–764.

60 Galpine JF, Brady C. Benign myalgic encephalomyelitis. Lancet 1957; 272(6972):757–758.

61 Petersen I et al. Risk and predictors of fatigue after infectious mononucleosis in a large primary-care cohort. Q J Med 2006; 99(1):49–55.

62 Behan PO, Bakheit AM. Clinical spectrum of postviral fatigue syndrome. Br Med Bull 1991; 47(4): 793–808.

63 Polman CH et al. Diagnostic criteria for multiple sclerosis: 2005 revisions to the "McDonald Criteria". Ann Neurol 2005; 58(6):840–846.

64 Ebers GC et al. A population-based study of multiple sclerosis in twins. N Engl J Med 1986; 315(26):1638–1642.

65 Courtney AM et al. Multiple sclerosis. Med Clin North Am 2009; 93(2):451–476,ix–x.

66 Scott TF, Kassab SL, Singh S. Acute partial transverse myelitis with normal cerebral magnetic resonance imaging: Transition rate to clinically definite multiple sclerosis. Mult Scler 2005; 11(4):373–377.

67 Weinshenker BG. Neuromyelitis optica is distinct from multiple sclerosis. Arch Neurol 2007; 64(6): 899–901.

68 Brat DJ et al. Surgical neuropathology update: A review of changes introduced by the WHO classification of tumours of the central nervous system, 4th edn. Arch Pathol Lab Med 2008; 132(6):993–1007.

69 Louis DN et al. WHO classification of tumours of the central nervous system, 4th edn. Lyon, France: IARC Press; 2007.

70 Rousseau A, Mokhtari K, Duyckaerts C. The 2007 WHO classification of tumors of the central nervous system – what has changed? Curr Opin Neurol 2008; 21(6):720–727.

71 Darnell RB, Posner JB. Paraneoplastic syndromes involving the nervous system. N Engl J Med 2003; 349(16):1543–1554.

72 Dalmau J et al. Anti-NMDA-receptor encephalitis: Case series and analysis of the effects of antibodies. Lancet Neurol 2008; 7(12):1091–1098.

73 Anderson NE, Barber PA. Limbic encephalitis – a review. J Clin Neurosci 2008; 15(9):961–971.

74 Rudnicki SA, Dalmau J. Paraneoplastic syndromes of the spinal cord, nerve, and muscle. Muscle Nerve 2000; 23(12):1800–1818.

75 Posner JB, Dalmau J. Paraneoplastic syndromes. Curr Opin Immunol 1997; 9(5):723–729.

76 Bennett JL et al. Neuro-ophthalmologic manifestations of a paraneoplastic syndrome and testicular carcinoma. Neurology 1999; 52(4):864–867.

77 Saiz A et al. Anti-Hu-associated brainstem encephalitis. J Neurol Neurosurg Psychiatry 2009; 80(4): 404–407.

78 Chiang YZ, Tjon Tan K, Hart IK. Lambert–Eaton myasthenic syndrome. Br J Hosp Med (Lond) 2009; 70(3):168–169.

79 Duddy ME, Baker MR. Stiff person syndrome. Front Neurol Neurosci 2009; 26:147–165.

80 Ferreyra HA et al. Management of autoimmune retinopathies with immunosuppression. Arch Ophthalmol 2009; 127(4):390–397.

81 Mehta SH, Morgan JC, Sethi KD. Paraneoplastic movement disorders. Curr Neurol Neurosci Rep 2009; 9(4):285–291.

82 Hadjivassiliou M et al. PET scan in clinically suspected paraneoplastic neurological syndromes: A 6-year prospective study in a regional neuroscience unit. Acta Neurol Scand 2009; 119(3):186–193.

83 Sarvazyan A et al. Cost-effective screening for breast cancer worldwide: Current state and future directions. Breast Cancer 2008; 1:91–99.

84 Young DF. Neurological complications of cancer chemotherapy. In: Silverstein A (ed). Neurological complications of therapy. New York: Futura Publishing; 1982:57–113.

85 Kannarkat G, Lasher EE, Schiff D. Neurologic complications of chemotherapy agents. Curr Opin Neurol 2007; 20(6):719–725.

86 Grolleau F et al. A possible explanation for a neurotoxic effect of the anticancer agent oxaliplatin on neuronal voltage-gated sodium channels. J Neurophysiol 2001; 85(5):2293–2297.

87 Jabbour E et al. Neurologic complications associated with intrathecal liposomal cytarabine given prophy-lactically in combination with high-dose methotrexate and cytarabine to patients with acute lymphocytic leukemia. Blood 2007; 109(8):3214–3218.

88 Schochet SS, Jr, Lampert PW, Earle KM. Neuronal changes induced by intrathecal vincristine sulfate. J Neuropathol Exp Neurol 1968; 27(4):645–658.

89 Berger PS. Neurological complications of radiotherapy. In: Silverstein A (ed). Neurological complications of therapy. New York: Futura Publishing; 1982:137–185.

90 Schlemmer HP et al. Differentiation of radiation necrosis from tumor progression using proton magnetic resonance spectroscopy. Neuroradiology 2002; 44(3):216–222.

91 Forsyth PA et al. Radiation necrosis or glioma recurrence: Is computer-assisted stereotactic biopsy useful? J Neurosurg 1995; 82(3):436–444.

92 Di Chiro G, Herdt JR. Angiographic demonstration of spinal cord arterial occlusion in postradiation myelomalacia. Radiology 1973; 106(2):317–319.

93 de Toffol B et al. Chronic cervical radiation myelopathy diagnosed by MRI. J Neuroradiol 1989; 16(3):251–253.

94 Wang PY, Shen WC, Jan JS. Serial MRI changes in radiation myelopathy. Neuroradiology 1995; 37(5):374–377.

95 Glantz MJ et al. Treatment of radiation-induced nervous system injury with heparin and warfarin. Neurology 1994; 44(11):2020–2027.

96 Happold C et al. Anticoagulation for radiation-induced neurotoxicity revisited. J Neurooncol 2008; 90(3):357–362.

97 Herpes simplex encephalitis. Lancet 1986; 1(8480):535–536.

98 Shoji H. Can we predict a prolonged course and intractable cases of herpes simplex encephalitis? Intern Med 2009; 48(4):177–178.

99 Dutt MK, Johnston ID. Computed tomography and EEG in herpes simplex encephalitis: Their value in diagnosis and prognosis. Arch Neurol 1982; 39(2):99–102.

100 Schroth G et al. Early diagnosis of herpes simplex encephalitis by MRI. Neurology 1987; 37(2):179–183.

101 Al-Shekhlee A, Kocharian N, Suarez JJ. Re-evaluating the diagnostic methods in herpes simplex encephalitis. Herpes 2006; 13(1):17–19.

102 Domingues RB et al. Diagnosis of herpes simplex encephalitis by magnetic resonance imaging and polymerase chain reaction assay of cerebrospinal fluid. J Neurol Sci 1998; 157(2):148–153.

103 Whitley RJ, Roizman B. Herpes simplex virus infections. Lancet 2001; 357(9267):1513–1518.

104 Kamei S et al. Evaluation of combination therapy using aciclovir and corticosteroid in adult patients with herpes simplex virus encephalitis. J Neurol Neurosurg Psychiatry 2005; 76(11):1544–1549.

105 Openshaw H, Cantin EM. Corticosteroids in herpes simplex virus encephalitis. J Neurol Neurosurg Psychiatry 2005; 76(11):1469.

106 Price RW. Neurological complications of HIV infection. Lancet 1996; 348(9025):445–452.

107 Clifford DB. AIDS dementia. Med Clin North Am 2002; 86(3):537–550,vi.

chapter 15

Further Reading, Keeping Up-to-date and Retrieving Information

It was not intended for this textbook to be a comprehensive discussion of neurology, but rather to put down on paper the simple concepts that have been developed over more than 30 years of teaching. The aim has always been to make the learning (and the practice) of clinical neurology more interesting and less intimidating for the non-neurologist (medical students, hospital medical officers, physician trainees, general physicians and general practitioners). Most of the chapters have been written from a symptom rather than a disease oriented approach and have discussed the more commonly encountered neurological disorders.

The basics of practising medicine will never change dramatically as a result of new technologies or the World Wide Web, but these will change the way health-care is delivered. This is not because of the technology itself or the attention it receives, but because patients will need and demand this kind of knowledge and expertise. Doctors of the 21st century must be ready and qualified to meet these expectations.

This chapter suggests techniques that can be employed to 'keep up-to-date' which, with the rapidly expanding knowledge base and the vast array of journals and web sites, at times seems an almost impossible task. It also contains recommendations for further reading, including other books that this author has constantly referred to for additional information.

KEEPING UP-TO-DATE

The amount of information available to the clinician is mindboggling. Typing the word 'stroke' into Google retrieves 49,000,000 hits! This is reduced to 1,580,000 for Google Scholar and 145,200 in PubMed. This has been referred to as 'information overload' [1].

As Glasziou pointed out, only 1 in 18 articles fulfil evidence-based medicine criteria, indicating that for the uninitiated there are vast numbers of potentially misleading papers in the literature. There are

> Although it is impossible to read every article this should not be used as an excuse to read none.

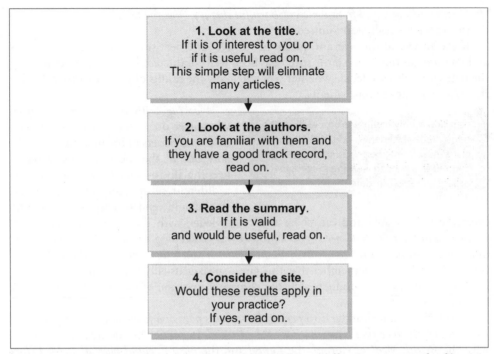

FIGURE 15.1 The McMaster group devised a simple and effective strategy for filtering papers

Adapted from *Clinical Epidemiology. A Basic Science for Clinical Medicine*, by DL Sackett, RB Haynes, P Tugwell, 1985, Little, Brown, p 370

a number of books [2, 3][2] and articles in journals [4–23] that discuss how to read the medical literature. Unfortunately, most medical practitioners never acquire the skills or have the time to read journal articles thoroughly. Most rely on information from colleagues, pharmaceutical company representatives, clinical scientific and education meetings, review articles and resources such as the online subscription service 'up-to-date' (http://www.upto date.com/home/index.html) to try and keep their knowledge current.

The McMaster group devised a simple and effective strategy for filtering papers [24]. They suggested the approach illustrated in Figure 15.1.

The next step depends on the nature of the paper:
- *Diagnostic test.* Was there an independent 'blind' comparison with a 'gold standard' of diagnosis?
- *Clinical course and prognosis.* Was there an 'inception cohort'?[3]
- *Determining aetiology.* Were the basic methods used to study causation strong?

---

2 A review of *How to read a paper* stated this is one of the bestselling texts on evidence-based medicine, used by healthcare professionals and medical students worldwide. Trisha Greenhalgh's ability to explain the basics of evidence-based medicine in an accessible and readable way means the book is an ideal introduction for all, from first-year students to experienced practitioners. This is a text that explains the meaning of critical appraisal and terms such as 'numbers needed to treat', 'how to search the literature', 'evaluate the different types of papers' and 'put the conclusions to clinical use'.
3 An inception cohort is where patients are identified at an early and uniform point in the course of the disease.

- *Distinguishing useful from useless or harmful therapy.* Was the assignment of patients to treatments really randomised?[4]

If the answer to the relevant question was 'yes', the next step is to read the patients and methods section to see if the study has been well conducted. In the end, after reading the paper you have to decide whether you will allow the results of this paper to influence the management of your patients.

> Learning is only beginning, not ending, the day a medical student graduates. All clinicians must for the benefit of their patients commit to a lifelong learning process in order to keep up-to-date.

Working with a group of colleagues who meet on a regular basis to discuss cases and papers in the literature is probably one of the most effective ways of keeping up-to-date. If each person has a different subspecialty area of interest they would tend to keep abreast of the literature in that area and can share their knowledge with the others. *Attendance at national and international meetings* is a second way of keeping abreast of the latest developments. *Pharmaceutical company sponsored guest speakers* at meetings is also common, but it is important to remember that this guest speaker usually has a point of view that is positive towards the products that the company markets; otherwise they would not be invited to speak.

Another useful technique is to *peruse the contents page of a journal for articles of interest, particularly those that have an associated editorial*. In particular, the three major journals, the *British Medical Journal*, the *Lancet* and the *New England Journal of Medicine*, may be scanned in this way to retrieve neurology-related and other articles of interest. The clinicopathological conferences in the *New England Journal of Medicine* are a wonderful source of information.[5]

Perhaps the most effective method of gaining new knowledge is retrieving information about a particular problem that you are dealing with at that time. Ready access to the Internet makes it possible to find relevant papers even during a consultation with the patient, e.g. when you wish to give the patient additional information. The Internet can help sort out a difficult diagnostic problem such as that discussed in Chapter 6, 'After the history and examination, what next?' Most frequently, the question that arises relates to the latest diagnostic test or criteria for a particular entity or the optimal treatment for a particular condition. It is not possible to retrieve and evaluate all this information at the time of consultation. A suggestion is to review the literature on a particular disease on a regular basis, adding to your database of knowledge by retaining the previous reviews.

A major problem is the growing number of institutions and companies vying to provide online information. It is almost impossible to choose between them. In essence all these entities are retrieving the same literature and trying to put it into a digestible form. It is suggested that you sample a few and find one that meets your needs before committing to a subscription.

---

4 If the natural history of a disease is unpredictable, and in particular if spontaneous remission can occur, the only way to assess whether a therapy is of benefit is to randomly allocate half of the patients to the active treatment and the other half to an alternative treatment or to a placebo.

5 The technique in this paragraph is used by the author who finds it an excellent method of keeping abreast of recent developments.

RETRIEVING USEFUL INFORMATION FROM THE INTERNET

Entrez–PubMed is the database used by most clinicians. A more detailed description on free-access and biomedical databases other than PubMed can be found in the article by Giglia [25].

Biomed–Central, the open access publisher, maintains a catalogue (http://databa ses.biomedcentral.com/browsecatalog) of more than 1000 databases. Some databases contain experimental data; others provide synopses of public information; and most are freely accessible. In the subject area there are options to search neurology or neuroscience (http://databases.biomedcentral.com/search), and under the content section the options include disease, experimental data, images, journal articles and links to other sources, to mention only a few.

Evidence-based medicine databases

There are many evidence-based medicine databases, but unfortunately most require payment for access.

- Abstracts can be viewed on the **Cochrane review** (http://www.cochrane.org/index. htm), but payment is required for the full article.
- **Netting the evidence** (http://www.shef.ac.uk/scharr/ir/netting) is a British-based website that is intended to facilitate evidence-based healthcare by providing support and access to helpful organisations and useful learning resources, such as an evidence-based virtual library, software and journals. The resources can be browsed by type, and a search facility is available.
- The aim of the **Turning research into practice (TRIP)** database (http://www. tripdatabase.com) is to allow health professionals to easily find the highest quality material available on the web – to help support evidence-based practice. This is a very interesting and user-friendly tool.
- The **QuickClinical (QC)** information retrieval system (http://www.chi.unsw.e du.au/chiweb.nsf/page/QuickClinical) is a new type of evidence-access technology that utilises intelligent search filter technology to model typical clinical tasks such as 'diagnosis' or 'prescribing' to ensure that only the most relevant evidence is retrieved. This means clinicians are more likely to search and, when they do search, are more likely to find information that changes their practice.
- The aim of the **Centre for Evidence Based Medicine** (http://www.cebm.net) is to develop, teach and promote evidence-based health care and provide support and resources to doctors and healthcare professionals to help maintain the highest standards of medicine.
- The **National Guideline Clearinghouse™ (NGC)** (http://www.ahrq.gov/) is a public resource for evidence-based clinical practice guidelines. NGC is an initiative of the Agency for Healthcare Research and Quality (AHRQ), US Department of Health and Human Services. NGC was originally created by AHRQ in partnership with the American Medical Association and the American Association of Health Plans (now America's Health Insurance Plans [AHIP]). It also offers synthesis of selected guidelines (http://www.guideline.gov/compare/synthesis.aspx) and expert commentary on issues (http://www.guideline.gov/resources/expert_commentary.aspx).
- **Clinicians Health Channel** (http://www.hcn.com.au/profiles/shared/componen t/use/) is sponsored by the Victorian Department of Health and is for the benefit of clinicians working in the Victorian public health sector. It provides access to journals, books, evidence-based practice resources, drug information resources and citation databases.

Searching strategies in PubMed and other search engines

The traditional approach to searching the literature has been with **PubMed** (http://www. ncbi.nlm.nih.gov/pubmed/), which is a service of the US National Library of Medicine and the National Institutes of Health. It is the integrated, text-based search-and-retrieval system used at The National Centre for Biotechnology Information (NCBI) for the major databases, including PubMed, Nucleotide and Protein Sequences, Protein Structures, Complete Genomes, Taxonomy and others.

There are tutorials available for using PubMed (http://www.nlm.nih.gov/bsd/disted/pubmed.html). There is also a PDF designed to print and tri-fold (http://nnlm.gov/training/resources/pmtri.pdf).

PubMed is the main database that most clinicians would use to retrieve the more scientifically valid information. On the top left side there is a dropdown box that contains other databases such as journals and OMIM (Online Mendelian Inheritance in Man). At OMIM you can search the individual chromosomes and also mitochondria just by ticking the box next to the relevant chromosome.

FINDING A NEUROLOGY JOURNAL
Simply change the dropdown box to journals and type in the word neurology and you will retrieve the links to 461 neurology journals! You can follow the links to the journal website by clicking on the NLM ID and then the URL (uniform resource locator) on the following page.

FINDING THAT PAPER YOU KNOW YOU HAVE SEEN
On numerous occasions you have a vague recollection of reading a particular paper and yet you cannot recall where. You may recall one of the authors, the journal or roughly when it was published. PubMed allows you to refine your search for a topic by author, journal and/or specific dates using the LIMITS tab.

FINDING PRACTICE GUIDELINES
Once again PubMed allows you to filter articles that are designated practice guidelines.

FINDING THE LATEST INFORMATION ON A PARTICULAR DISEASE
Use the PubMed database and type in the 'for' section the item of interest. To limit the results to possibly more useful articles use the LIMITS tab. Editorials, randomised controlled trials, clinical trials, meta-analyses and reviews can all be selected. Unfortunately, the word 'review' is included in so many papers it often retrieves numerous and at times irrelevant references that are not true reviews of the subject of interest.

Related references
Another very useful function of PubMed is the related references link. If, as you peruse the initial list of references, you see a particular article that seems to be close to what you want, click the related references (on the right side of the page) and see many other possibly relevant papers.

Exporting references to a reference manager
It is possible to export the references into a reference management program such as *Endnotes* or *Reference Manager*. To export to *Endnotes* the references need to be converted to

text files (*.txt).[6] The text file is saved onto the disc. In the *Endnotes* program go to file and select the import option. Set the import option to 'PubMed (NLM)', duplicates to 'discard duplicates' and text translation to 'no translation'. Then simply select 'import' and choose the directory where the text file is to be saved. Inside the individual reference you can link to a downloaded PDF.

PubMed and MedlinePlus allow searching by topics, authors or journals. The evolution of *ontological derivation* (a systematic arrangement of all of the important categories of objects or concepts that exist in some field of discourse, showing the relations between them) and *semantic search engines* (which improve online searching by using data from semantic networks) is changing the way searches are performed and adds a deeper layer of complexity to the interrogation of the wealth of defined medical knowledge. A semantic network is a network that represents semantic relationships between the concepts and the interpretations of a word, sentence or other language form to disambiguate queries and web text in order to generate more relevant results. Semantics is the branch of the science of language concerned with meaning.

ALTERNATIVE SEARCH ENGINES USING THE SEMANTIC WEB
Most of the alternative search engines rely on answering a question, but also on phrases and keywords. There are many semantic-based alternative search engines; only a few will be discussed here.

GoPubMed
GoPubMed (http://www.gopubmed.org) retrieves PubMed abstracts for your search query and sorts relevant information into categories. It lists the title of the article, and there is the ability to look at the abstract or link to a specific article by selecting the author icon or to go to the journal by selecting the journal icon. This is often useful as it is not uncommon for two or more related articles to be printed in the same volume. Other functions in GoPubMed include:
- *What* collates abstracts according to the concept hierarchies of GO and MeSH – providing a combined search across the fields of molecular biology and medicine.
- *Where* provides information about geographic localisation of people, research centres and universities, as well as journals in which retrieved papers were published. The journals are separated into top high impact and more top journals. There is an option to search for a specific journal and to look at reviews only.
- *When* is the citations time machine. You can see articles published today, last week, last month, last year, during the last 5 years or specify a date.

SearchMedica
This is a great 'professional medical search' resource. SearchMedica (http://www.searchmedica.com) is a search engine that scans reputable journals, systematic reviews and evidence-based articles to provide search results. Although SearchMedica displays fewer results than standard search engines, it is accurate, clinically relevant and surprisingly comprehensive. There are options to scan the entire Web or just

---

6 In 2009 PubMed altered the way files are handled. Currently on the right side of the page is a 'Send To' tab; click on this, choose 'File' (there are other options such as 'Clipboard', 'E-mail', 'Collections' and 'Order') and then select 'Medline' under format. It is possible to sort the references by recently added, first author, last author, journal, publication date or title using the 'Sort By' tab. Selecting 'Create file' brings up another dialogue box asking if you wish to save or open the file; select 'Save' and save the file pubmed_result.txt into the relevant directory on your computer.

recommended medical sites and an option to choose mental/nervous system. The limitation is that there are a restricted number of users and it is not always possible to access this website.

Hakia–PubMed

Hakia (http://www.hakia.com) is a true general semantic Web search engine and believes that searchers suffer from information pollution! Hakia semantic technologies have developed a dedicated semantic medical search of PubMed (that has moved away from the popularity-ranked results) to provide credible and relevant search results (http://pubmed.hakia.com/). Credible sites are those that have been vetted by librarians and other information professionals.

Webicina

Webicina (http://www.webicina.com) was designed to help doctors from all the medical specialties, and patients as well, to get closer to the Web 2.0-based world. E-patients are tech-savvy members of the community trying to find reliable medical information on the web who want to communicate with their doctors via e-mail or skype and store their medical files online. The number of e-patients is growing rapidly while the number of web-savvy doctors is not.

The problem with all search engines is that none is able at this stage to sort the wheat from the chaff. They cannot differentiate between papers that should influence management and those that should be ignored. Although evidence-based medicine is the ideal, in many instances there simply is NO evidence one way or another to guide treatment. Under these circumstances the pros and cons of the treatment you elect to recommend need to be discussed with the patient.

GENERAL NEUROLOGY WEBSITES

- **Cochrane Collaboration** (http://www.cochrane.org/index.htm). The aim of the Cochrane Collaboration is improving healthcare decision making globally, through systematic reviews of the effects of healthcare interventions. Unfortunately, many reviews conclude that there is insufficient evidence and that further studies are needed.
- **European Federation of Neurological Societies (EFNS)** (http://www.efns.org/content_old.php?myaction=viewsub-1-1-6). The EFNS represents the national neurological societies of 40 European countries.
- **Internet Drug Index** (http://www.rxlist.com/). This provides an alphabetical list of drugs, a pill identifier and an explanation of diseases, conditions and tests.
- **World Federation of Neurology (WFN)** (http://www.wfneurology.org/). The WFN is the international body representing the specialty of neurology in more than 100 countries/regions of the globe. The WFN has these neurological societies as its members, and their individual members are in turn WFN members through the association. The purpose of the WFN is to improve human health worldwide by promoting prevention and the care of persons with disorders of the entire nervous system by:
  - fostering the best standards of neurological practice
  - educating, in collaboration with neuroscience and other international public and private organisations
  - facilitating research through its research groups.

COUNTRY-BASED NEUROLOGY WEBSITES

North American websites
- American Academy of Neurology, http://www.aan.com/
- American Neurological Association, http://www.aneuroa.org/
- Canadian Neurological Sciences Federation, http://www.ccns.org/
- National Institutes of Health – Brain and Nervous System, http://health.nih.gov/search.asp/3

European websites
- European Federation of Neurological Societies, http://www.efns.org/content_old.php?myaction=viewsub-1-1-6# (This URL will link to the neurological societies of 40 countries.)

Asia and Pacific websites
- Asia ASEAN Neurological Association, http://www.asean-neurology.org/
- Australian and New Zealand Association of Neurologists, http://www.anzan.org.au/index.asp
- Hong Kong Neurological Society, http://www.ns.org.hk/
- Japanese Society of Psychiatry and Neurology, http://www.jspn.or.jp/english/index.html
- Korean Neurological Association, http://www.neuro.or.kr/eng/
- Malaysian Society of Neurosciences, http://www.neuro.org.my/
- Neurological Society of India, http://www.neurosocietyindia.com/
- Neurological Society of Thailand, http://thaineurology.com/index.html
- Pakistan Neurological Society, http://www.pakns.org/
- Philippine Neurological Association, http://www.pna.org.ph/
- Singapore Clinical Neuroscience Society, http://cnssingapore.blogspot.com/

WEBSITES RELATED TO THE MORE COMMON NEUROLOGICAL PROBLEMS

Clinical trials
The following are very useful and readily accessible resources.
- The National Institutes of Health has a website (http://www.clinicaltrials.gov/) dedicated to clinical trials that has in excess of 70,000 registered trials. These can be searched by topic and country, e.g. headache, stroke etc. The website comments on whether the trial is recruiting or not and whether completed. Links are provided to the most up-to-date information, including when the results have been published linked to abstracts on PubMed.
- It also has a website dedicated to *neurological disorders* listed alphabetically (http://www.ninds.nih.gov/index.htm).
- There is a section dedicated to *patient resources* also listed alphabetically (http://www.ninds.nih.gov/find_people/voluntary_orgs/organizations_index.htm).

Cerebral vascular disease
- American Stroke Association, http://www.strokeassociation.org/presenter.jhtml?identifier=1200037
- Stroke Trials Registry, http://www.strokecenter.org/trials/

- Washington University Internet Stroke Centre, http://www.strokecenter.org/prof/
- Cochrane Library Stroke Reviews, http://www.cochrane.org/reviews/en/topics/93_reviews.html

Epilepsy
- International General Epilepsy Sites, http://www.epinet.org.au
- International League against Epilepsy, http://www.ilae-epilepsy.org/
- Scottish Intercollegiate Guidelines Network, http://www.sign.ac.uk/guidelines/fulltext/70/index.html; PDF version, http://www.sign.ac.uk/pdf/sign70.pdf
- American Epilepsy Society, http://www.aesnet.org/
- Epilepsy Society of Australia, http://www.epilepsy-society.org.au/pages/index.php, http://www.epilepsyaustralia.org/

EPILEPSY TREATMENT GUIDELINES
- American Epilepsy Society Guidelines and Practice Parameters, http://www.aesnet.org/go/practice/guidelines/guidelines-and-practice-parameters
- American Academy of Neurology Practice Guidelines on the Use of Newer Seizure Medicines in New Onset Epilepsy, http://aan.com/professionals/practice/pdfs/patient_ep_onset_c.pdf
- Practice Guideline on the Use of the Newer Seizure Medicines in Refractory Epilepsy, http://aan.com/professionals/practice/pdfs/patient_ep_refract_c.pdf

AVAILABLE TREATMENTS FOR REFRACTORY EPILEPSY
- American Academy of Neurology Treatments for Patients with Refractory Epilepsy, http://aan.com/professionals/practice/pdfs/patient_ep_treatment_b.pdf
- Canada-Ontario New Epilepsy Treatment Guidelines, http://www.epilepsyontario.org/client/EO/EOWeb.nsf/web/New+Epilepsy+Treatment+Guidelines
- National Institute for Health and Clinical Excellence (NICE) (UK), http://www.nice.org.uk/guidance/index.jsp?action=byID&r=true&o=10954

Headache
- American Headache Society, http://www.achenet.org/resources/information/index.asp
- The Migraine Trust, http://www.migrainetrust.org
- The National Headache Foundation, http://www.headaches.org
- National Institute of Neurological Disorders and Stroke, http://www.ninds.nih.gov/disorders/migraine/migraine.htm

Parkinson's and movement disorders
- National Institute of Neurological Disorders and Stroke, http://www.ninds.nih.gov/disorders/parkinsons_disease/parkinsons_disease.htm
- Parkinson's Disease Foundation (USA), http://www.pdf.org/
- Parkinson's Disease Society (UK), http://www.parkinsons.org.uk/
- Tourette syndrome, http://www.tsa-usa.org/

Multiple sclerosis
- Multiple Sclerosis Society (UK), http://www.mssociety.org.uk/for_professionals/resources/official_documen.html

- National Multiple Sclerosis Society (USA), http://www.nationalmssociety.org/index. aspx
- MS Australia, http://www.msaustralia.org.au/

Neurophysiology
- American Association of Neuromuscular and Electrodiagnostic Medicine, http://www.aanem.org/
- British Society for Clinical Neurophysiology, http://www.bscn.org.uk/

MAJOR NEUROLOGY JOURNAL WEBSITES

The major general medical journals listed below frequently have neurology-related editorials, original research, review articles and neurology cases or clinical pathological conferences.

The most significant website is of course PubMed (http://www.ncbi.nlm.nih.gov/sites/entrez?db=pubmed), supported by the US National Library of Medicine and the National Institutes of Health in the USA.

General journal websites with neurology content
- *The Lancet* (UK), http://www.thelancet.com/
- *Lancet Neurology* (UK), http://www.thelancetneurology.com/
- *British Medical Journal* (UK), http://www.bmj.com/
- *New England Journal of Medicine*, http://content.nejm.org/

Specific neurology journal websites
The journals marked with an asterisk (*) were rated as the top 5 in a questionnaire of members of the World Federation of Neurology [26].
- *Acta Neurologica Scandinavica* (Sweden), http://www.wiley.com/bw/journal.asp?ref=0001-6314&site=1
- *Annals of Indian Academy of Neurology* (India), http://www.annalsofian.org/
- *Annals of Neurology** (USA), http://www3.interscience.wiley.com/journal/76507645/home?CRETRY=1&SRETRY=0
- *Archives of Neurology* (USA), http://archneur.ama-assn.org/
- *Brain** (UK), http://brain.oxfordjournals.org/
- *Cerebrovascular Diseases*, http://www.online.karger.com/ProdukteDB/produkte.asp?Aktion=JournalHome&ProduktNr=224153
- *Chinese Journal of Cerebrovascular Diseases*, http://chinanew.eastview.com/kns50/Navi/item.aspx?NaviID=1&BaseID=NXGB&NaviLink=%e4%b8%ad%e5%9b%bd%e8%84%91%e8%a1%80%e7%ae%a1%e7%97%85%e6%9d%82%e5%bf%97
- *Chinese Journal of Neurology*, http://zhsjk.periodicals.net.cn/ http://chinanew.eastview.com/kns50/Navi/item.aspx?NaviID=1&BaseID=ZHSJ&NaviLink=%e4%b8%ad%e5%8d%8e%e7%a5%9e%e7%bb%8f%e7%a7%91%e6%9d%82%e5%bf%97
- *Epilepsia (USA)*, http://www.wiley.com/bw/journal.asp?ref=0013-9580
- *European Journal of Neurology*, http://www.wiley.com/bw/journal.asp?ref=1351-5101
- *Headache (USA)*, http://www.wiley.com/bw/journal.asp?ref=0017-8748

- *Journal of Clinical Neuroscience* (Australia), http://www.elsevier.com/wps/find/journal description.cws_home/623056/description#description
- Journal of Neurology, Neurosurgery, and Psychiatry (UK), http://jnnp.bmj.com/
- *Journal of the Neurological Sciences* (USA), http://www.elsevier.com/wps/find/journal description.cws_home/506078/description#description
- *Journal für Neurologie, Neurochirurgie und Psychiatrie* (Austria), http://www.kup.at/ journals/neurologie/index.html
- *Journal of Neurotrauma** (USA), http://www.liebertpub.com/products/product.aspx? pid=39
- *Movement Disorders* (USA), http://www3.interscience.wiley.com/journal/76507419/ home
- *Multiple Sclerosis* (USA), http://msj.sagepub.com/
- *Neurology** (USA), http://www.neurology.org/
- *Neurology Asia*, http://neurologyasia.org/journal.php
- *Neurology, Neurophysiology and Neuroscience* (USA), http://www.neurojournal.com/ index
- *Pakistan Journal of Neurology*, http://www.pakmedinet.com/PJNeuro
- *Stroke** (USA), http://stroke.ahajournals.org/

RESOURCES FOR PATIENTS

There are literally thousands of disease-oriented consumer organisations around the world striving to raise money for research into their particular ailment of interest and also aiming to keep their members abreast of the latest developments. The American Academy of Neurology produces regular practice guidelines for both the treating clinician and the patient.

Probably one of the most authoritative is the site sponsored by the United States National Library of Medicine and the National Institutes of Health titled **MedlinePlus** (http://medlineplus.gov/). MedlinePlus website states that it 'brings together authoritative information from National Library of Medicine (NLM), the National Institutes of Health (NIH), and other government agencies and health-related organisations. Preformulated MEDLINE searches are included in MedlinePlus and give easy access to medical journal articles. MedlinePlus also has extensive information about drugs, an illustrated medical encyclopaedia, interactive patient tutorials, and latest health news. The help topics section links to the National Institute of Neurological Disorders and Stroke website. It also provides health information in over 40 languages (http://www. nlm.nih.gov/medlineplus/languages/languages.html).

RECOMMENDED BOOKS

Medical practitioners often possess large numbers of medical books, most of which they never read and to some of which they occasionally refer. The problem with textbooks is that most of the information is rapidly out of date; this is particularly the case with investigations and treatment.

Although this book has primarily been written for students and the non–neurologist, it is also potentially suitable for the neurology trainee in the early stages of training. What follows is a list of books (not in any particular order) that this author has collected and enjoyed reading. Many have been useful resources to which he has constantly referred.

Gray's Anatomy, 40th edn, Susan Standring, Churchill Livingstone. This is a book that one refers to when very detailed neuroanatomy is required.

Mechanism and Management of Headache. 7th edn, J Lance, PJ Goadsby, Elsevier Butterworth–Heinemann, 2004. One of those books to which you will constantly refer.

Aids to the Examination of the Peripheral Nervous System, 4th edn, Brain, WB Saunders Company, 2000. This is a thin paperback book that should be on every desktop. It shows how to examine each muscle, the nerve and nerve root supply and contains excellent illustrations of the individual nerves supplying muscles, the sensory supply to the skin of the nerves and the nerve roots (dermatomes).

Seizures and Epilepsy, J Engel, Jr, FA Davis Company, 1989. An excellent clinical textbook on the subject of epilepsy.

The Diagnosis of Stupor and Coma, Fred Plum, Jerome Posner, Oxford University Press, 2007. One of the neurological classics with a superb description of how to examine the comatose patient and how to use those findings to establish the cause of the coma.

Neurological Aspects of Substance Abuse, 2nd edn, JCM Brust, Elsevier Butterworth–Heinemann, 2004. An excellent reference source for dealing with patients admitted with complications from using recreational drugs.

Cerebrospinal Fluid in Diseases of the Nervous System, 2nd edn, RA Fishman, WB Saunders Company, 1992. An invaluable resource to check the cerebrospinal fluid abnormalities in particular diseases.

McAlpine's Multiple Sclerosis, 1st edn, WB Matthews, ED Acheson, JR Batchelor, RO Weller, Churchill Livingstone, 1985.

McAlpine's Multiple Sclerosis, 4th edn, A Compstan, I McDonald, J Noseworthy, H Lassmnaa, D Miller, K Smith, H Wekerle, C Confravreux, Churchill Livingstone, 2005. Both these books are excellent resources on multiple sclerosis.

Neurological Complications of Therapy, A Silverstein (ed), Futura Publishing Company, 1982. Although old nothing has been written that has replaced it. This book has excellent chapters on the neurological complications of chemotherapy and radiotherapy.

Principles and Practice of Movement Disorders, S Fahn S, J Jankovic, Churchill Livingstone, Elsevier, 2007. Written by two world experts who have clearly seen many patients with movement disorders. Described by a colleague with subspecialty interest in this area as the best book he has ever read on the subject.

Neurological Complications of Renal Disease, CF Bolton, GB Young, Butterworth Publishers, 1990. An excellent description of the neurological complications of renal disease.

Handbook of Neurologic Rating Scales, RM Herndon (ed), Demos Vermande, 1997. Describes and discusses the neurological rating scales applicable to many disorders of the nervous system.

Primer on the Autonomic Nervous System, D Robertson, I Biaggioni, G Burnstock, PA Low, Elsevier Academic Press, 2004. This has been written by one of the world's authorities on the autonomic nervous system.

AIDS and the Nervous System, 1st edn, ML Rosenblum, RM Levy, DE Bresdesen, Raven Press, 1988; 2nd edn, JR Berger, RM Levy, 1997. Excellent description of the approach to the patient with AIDS and neurological symptoms.

The Clinical Practice of Critical Care Neurology, E Wijdicks, Oxford University Press, 2003. An excellent book to aid the neurologist who is called upon to see patients in the intensive care unit.

Neurologic Catastrophes in the Emergency Department, E Wijdicks, Butterworth–Heinemann, 1999. A useful book for every neurologist attached to a hospital who has to attend the accident and emergency department.

Infectious Diseases of the Central Nervous System, KL Tyler, JB Martin, (Contemporary Neurology Series), FA Davis Co., 1993.

Posterior Circulation Disease: Clinical Findings, Diagnosis, and Management, LR Kaplan, Blackwell Science, 1996.

Peripheral Neuropathy, 4th edn, P Dyck, PK Thomas (eds), Elsevier Saunders, 2005.

The Treatment of Epilepsy – Principles and Practice, 3rd edn, E Wyllie (ed), Lippincott Williams & Wilkins, 2001.

Cranial Neuroimaging and Clinical Neuroanatomy, H-J Kretschmann, W Weinrich, Georg Thieme Verlag, 2004.

Handbook of Epilepsy Treatment, 2nd edn, SD Shorvon, Blackwell Science, 2005.

Handbook of Clinical Neurology, PJ Vinken, GW Bruyn, HL Klawans (eds), Elsevier, 1986. This is the encyclopaedia of clinical neurology, currently into the revised edition. Each chapter is very detailed and a good place to look for those neurological oddities. (An example is the patient with severe muscle hypertrophy such that he was bursting out of his clothes. This author consulted the handbook and was able to find the cause of the patient's problem: it was hypothyroidism.)

General neurology books

There are a number of excellent textbooks of general neurology; the author does not own all of these but reviews in the literature have been very positive.

Neurology in Clinical Practice, W Bradley et al, Butterworth–Heinemann

Practical Neurology, J Biller, Lippincott, Williams & Wilkins

Textbook of Clinical Neurology, C Goetz, WB Saunders Company
Merritt's Neurology, RL Lewis, HH Merritt, Lippincott, Williams & Wilkins
Harrison's Neurology in Clinical Practice, S Hauser, McGraw Hill
Neurological Differential Diagnosis, J Patten, Springer–Verlag
Adams and Victor's Manual of Neurology, 7th edn, M Victor, AH Ropper, McGraw–Hill
Introductory Neurology, JG McLeod, JW Lance, L Davies, Blackwell Science

REFERENCES

1 Glasziou PP. Information overload: What's behind it, what's beyond it? Med J Aust 2008; 189(2):84–85.
2 Greenhalgh T. How to read a paper: The basics of evidence based medicine, 2nd edn. London: BMJ Books; 2001.
3 Sackett DL et al. Evidence-based medicine: How to practise and teach EBM. Toronto: Churchill Livingstone; 2000.
4 Richardson WS et al. Users' guides to the medical literature: XXIV. How to use an article on the clinical manifestations of disease. Evidence-Based Medicine Working Group. JAMA 2000; 284(7):869–875.
5 Giacomini MK, Cook DJ. Users' guides to the medical literature: XXIII. Qualitative research in health care B. What are the results and how do they help me care for my patients? Evidence-Based Medicine Working Group. JAMA 2000; 284(4):478–482.
6 Giacomini MK, Cook DJ. Users' guides to the medical literature: XXIII. Qualitative research in health care A. Are the results of the study valid? Evidence-Based Medicine Working Group. JAMA 2000; 284(3): 357–362.
7 McGinn TG et al. Users' guides to the medical literature: XXII. How to use articles about clinical decision rules. Evidence-Based Medicine Working Group. JAMA 2000; 284(1):79–84.
8 Hunt DL, Jaeschke R. McKibbon KA. Users' guides to the medical literature: XXI. Using electronic health information resources in evidence-based practice. Evidence-Based Medicine Working Group. JAMA 2000; 283(14):1875–1879.
9 Bucher HC et al. Users' guides to the medical literature: XIX. Applying clinical trial results. A. How to use an article measuring the effect of an intervention on surrogate end points. Evidence-Based Medicine Working Group. JAMA 1999; 282(8):771–778.
10 Randolph AG et al. Users' guides to the medical literature: XVIII. How to use an article evaluating the clinical impact of a computer-based clinical decision support system. JAMA 1999; 282(1):67–74.
11 Barratt A et al. Users' guides to the medical literature: XVII. How to use guidelines and recommendations about screening. Evidence-Based Medicine Working Group. JAMA 1999; 281(21):2029–2034.
12 Guyatt GH et al. Users' guides to the medical literature: XVI. How to use a treatment recommendation. Evidence-Based Medicine Working Group and the Cochrane Applicability Methods Working Group. JAMA 1999; 281(19):1836–1843.
13 Richardson WS et al. Users' guides to the medical literature: XV. How to use an article about disease probability for differential diagnosis. Evidence-Based Medicine Working Group. JAMA 1999; 281(13): 1214–1219.
14 Dans AL et al. Users' guides to the medical literature: XIV. How to decide on the applicability of clinical trial results to your patient. Evidence-Based Medicine Working Group. JAMA 1998; 279(7):545–549.
15 O'Brien BJ et al. Users' guides to the medical literature: XIII. How to use an article on economic analysis of clinical practice. B. What are the results and will they help me in caring for my patients? Evidence-Based Medicine Working Group. JAMA 1997; 277(22):1802–1806.
16 Drummond MF et al. Users' guides to the medical literature: XIII. How to use an article on economic analysis of clinical practice. A. Are the results of the study valid? Evidence-Based Medicine Working Group. JAMA 1997; 277(19):1552–1557.
17 Guyatt GH et al. Users' guides to the medical literature: XII. How to use articles about health-related quality of life. Evidence-Based Medicine Working Group. JAMA 1997; 277(15):1232–1237.
18 Naylor CD, Guyatt GH. Users' guides to the medical literature: XI. How to use an article about a clinical utilization review. Evidence-Based Medicine Working Group. JAMA 1996; 275(18):1435–1439.
19 Naylor CD, Guyatt GH. Users' guides to the medical literature: X. How to use an article reporting variations in the outcomes of health services. The Evidence-Based Medicine Working Group. JAMA 1996; 275(7):554–558.
20 Guyatt GH et al. Users' guides to the medical literature: IX. A method for grading health care recommendations. Evidence-Based Medicine Working Group. JAMA 1995; 274(22):1800–1804.
21 Wilson MC et al. Users' guides to the medical literature: VIII. How to use clinical practice guidelines. B. what are the recommendations and will they help you in caring for your patients? The Evidence-Based Medicine Working Group. JAMA 1995; 274(20):1630–1632.
22 Hayward RS et al. Users' guides to the medical literature: VIII. How to use clinical practice guidelines. A. Are the recommendations valid? The Evidence-Based Medicine Working Group. JAMA 1995; 274(7):570–574.

23 Richardson WS, Detsky AS. Users' guides to the medical literature: VII. How to use a clinical decision analysis. B. What are the results and will they help me in caring for my patients? Evidence Based Medicine Working Group. JAMA 1995; 273(20):1610–1613.

24 Sackett DL, Haynes RB, Tugwell P. Clinical epidemiology: A basic science for clinical medicine. Little, Brown; 1985: 370.

25 Giglia E. Beyond PubMed. Other free-access biomedical databases. Eur Medicophys 2007; 43(4): 563–569.

26 Yue W, Wilson CS, Boller F. Peer assessment of journal quality in clinical neurology. J Med Libr Assoc 2007; 95(1):70–76.

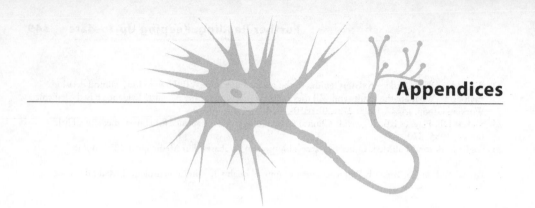

Appendices

The Mini-Mental State Examination

(Chapter 5)

Maximum score	Score	Item
		Orientation
5	( )	What is the year, season, date, day, month?
5	( )	Where are we: state, country, town, hospital, floor?
		Registration
3	( )	Name 3 objects, 1 second to say each. Then ask the patient to name the 3 after you have said them. Give 1 point for each correct answer. Then repeat them until the patient learns all 3. Count the number of trials and record. Trials ( )
		Attention and calculation
5	( )	Ask the patient to begin with 100 and count backwards by 7. Stop after 5; subtraction is 93, 86, 79, 72, 65. Score the total number of correct answers. If the patient cannot or will not perform this task, ask the patient to spell the word 'world' backwards. The score is the number of letters in correct order.
		Recall
3	( )	Ask the patient to name the 3 objects above. Give 1 point for each correct answer.
		Language

9	( )	• Name a pencil, and a watch. (2 points)
		• Repeat the following 'no ifs, ands or buts'. (1 point)
		• Follow a 3-stage command: take a piece of paper in the right hand, fold it in half and put it on the desk. (3 points)
		• Read and obey the following:
		  ◦ close your eyes (1 point)
		  ◦ write a sentence (1 point)
		  ◦ copy a design (1 point)

Total score	?/30	

Assess the level of consciousness along a continuum: alert → drowsy → stupor → coma

Instructions for administering the Mini-Mental State Examination

ORIENTATION

Ask for the date and where they are. Then ask specifically for parts omitted, for example, 'Can you also tell me what season it is?' (1 point for each correct answer)

Ask in turn: 'Can you tell me the name of this hospital (town, country etc)? (1 point for each correct answer)

REGISTRATION

Ask the patient if you may test their memory. Then say the names of 3 unrelated objects, clearly and slowly, about 1 second for each. After you have said all 3, ask the patient to repeat them. This first repetition determines the score (0–3), but keep saying them until they can repeat all 3, up to 6 trials. If they do not eventually learn all 3, recall cannot be meaningfully tested.

ATTENTION AND CALCULATION

Ask the patient to begin with 100 and count backwards by 7, and stop after 5 subtractions (93, 86, 79, 72, 65). Score the total number of correct answers. If the patient cannot or will not perform this task, ask him/her to spell the word 'world' backwards. The score is the number of letters in correct order. For example, DLROW = 5, DLORW = 3.

RECALL

Ask the patient if they can recall the 3 words you previously asked them to remember. (Score 0–3)

LANGUAGE

Naming: Show a wrist watch and ask the patient what it is. Repeat for a pencil.
(Score 0–2)

Repetition: Ask the patient to repeat the sentence after you. Allow only one trial.
(Score 0 or 1)

Three-stage command: Give the patient a piece of plain blank paper and ask them to take the piece of paper in the right hand, fold it in half and place it back on the desk.
Score 1 point for each part correctly executed.

Reading: On a blank piece of paper print the sentence 'Close your eyes', in letters large enough for the patient to see clearly. Ask the patient to read it and do what it says.
Score 1 point only if the patient actually closes the eyes.

Writing: Offer a blank piece of paper and ask the patient to write a sentence for you. Do not dictate a sentence; it is to be written spontaneously. It must contain a subject and a verb and be sensible. Correct grammar and punctuation are not necessary.

Copying: On a clean piece of paper, draw intersecting pentagons with each side about 1 inch, and ask the patient to copy it exactly as it is. All 10 angles must be present and must intersect to score 1 point. Tremor and rotation are ignored.

Benign Focal Seizures of Childhood

(Chapter 8)

Rolandic epilepsy

These are focal seizures consisting of unilateral facial sensory–motor symptoms. Motor manifestations are clonic contractions sometimes concurrent with ipsilateral tonic deviation of the mouth and the lower lip and may spread to the ipsilateral hand (same side as face is affected). The sensory symptoms consist of numbness or paraesthesiae (tingling, prickling or freezing) inside the mouth, associated with strange sounds, such as death rattle, gargling, grunting and guttural sounds. The speech is affected by anarthria, with the child being unable to utter a single intelligible word and attempting to communicate with gestures. There may or may not be impaired consciousness, but many of these seizures occur during sleep and the child awakes hemiparetic and anarthric [1].

Although rolandic seizures are usually brief, lasting for 1–3 minutes, opercular status epilepticus may persist for hours to months and consists of ongoing unilateral or bilateral contractions of the mouth, tongue or eyelids, positive or negative subtle perioral or other myoclonus, dysarthria, speech arrest, difficulties in swallowing, buccofacial apraxia and hypersalivation [1].

Panayiotopoulos syndrome

The first apparent ictal symptom is usually nausea and/or vomiting, but this may also occur long after the onset of other manifestations. Pallor, urinary and/or faecal incontinence, hypersalivation, difficulty breathing and even cyanosis are other autonomic manifestations. The seizures are usually lengthy, lasting more than 6 minutes, and almost half of them last for 30 minutes to many hours, thus constituting autonomic status epilepticus [1].

Idiopathic childhood occipital epilepsy of gastaut

Seizures are usually frequent and brief and manifest with elementary visual hallucinations, blindness or both [1]. Elementary visual hallucinations are frequently the first and often the only seizure symptom and consist mainly of small multicoloured circular patterns that often appear in the periphery of a visual field, becoming larger and multiplying during the course of the seizure, frequently moving towards the other side. Unlike in migraine, the visual disturbance develops rapidly within seconds. Ictal blindness is probably the second most common symptom after visual hallucinations. It is sudden and usually total. Complex visual hallucinations, such as faces and figures, and visual illusions, such as micropsia (objects appear undersize), palinopsia (the hallucinatory persistence of an object after the viewer has turned away) and metamorphopsia (images appear distorted in various ways), occur in < 10% of patients and mainly after the appearance of elementary visual hallucinations [1].

Post-ictal headache, mainly diffuse, but also severe, unilateral, pulsating and indistinguishable from migraine headache, occurs in half the patients, in 10% of whom it may be associated with nausea and vomiting. This occurs immediately, or 5–10 minutes after the end of the visual hallucinations. The duration and severity of the headache appears to be proportional to the duration and severity of the preceding seizure although it may also occur after brief simple visual seizures.

REFERENCES
1 Panayiotopoulos CP, et al: Benign childhood focal epilepsies: Assessment of established and newly recognized syndromes, *Brain* 131(Pt 9):2264–2286, 2008.

Currently Recommended Drugs for Epilepsy

(Chapter 8)

The following recommendations are based on the guidelines of the American Epilepsy Society [1, 2], the International League Against Epilepsy [3], the European Federation of Neurological Societies [4], tshe Cochrane database [5] and the SANAD trial [6, 7].

General principles

- Formulations of antiepileptic drugs (AEDs) are not interchangeable and generic substitution should not be employed.
- Lamotrigine and oxcarbazepine seem to be better tolerated and may produce fewer long-term side effects and adverse interactions.
- Lamotrigine may have advantages in young women, adolescents and the elderly as it is well tolerated, does not cause weight gain, has a favourable cognitive and behavioural profile and does not induce the metabolism of lipid-soluble drugs (such as the hormonal components of the oral contraceptive agents).
- Side effects may also occur as a result of drug interactions, and the MIMS interact program should be used to check potential drug interactions prior to prescribing an anticonvulsant.

The SANAD study [6, 7], a pragmatic randomised clinical trial found that:

- Carbamazepine is the drug of choice for partial or focal seizures.
- Valproic acid is the drug of choice for generalised seizures.

New onset epilepsy

GENERALISED ONSET TONIC–CLONIC SEIZURES

Carbamazepine, phenytoin and valproic acid have the most evidence to support their use, but the newer AEDs such as lamotrigine, oxcarbazepine, phenobarbital, topiramate are efficacious in adults, and carbamazepine, phenobarbital, phenytoin, topiramate and valproic acid are efficacious in children.

ABSENCE SEIZURES

Drugs of choice are ethosuximide, lamotrigine and valproic acid.

Carbamazepine, oxcarbazepine, phenytoin, gabapentin and tiagabine may precipitate or aggravate absence seizures.

JUVENILE MYOCLONIC EPILEPSY

There is no evidence to guide drug of first choice.

Valproic acid is regarded by some authorities as the drug of choice [1]. Clonazepam can suppress the myoclonic but not the tonic–clonic seizures, which is a disadvantage as it removes the warnings jerks of a tonic–clonic seizure [8].

Carbamazepine, oxcarbazepine, phenytoin, gabapentin and tiagabine may precipitate or aggravate absence and myoclonic seizures.

PARTIAL WITH OR WITHOUT SECONDARY GENERALISED SEIZURES

Carbamazepine, phenytoin, valproic acid, gabapentin, lamotrigine, topiramate and oxcarbazepine have efficacy as monotherapy in newly diagnosed adolescents and adults with either partial or mixed seizure disorders.

Refractory epilepsy

Control of seizures is inadequate in more than 30% of patients with epilepsy and in patients who have many seizures prior to commencing therapy, and only a small percentage of patients will become seizure-free if they fail to respond to the first drug. The seizure-free rate for monotherapy is the same with established as with new drugs [9].

Limited evidence suggests that lamotrigine and topiramate are also effective for adjunctive treatment of idiopathic generalised epilepsy in adults and children, as well as treatment of the Lennox–Gastaut syndrome. Gabapentin, lamotrigine, topiramate, tiagabine, oxcarbazepine, levetiracetam and zonisamide are appropriate for adjunctive treatment of refractory partial seizures in adults. Gabapentin, lamotrigine, oxcarbazepine and topiramate are for the treatment of refractory partial seizures in children.

Status epilepsy

Intravenous (IV) lorazepam is the drug of choice in both adults [10] and children [5]. Others include IV diazepam or IV phenytoin. If IV access is not available, 30 mg diazepam intrarectal gel can be used as an alternative [10].

In recent years IV valproic acid and IV levetiracetam have become available. Small studies suggest that IV levetiracetam [11] and IV valproic acid [12] may be effective in benzodiazepine refractory status epilepsy, but as yet there are no large randomised controlled trials.

Side effects of the antiepileptic drugs

Patients are often horrified and some are terrified when they are given a list of the potential side effects of drugs. It is important to stress to patients that drugs remain on the market because there are more patients who benefit than those who experience side effects. In general, side effects commence soon after therapy is initiated.

The commonest side effects related to all the drugs would include dizziness and ataxia with excess doses.

One very important drug interaction is the interaction between valproic acid and lamotrigine. Lamotrigine increases the serum levels of valproic acid and, therefore, the lamotrigine dose needs to be increased very slowly, commencing with 25 mg every 2nd day for 2 weeks, then 25 mg daily for 2 weeks and then increasing more rapidly as needed.

The following table lists the more common and potentially most serious side effects as compiled from the MIMS database [13].

TABLE C.1	Antiepileptic drugs and their more common and potentially most serious side effects
Antiepileptic drug	**Side effects**
Phenytoin	• Gum hyperplasia • Hirsutism • Coarse features • Osteomalacia
Carbamazepine and oxcarbamazepine	• Skin rash (rarely, Stevens–Johnson syndrome) • Drowsiness and fatigue • Hepatic toxicity • Blood dyscrasias
Valproic acid	• Weight gain • Hair loss (reversible even if drug is continued) • Hyponatraemia (syndrome of inappropriate antidiuretic hormone, SIADH) • Hepatic toxicity • Blood dyscrasias • Congenital malformations (spina bifida)
Ethosuximide	• Drowsiness • Skin rash • Blood dyscrasias • Personality changes • Dependence
Phenobarbitone	• Drowsiness • Bradycardia • Hypotension • Dependence • Osteoporosis • Blood dyscrasias
Clonazepam	• Drowsiness • Depression • Dependence • Behavioural disturbances (agitation, aggression)
Gabapentin	• Drowsiness and fatigue • Weight gain • Leucopenia • Dry mouth • Gastrointestinal upset
Levetiracetam	• Drowsiness and fatigue • Headache • Memory impairment • Aggression, confusion, irritability and suicidal thoughts • Blood dyscrasias (thrombocytopenia)

TABLE C.1 Antiepileptic drugs and their more common and potentially most serious side effects—*cont'd*

Antiepileptic drug	Side effects
Lamotrigine	• Skin rash (including Stevens–Johnson syndrome and toxic epidermal necrolysis) • Fever • Blood dyscrasias • Hepatic dysfunction
Pregabalin	• Drowsiness • Confusion and hallucinations • Weight gain • Tremor • Gastrointestinal upset • Pancreatitis • Rhabdomyolysis • Renal failure
Tiagabine	• Drowsiness • Restlessness • Exacerbation of seizures • Tremor
Topiramate	• Drowsiness and fatigue • Depression and suicidal thoughts • Personality changes • Anorexia and weight loss • Blood dyscrasias (leucopenia)
Vigabatrin	• Drowsiness and fatigue • Depression • Visual field defects • Weight gain • Gastrointestinal upset

REFERENCES

1 French JA, et al: Efficacy and tolerability of the new antiepileptic drugs. II: Treatment of refractory epilepsy: Report of the Therapeutics and Technology Assessment Subcommittee and Quality Standards Subcommittee of the American Academy of Neurology and the American Epilepsy Society, *Neurology* 62(8): 1261–1273, 2004.

2 French JA, et al: Efficacy and tolerability of the new antiepileptic drugs. I: Treatment of new onset epilepsy: Report of the Therapeutics and Technology Assessment Subcommittee and Quality Standards Subcommittee of the American Academy of Neurology and the American Epilepsy Society, *Neurology* 62(8): 1252–1260, 2004.

3 Glauser T, et al: ILAE treatment guidelines: Evidence-based analysis of antiepileptic drug efficacy and effectiveness as initial monotherapy for epileptic seizures and syndromes, *Epilepsia* 47(7):1094–1120, 2006.

4 Meierkord H, et al: EFNS guideline on the management of status epilepticus, *Eur J Neurol* 13(5):445–450, 2006.

5 Appleton R, Macleod S, Martland T: Drug management for acute tonic–clonic convulsions including convulsive status epilepticus in children, *Cochrane Database Syst Rev* (3), 2008:CD001905.

6 Marson AG, et al: The SANAD study of effectiveness of valproate, lamotrigine, or topiramate for generalised and unclassifiable epilepsy: An unblinded randomised controlled trial, *Lancet* 369(9566):1016–1026, 2007.

7 Marson AG, et al: The SANAD study of effectiveness of carbamazepine, gabapentin, lamotrigine, oxcarbazepine, or topiramate for treatment of partial epilepsy: An unblinded randomised controlled trial, *Lancet* 369(9566):1000–1015, 2007.

8 Obeid T, Panayiotopoulos CP: Clonazepam in juvenile myoclonic epilepsy, *Epilepsia* 30(5):603–606, 1989.

9 Kwan P, Brodie MJ: Early identification of refractory epilepsy, *N Engl J Med* 342(5):314–319, 2000.

10 Prasad K, et al: Anticonvulsant therapy for status epilepticus, *Cochrane Database Syst Rev* (4), 2005:CD003723.

11 Knake S, et al: Intravenous levetiracetam in the treatment of benzodiazepine refractory status epilepticus, *J Neurol Neurosurg Psychiatry* 79(5):588–589, 2008.

12 Agarwal P, et al: Randomized study of intravenous valproate and phenytoin in status epilepticus, *Seizure* 16(6):527–532, 2007.

13 MIMS. Available: http://www.mims.com.au/index.php?option=com_content&task=view&id=98&Itemid=133 (14 Dec 2009).

Treatment of Migraine

(Chapter 9)

TABLE D.1 Acute treatment for migraine

Agent	Route	Dose
Acetylsalicylic acid	Oral	650–1300 mg QQH*
Ibuprofen	Oral	400–800 mg QID*
Naproxyn	Oral	275–550 mg QID
Rizatriptan	Oral	10 mg
Eletriptan	Oral	80 mg
Almotriptan	Oral	12.5 mg
Sumatriptan	Oral	50–100 mg (repeat twice in 24 hours)
Sumatriptan	S/C	6 mg (repeat once in 24 hours)
Sumatriptan	IN	10 mg and 20 mg/0.1 mL (into 1 nostril)
Naratriptan	Oral	2.5 mg
Zolmatriptan	Oral	2.5 mg
Cafergot	Oral	1–2 mg
Cafergot	Rectal	2 mg (max 3 doses/24 hours)
Ergotamine	Oral	1–2 mg (repeat 1 hour max 3 doses/24 hours)
Dihydroergotamine	S/C, IM,IV	0.5–1.0 mg (repeat at 1 hour, max 4 mg/24 hours)
Chlorpromazine	IM, IV	50 mg IM or 0.1 mg/kg over 20 minutes, repeat after 15 minutes (pre-treat with IV normal saline)
Butorphanol	IN	1 mg in 1 nostril (repeat 3–5 hours later)
Metoclopramide	IV	10 mg
Prochlorperazine	Rectal	25 mg (max 3 doses/24 hours)
Dexamathasone	IV	10–20 mg

IM = intramuscular; IN =intranasal; IV = intravenous; max = maximum; QID = 6 hourly; QQH = 4 hourly; S/C = subcutaneous

*± Metoclopramide (oral or IV) 10 mg or domperidone (oral) 10–20 mg [1–6]

TABLE D.2 Prophylactic therapy for migraine

Agent	Dose	Maximum daily dose
Serotinin receptor antagonists		
Methysergide	1–2 mg TDS	8 mg (max 5 months, 1 month off)
Pizotifen	0.5 mg	1.5 mg
Tricyclic antidepressants		
Amitriptyline	10–150 mg	150 mg
Nortriptyline	10–150 mg	150 mg
Beta-blockers		
Propranolol	40–240 mg/day	240 mg
Atenolol	50–150 mg/day	150 mg
Metopropol	100–200 mg/day	200 mg
Anticonvulsants		
Valproic acid	500–1500 mg	1500 mg
Topirimate	25 mg initially	200 mg
Calcium channel blockers		
Verapamil	240–320 mg	320 mg
Flunarizine	5–10 mg	10 mg

max = maximum; mg = milligram; TDS = transdermyl

REFERENCES

1 Schoenen J, Jacquy J, Lenaerts M: Effectiveness of high-dose riboflavin in migraine prophylaxis. A randomized controlled trial, *Neurology* 50(2):466–470, 1998.
2 MacLennan SC, et al: High-dose riboflavin for migraine prophylaxis in children: A double-blind, randomized, placebo-controlled trial, *J Child Neurol* 23(11):1300–1304, 2008.
3 Dodick DW, et al: Topiramate versus amitriptyline in migraine prevention: A 26-week, multicenter, randomized, double-blind, double-dummy, parallel-group noninferiority trial in adult migraineurs, *Clin Ther* 31(3):542–559, 2009.
4 Louis P, Spierings EL: Comparison of flunarizine (Sibelium) and pizotifen (Sandomigran) in migraine treatment: A double-blind study, *Cephalalgia* 2(4):197–203, 1982.
5 Pryse-Phillips WE, et al: Guidelines for the diagnosis and management of migraine in clinical practice. Canadian Headache Society, *CMAJ* 156(9):1273–1287, 1997.
6 Evers S, et al: EFNS guideline on the drug treatment of migraine – report of an EFNS task force, *Eur J Neurol* 13(6):560–572, 2006.
7 Geraud G, Compagnon A, Rossi A: Zolmitriptan versus a combination of acetylsalicylic acid and metoclopramide in the acute oral treatment of migraine: A double-blind, randomised, three-attack study, *Eur Neurol* 47(2):88–98, 2002.
8 Sorge F, Marano E: Flunarizine v. placebo in childhood migraine. A double-blind study, *Cephalalgia* 5(Suppl 2):145–148, 1985.
9 Diener HC, et al: Efficacy, tolerability and safety of oral eletriptan and ergotamine plus caffeine (Cafergot) in the acute treatment of migraine: A multicentre, randomised, double-blind, placebo-controlled comparison, *Eur Neurol* 47(2):99–107, 2002.
10 Ferrari MD, et al: Oral triptans (serotonin 5-HT(1B/1D) agonists) in acute migraine treatment: A meta-analysis of 53 trials, *Lancet* 358(9294):1668–1675, 2001.

Epidemiology and Primary Prevention of Stroke

(Chapter 10)

The prevalence of stroke almost doubles for each 10 years after the age of 55 [1, 2]. A family history of stroke/TIA increases the risk by 1.4–2.4 times (95% CI 0.60–6.03) [3]. The relative risk of stroke with a paternal history is 2.4 (95% CI 0.96–6.03), while with a maternal history it is 1.4 (95% CI 0.60–3.25) [3]. The relative risk of stroke with the other currently recognised risk factors is shown in Table E.1. *The prevalence of hypertension, diabetes and smoking makes these risk factors the most significant, although smoking is less significant because of reduced incidence.*

TABLE E.1 Influence of risk factors on the relative risk of stroke

Risk factor	Prevalence (%)	Relative risk of stroke
Hypertension	20–60	1–4*
Cigarette smoking	12–18	1.8
Diabetes	5–27	1.8–6
Non-valvular atrial fibrillation	1.5–23.5**	2.6–4.5
Dyslipidaemia	15	1.5–2.5
Coronary artery disease	5.6–8.4	1.55–1.73
Asymptomatic carotid stenosis	2–7	2.0

*The influence of hypertension diminishes with increasing age; the relative risk is 4 at the age of 50, 3 at 60, 2 at 70, 1.8 at 80 and 1.0 at 90 years of age.
**The prevalence of atrial fibrillation increases dramatically after the age of 80; the incidence is 1.5 at 50–59, 2.8 at 60–69, 9.9 at 70–79 and 23.5 at 80–89 years of age. Hypertension, smoking and alcohol abuse are risk factors for subarachnoid haemorrhage [4]. Increasing age, hypertension, high alcohol intake and male sex are risk factors for intracerebral haemorrhage [5].

The risk of stroke related to atrial fibrillation can be estimated using the $CHADS_2$ score [6] or the score derived from the Framingham study [7]. How to calculate the $CHADS_2$ score is shown in Table E.2, and the correlation between the score and stroke risk is given in Table E.3.

Primary prevention refers to the institution of therapy for those risk factors that can be modified. A large number of risk factors have been identified as predisposing to an increased risk of cerebral vascular disease. Some, such as genetic predisposition and ageing, cannot be modified. Hypertension and atrial fibrillation are the two most significant risk factors for which primary prevention is most effective.

TABLE E.2 CHADS$_2$ score – points allocated for each of the five entities that make up the score

	Condition	Points
C	Congestive heart failure (in last 3 months)	1
H	Hypertension (untreated or treated)	1
A	Age > 75 years	1
D	Diabetes	1
S2	Prior stroke or TIA	2

TABLE E.3 The annual risk of stroke in patients with atrial fibrillation using the CHADS$_2$ criteria [6]*

CHADS$_2$ score	Stroke risk %	95% CI
0	1.9	1.2–3.0
1	2.8	2.0–3.8
2	4.0	3.1–5.1
3	5.9	4.6–7.3
4	8.5	6.3–11.1
5	12.5	8.2–17.5
6	18.2	10.5–27.4

*This is very useful in terms of explaining risk versus benefit of treatment with anticoagulants.

Risk factors for stroke
- Hypertension
- Atrial fibrillation
- Hyperlipidaemia
- Diabetes
- Obesity
- Smoking
  Lifestyle modifications are encouraged for all and include:
1 Weight reduction if overweight
2 Limitation of alcohol intake
3 Increased aerobic physical activity (30–45 minutes daily)
4 Reduction of sodium intake (< 2.34 g)
5 Maintenance of adequate dietary potassium (> 120 mmol/dL)
6 Smoking cessation
7 Dietary Approaches to Stop Hypertension (DASH) diet (rich in fruit, vegetables and low-fat dairy products and reduced in saturated and total fat) [8, 9].

HYPERTENSION
The link between hypertension and stroke was identified in the early 1960s by insurance companies [10]. The relative risk of death due to vascular lesions of the nervous system was found to be 1.6 for a blood pressure (BP) of 130–147/83–92 mmHg, rising to as

high as 6.2 for a BP of 148–177/93–102 mmHg. As early as 1967 [11], it was shown that treatment of patients with a diastolic BP in excess of 115 mmHg resulted in a relative risk reduction of 83% and an absolute risk reduction of 36% with number needed to treat of only 3.3!

The definition of what constitutes hypertension has evolved as further studies on the effect of treatment with different levels of BP have been undertaken. At one stage a normal systolic BP was considered to be 100 plus the age of the patient! The Progress Study [12] demonstrated a benefit from lowering the BP in patients who would not have been considered to have hypertension at the time of the study. Current recommendations suggest a BP < 140/90 mmHg. However, many elderly patients will not be able to tolerate the medications required to achieve this level, nor will they achieve this level of BP [9].

TREATMENT of HYPERTENSION

Lowering BP to optimal levels appears to be more important than specific drug selection. At least five classes of drugs, thiazide and thiazide-type diuretics, angiotensin-converting enzyme inhibitors, angiotensin receptor blockers, beta-blockers and calcium antagonists, have been proven to reduce mortality. Combination therapy is needed in many if not most patients to achieve optimal BP control; sometimes as many as two or three drugs are required [8]. Many elderly patients may not be able to tolerate the drugs or a BP < 140/90 mmHg, and it may be necessary to compromise and accept the lowest possible BP.

ATRIAL FIBRILLATION

The annual risk of stroke can be calculated from the $CHADS_2$ score (see Tables E.2 and E.3). Anticoagulation is recommended for patients with atrial fibrillation who have valvular heart disease (particularly those with mechanical heart valves) and antithrombotic therapy in patients with non-valvular atrial fibrillation with a $CHADS_2$ score of 2 (annual risk of stroke ≥ 4%) or greater, provided there are no contraindications [13]. Others would argue that, although patients with a $CHADS_2$ score of 2 or more derive greater benefit, even patients with a $CHADS_2$ score of 1 benefit from oral anticoagulant therapy with a low risk of haemorrhage [14]. Anticoagulation reduces the risk of stroke by as much as 60–70% [15]. Even after the risk of stroke is explained to patients, a number will simply refuse to use anticoagulants.

Some would argue that many of the factors that are purported to be barriers to anticoagulant therapy in older persons with atrial fibrillation probably should not influence the choice of stroke prophylaxis in these patients [16]. Impaired cognitive function is only a contraindication if the patient's medication cannot be supervised. A risk of falls is also a relative not an absolute contraindication. Although intracranial bleeding occurs in patients on anticoagulants, in patients at high risk of stroke the benefit outweighs the risk [17]. In patients with a high annual risk of stroke, for example a $CHADS_2$ score of 3 or more, the slight increased risk associated with anticoagulation is outweighed by the significant reduction in the subsequent risk of stroke. There is little or conflicting evidence that increasing age, propensity to falls, activities that may predispose to trauma and prior gastrointestinal bleeding influence anticoagulant-related bleeding. The level of anticoagulation, not the use of anticoagulation, is the factor that influences the risk of intracranial bleeding [18].

The only absolute contraindications to the use of anticoagulants are an underlying risk of bleeding, for example severe alcoholic liver disease with an elevated PT INR, epistaxis (which can easily be remedied prior to the commencement of anticoagulation), active peptic ulcer disease or gastrointestinal bleeding of any cause. If the bleeding source can be defined and treated, anticoagulation could then be commenced.

TREATMENT of ATRIAL FIBRILLATION

Coumadin (warfarin) is recommended for all patients with non-valvular atrial fibrillation and a CHADS2 score of 2 or more, provided there are no contraindications [13]. The absolute and relative contraindications have been discussed in the text. The PT INR should be maintained somewhere between 2.0 and 3.0. Although a higher level of anticoagulation at 3.0–3.5 has been recommended in patients with a mechanical heart valve [20], subsequent studies using moderate- and low-dose warfarin have suggested that lower intensity anticoagulation may be as effective and reduce the risk of haemorrhagic complications in this group of patients [21–23].

Warfarin is a very difficult drug to use because, in a number of patients, the PT INR fluctuates wildly, requiring careful monitoring and frequent blood tests. NO patient should go longer than 4 weeks between tests of PT INR. It is hoped that trials currently underway using thrombin or factor Xa inhibitors will replace warfarin. Recently, dabigatran 110 mg was shown to be equivalent to warfarin while 150 mg was associated with a lower rate of stroke and systemic embolism but an equivalent rate of major haemorrhage [24].

ASYMPTOMATIC CAROTID STENOSIS

The 5-year risk of stroke in patients with asymptomatic carotid stenosis is 11.8% for all strokes and 6.1% for fatal or disabling strokes [25]. Thus, the risk of severe or disabling stroke is very low (1.2% per annum).

MANAGEMENT of ASYMPTOMATIC CAROTID STENOSIS

In asymptomatic carotid stenosis the absolute risk reduction with carotid endarterectomy (CEA) over 5 years is similar to that of symptomatic patients with a moderate degree of stenosis (50–69%). In asymptomatic patients with a stenosis of 50–69%, it was 5.8% in the Asymptomatic Carotid Atherosclerosis Study (ACAS) [26] and 6% in the Asymptomatic Carotid Surgery Trial (ACST) [25], i.e. approximately 1% per year.

An acceptable stroke complication rate of endarterectomy for patients with asymptomatic stenosis is < 3%. There is no evidence that complication rates of CEA are lower in recent years; on the contrary, they may be a little higher than those reported in the randomised controlled trials. This may reflect the older age of patients undergoing endarterectomy [27].

The European Society of Vascular Surgeons (ESVS) published guidelines recommend [28]:

- CEA in asymptomatic men < 75 years old with 70–99% stenosis if the perioperative stroke/death risk is < 3%.
- The benefit in women with an asymptomatic stenosis is significantly less than in men; CEA should therefore be considered only in younger, fit women.
- Aspirin at a dose of 75–325 mg daily and statins should be given before, during and following CEA.
- Carotid artery stenting (CAS) is recommended for high-risk patients only and is discussed in the section dealing with secondary prevention.

The Cochrane review suggests that endarterectomy is still the treatment of choice [29].

---

1 The name warfarin stems from the acronym WARF, for Wisconsin Alumni Research Foundation + the ending –arin, indicating its link with coumarin, the first naturally occurring anticoagulant discovered in mouldy sweet clover [19].

HYPERLIPIDAEMIA

High total cholesterol and low high-density lipoprotein (HDL) cholesterol increase the risk of stroke twofold and treatment can result in a significant risk reduction [30].

TREATMENT of HYPERLIPIDAEMIA

In general, increasing levels of total cholesterol are associated with higher rates of ischaemic stroke. Low HDL is a risk factor for ischaemic stroke in men, but more data are needed to determine its effect in women. Lipid-modifying medications can substantially reduce the risk of stroke in high-risk patients such as those with coronary heart disease. Additional studies are needed to clarify the risk associated with lipoproteins in women and the effect of treatment in older persons (> 70–75 years of age) [9].

There are a large number of statins that have been studied in patients with atherosclerotic vascular disease. High-dose atorvastatin (80 mg) resulted in a modest 5-year absolute reduction in risk of 2.2% (adjusted hazard ratio, 0.84; 95% confidence interval, 0.71–0.99; P=0.03; unadjusted P=0.05) in patients with high cholesterol and cerebral ischaemia but without known coronary artery disease [31].

Recent data demonstrate that apolipoprotein B (apo B) is a better measure of circulating LDL particle number (LDL-P) and is a more reliable indicator of risk than LDL-C. It has been recommended that measurement of apo B should be added to the routine assessment of patients at risk [32].

It has been assumed that the reduction in risk demonstrated in the statin trials reflects the reduction in the cholesterol, but this may not be the case. Rosuvastatin 20 mg/day has been shown to reduce myocardial infarction, stroke, arterial revascularisation, hospitalisation for unstable angina or death from cardiovascular causes in patients with high-sensitivity C-reactive protein (CRP) levels of 2.0 mg/L or higher in the absence of an elevated cholesterol (a low-density glycoprotein cholesterol level < 3.4 mmol/L). The hazard ratio for stroke was 0.18 in the treatment group and 0.34 in the control group (hazard ratio, 0.52; 95% CI, 0.34–0.79; P = 0.002) [33]. This finding has prompted a call for the treatment of patients with an elevated high-sensitivity CRP to be treated with statin therapy even in the absence of an elevated low-density lipoprotein cholesterol [34]. This policy has not been implemented at the time of writing.

DIABETES

The relative risk of stroke with diabetes is 1.8–6 [35] and currently there is no proof that tight control of diabetes reduces the risk. Tight glycaemic control in diabetic patients has a significant benefit on the other long-term complications and is therefore recommended in patients with cerebral vascular disease, despite the lack of proof of benefit.

OBESITY

The relative risk of stroke with obesity is 1.75–2.37 [36]. The benefit of treatment is unknown and largely relates to the difficulty patients experience with weight reduction. Weight reduction has been shown to lower BP and this would lead to a reduction in the incidence of stroke [37].

All patients should be encouraged to lose weight and the patient and their spouse should be seen by a dietician. A more pragmatic approach might be to accept that, if attempts to lose weight make both the patient and their family utterly miserable, it is probably wise to encourage a more modest amount of weight reduction or accept that it is not possible.

SMOKING

Smoking increases the risk of stroke 1.8-fold and there is relative risk reduction of 50% within 1 year; 5 years after cessation of smoking the risk is back to a baseline level [38].

REFERENCES

1 Gunarathne A, et al: Secular trends in the cardiovascular risk profile and mortality of stroke admissions in an inner city, multiethnic population in the United Kingdom (1997–2005), *J Hum Hypertens* 22(1):18–23, 2008.

2 Brown RD, et al: Stroke incidence, prevalence, and survival: Secular trends in Rochester, Minnesota, through 1989, *Stroke* 27(3):373–380, 1996.

3 Kiely DK, et al: Familial aggregation of stroke. The Framingham Study, *Stroke* 24(9):1366–1371, 1993.

4 Teunissen LL, et al: Risk factors for subarachnoid hemorrhage: A systematic review, *Stroke* 27(3):544–549, 1996.

5 Ariesen MJ, et al: Risk factors for intracerebral hemorrhage in the general population: A systematic review, *Stroke* 34(8):2060–2065, 2003.

6 Gage BF, et al: Validation of clinical classification schemes for predicting stroke: Results from the National Registry of Atrial Fibrillation, *JAMA* 285(22):2864–2870, 2001.

7 Wang TJ, et al: A risk score for predicting stroke or death in individuals with new-onset atrial fibrillation in the community: The Framingham Heart Study, *JAMA* 290(8):1049–1056, 2003.

8 Chobanian AV, et al: Seventh report of the Joint National Committee on Prevention, Detection, Evaluation, and Treatment of High Blood Pressure, *Hypertension* 42(6):1206–1252, 2003.

9 Goldstein LB, et al: Primary prevention of ischemic stroke: A guideline from the American Heart Association/American Stroke Association Stroke Council: Cosponsored by the Atherosclerotic Peripheral Vascular Disease Interdisciplinary Working Group; Cardiovascular Nursing Council; Clinical Cardiology Council; Nutrition, Physical Activity, and Metabolism Council; and the Quality of Care and Outcomes Research Interdisciplinary Working Group: The American Academy of Neurology affirms the value of this guideline, *Stroke* 37(6):1583–1633, 2006.

10 Metropolitan Life Insurance Company: *Blood pressure: Insurance experience and its implications*, New York, 1961, Metropolitan Life Insurance Company.

11 Veterans Administration Cooperative Study Group on Antihypertensive Agents: Effects of treatment on morbidity in hypertension. Results in patients with diastolic blood pressures averaging 115 through 129 mm Hg, *JAMA* 202(11):1028–1034, 1967.

12 Progress Study Group: Randomised trial of a perindopril-based blood-pressure-lowering regimen among 6,105 individuals with previous stroke or transient ischaemic attack, *Lancet* 358(9287):1033–1041, 2001.

13 Singer DE, et al: Antithrombotic therapy in atrial fibrillation: American College of Chest Physicians Evidence-Based Clinical Practice Guidelines (8th edn), *Chest* 133(6 Suppl):546S–592S, 2008.

14 Healey JS, et al: Risks and benefits of oral anticoagulation compared with clopidogrel plus aspirin in patients with atrial fibrillation according to stroke risk: The atrial fibrillation clopidogrel trial with irbesartan for prevention of vascular events (ACTIVE-W), *Stroke* 39(5):1482–1486, 2008.

15 Go AS, et al: Anticoagulation therapy for stroke prevention in atrial fibrillation: How well do randomized trials translate into clinical practice? *JAMA* 290(20):2685–2692, 2003.

16 Man-Son-Hing M, Laupacis A: Anticoagulant-related bleeding in older persons with atrial fibrillation: Physicians' fears often unfounded, *Arch Intern Med* 163(13):1580–1586, 2003.

17 Man-Son-Hing M, et al: Choosing antithrombotic therapy for elderly patients with atrial fibrillation who are at risk for falls, *Arch Intern Med* 159(7):677–685, 1999.

18 Gage BF, et al: Incidence of intracranial hemorrhage in patients with atrial fibrillation who are prone to fall, *Am J Med* 118(6):612–617, 2005.

19 WAR Foundation: *Warfarin*, Jul 2009:Available: http://www.spiritus-temporis.com/warfarin/history.html.

20 Smith AG: Guidelines on oral anticoagulation: Second edition, *J Clin Pathol* 44(1):86, 1991.

21 Saour JN, et al: Trial of different intensities of anticoagulation in patients with prosthetic heart valves, *N Engl J Med* 322(7):428–432, 1990.

22 Pengo V, et al: A comparison of a moderate with moderate-high intensity oral anticoagulant treatment in patients with mechanical heart valve prostheses, *Thromb Haemost* 77(5):839–844, 1997.

23 Acar J, et al: AREVA: Multicenter randomized comparison of low-dose versus standard-dose anticoagulation in patients with mechanical prosthetic heart valves, *Circulation* 94(9):2107–2112, 1996.

24 Connolly SJ, et al: Dabigatran versus warfarin in patients with atrial fibrillation, *N Engl J Med* 361(12):1139–1151, 2009.

25 Halliday A, et al: Prevention of disabling and fatal strokes by successful carotid endarterectomy in patients without recent neurological symptoms: Randomised controlled trial, *Lancet* 363(9420):1491–1502, 2004.

26 Executive Committee for the Asymptomatic Carotid Atherosclerosis Study: Endarterectomy for asymptomatic carotid artery stenosis, *JAMA* 273(18):1421–1428, 1995.

27 Rerkasem K, Rothwell PM: Temporal trends in the risks of stroke and death due to endarterectomy for symptomatic carotid stenosis: An updated systematic review, *Eur J Vasc Endovasc Surg* 37(5):504–511, 2009.

28 Liapis CD, et al: ESVS guidelines. Invasive treatment for carotid stenosis: Indications, techniques, *Eur J Vasc Endovasc Surg* 37(4 Suppl):1–19, 2009.

29 Coward LJ, Featherstone RL, Brown MM: Safety and efficacy of endovascular treatment of carotid artery stenosis compared with carotid endarterectomy: A Cochrane systematic review of the randomized evidence, *Stroke* 36(4):905–911, 2005.

30 National Institutes of Health ATP III: *Detection, evaluation, and treatment of high blood cholesterol in adults*, Bethesda, Maryland, 2002, National Institutes of Health.

31 Amarenco P, et al: High-dose atorvastatin after stroke or transient ischemic attack, *N Engl J Med* 355(6):549–559, 2006.

32 Contois JH, et al: Apolipoprotein B and cardiovascular disease risk: Position statement from the AACC Lipoproteins and Vascular Diseases Division Working Group on Best Practices, *Clin Chem* 55(3):407–419, 2009.

33 Ridker PM, et al: Rosuvastatin to prevent vascular events in men and women with elevated C-reactive protein, *N Engl J Med* 359(21):2195–2207, 2008.

34 Watson KE: The JUPITER trial: How will it change clinical practice? *Rev Cardiovasc Med* 10(2):91–96, 2009.

35 Force UPST: *Guide to clinical preventive services*, 2nd edn, Baltimore, 1996, Williams & Wilkins.

36 Welin L, et al: Risk factors for coronary heart disease during 25 years of follow-up. The study of men born in 1913, *Cardiology* 82(2–3):223–228, 1993.

37 Neter JE, et al: Influence of weight reduction on blood pressure: A meta-analysis of randomized controlled trials, *Hypertension* 42(5):878–884, 2003.

38 Wolf PA, et al: Cigarette smoking as a risk factor for stroke. The Framingham Study, *JAMA* 259(7): 1025–1029, 1988.

Current Criteria for Tissue Plasminogen Activator (t-PA) in Patients with Ischaemic Stroke*

(Chapter 10)

- Diagnosis of ischaemic stroke causing measurable neurological deficit
- The neurological signs should not be clearing spontaneously
- The neurological signs should not be minor and isolated
- Caution should be exercised in treating a patient with major deficits
- The symptoms of stroke should not be suggestive of subarachnoid haemorrhage
- Onset of symptoms < 4.5 hours before commencing treatment
- No head trauma or prior stroke in the previous 3 months
- No myocardial infarction in the previous 3 months
- No gastrointestinal or urinary tract haemorrhage in the previous 21 days
- No major surgery in the previous 14 days
- No arterial puncture at a non-compressible site in the previous 7 days
- No history of previous intracranial haemorrhage
- Blood pressure not elevated (systolic < 185 and diastolic < 110 mmHg)
- No evidence of active bleeding or acute trauma (fracture) on examination
- Not taking an oral anticoagulant or, if anticoagulant being taken, INR < 1.8
- If receiving heparin in previous 48 hours, aPTT must be in normal range
- Platelet count > 100 000/mm^3
- Blood glucose concentration > 50 mg/dL (2.7 mmol/L)
- No seizure with post-ictal residual neurological impairments
- CT does not show multilobar infarction (hypodensity > 1/3 cerebral hemisphere)
- The patient or family members understand the potential risks and benefits from treatment

---

INR = international normalised ratio; aPTT = activated partial thromboplastin
*Adapted from Table 11 in the 'Guidelines for the early management of adults with ischemic stroke' [1]

REFERENCES

1 Adams HP, Jr. et al: Guidelines for the early management of adults with ischemic stroke: A guideline from the American Heart Association/American Stroke Association Stroke Council, Clinical Cardiology Council, Cardiovascular Radiology and Intervention Council, and the Atherosclerotic Peripheral Vascular Disease and Quality of Care Outcomes in Research Interdisciplinary Working Groups: The American Academy of Neurology affirms the value of this guideline as an educational tool for neurologist. *Stroke* 38(5):1655–1711, 2007.

Barwon Health Dysphagia Screen

(Chapter 10)

All patients admitted with stroke or with TIA symptoms need to be screened for dysphagia before being given food or drink. Failure of the screen indicates dysphagia. The screen is to be completed by a speech pathologist, a doctor or competency assessed nurse.

Note: A speech pathologist is available via pager 0800–1600 Mon/Fri and 0800–1030 Sat/Sun to review if screen failed.

STROKE 121 DYSPHAGIA SCREEN

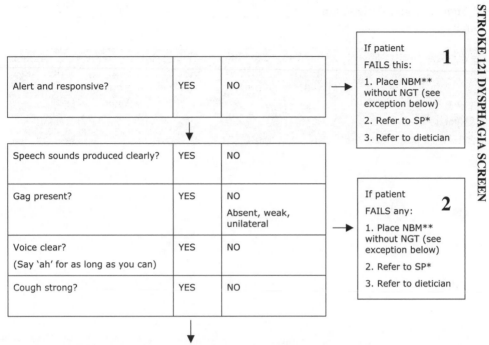

Alert and responsive?	YES	NO	
Speech sounds produced clearly?	YES	NO	
Gag present?	YES	NO Absent, weak, unilateral	
Voice clear? (Say 'ah' for as long as you can)	YES	NO	
Cough strong?	YES	NO	

If patient FAILS this: **1**
1. Place NBM** without NGT (see exception below)
2. Refer to SP*
3. Refer to dietician

If patient FAILS any: **2**
1. Place NBM** without NGT (see exception below)
2. Refer to SP*
3. Refer to dietician

Position the patient in an upright position at 90° so that he/she can sip some water.

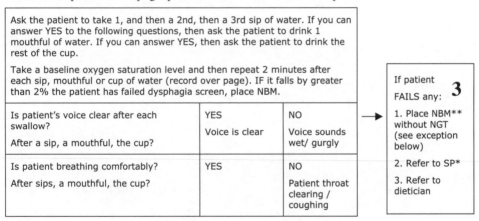

Ask the patient to take 1, and then a 2nd, then a 3rd sip of water. If you can answer YES to the following questions, then ask the patient to drink 1 mouthful of water. If you can answer YES, then ask the patient to drink the rest of the cup.

Take a baseline oxygen saturation level and then repeat 2 minutes after each sip, mouthful or cup of water (record over page). IF it falls by greater than 2% the patient has failed dysphagia screen, place NBM.

Is patient's voice clear after each swallow? After a sip, a mouthful, the cup?	YES Voice is clear	NO Voice sounds wet/ gurgly
Is patient breathing comfortably? After sips, a mouthful, the cup?	YES	NO Patient throat clearing / coughing

If patient FAILS any: **3**
1. Place NBM** without NGT (see exception below)
2. Refer to SP*
3. Refer to dietician

* SP = speach pathologist

** NBM = nil by mouth

Screen pass (all yes answers): patient can commence a full ward diet and thin fluids.

Screen fail exception: If oral drugs cannot be withheld or be given by an alternative route (Pharmacy has a list of alternatives for dysphagic patients) then a Flexiflow NGT size 10 or 12 should be inserted primarily for drug administration, its position checked by chest X-ray and management orders written on admission NGT inserted for medications: YES ( ) NO ( )

Continue to monitor for signs of dysphagia as described in the 'Dysphagia Screening After Stroke' learning package

Signature and designation _____Date: _____
Time: _____

Parameter	Baseline	2 minutes post 1st sip water	2 minutes post 2nd sip water	2 minutes post 3rd sip water	2 minutes post mouthful water	2 minutes post cup water
Oxygen Saturation						

Nerve Conduction Studies and Electromyography

(Chapter 11)

Nerve conduction studies (NCS) are like any other test in that they have a sensitivity and specificity and positive and negative predictive values. NCS can help confirm a diagnosis and provide an objective measure of severity and can help in determining subsequent treatment and response to treatment.

What to tell the patient to expect

Many patients are very worried about NCS and electromyography (EMG), and it does not help if no explanation of what to expect is provided at the time of ordering the test. An explanation should always be, and usually is, provided at the time of the actual test. NCS are performed by taping a disc (recording electrode) to the skin over the surface of the muscle and then applying a stimulating electrode and administering a small, safe, but at times uncomfortable, electrical impulse several times at different sites along the various nerves. NOT all patients undergoing NCS will have a needle inserted into a muscle. This is done when performing EMG. Figures H.1 and H.2 can be used to show patients what to expect.

How to interpret NCS and EMG reports

Most practitioners not familiar with NCS will simply read the conclusion. Neurophysiologists frequently use abbreviations that are confusing to the uninitiated. Table H.1 contains a list of the common terms and abbreviations used in NCS and EMG reports.

NCS reflect the degree of damage to the nerve and as such initially may be entirely normal or demonstrate minor and non-diagnostic abnormalities when the symptoms are either intermittent in nature or of recent onset. Repeat test-

Normal NCS do not exclude a diagnosis when symptoms are intermittent in nature or of recent onset.

ing some 3–6 months later will often demonstrate worsening and be more conclusive. Patients with symptoms of carpal tunnel syndrome of only a few weeks duration often have normal NCS, as do patients in the first 1 or 2 weeks of acute inflammatory demyelinating peripheral neuropathy.

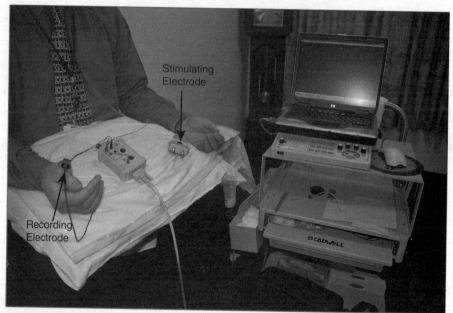

FIGURE H.1 NCS set-up: The surface electrode is placed over the muscle (in this case the APB) and the stimulating electrode is placed over the nerve (not shown here) and a DC electrical impulse is applied to the nerve

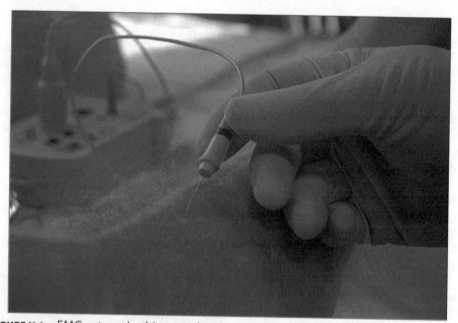

FIGURE H.2 EMG set-up: In this case the concentric needle electrode is inserted in the tibialis anterior muscle

When to order NCS and EMG

- Probably the most useful application of electrophysiology is in carpal tunnel syndrome [1] where the sensitivity is high [2] and the response to surgery can be anticipated based on the severity of the findings [3]. In carpal tunnel syndrome

TABLE H.1   Common terms used in electromyography (*) and nerve conduction studies

Term	Explanation
Distal motor latency (DML)	The latency between the distal point of stimulation of the nerve and the recording electrode on the surface of the muscle
Motor nerve conduction velocity (MNCV)	The conduction velocity between two points of stimulation along the motor nerve
Sensory nerve conduction velocity (SNCV)	The conduction velocity along the sensory nerve
Sensory nerve action potential (SNAP)	The response on stimulating the sensory nerve
Compound motor action potential (CMAP)	The response recorded over the muscle when stimulating the motor nerve
Single fibre electromyography (SFEMG)	Using a very fine needle to record the response in a single muscle fibre, particularly useful in myasthenia gravis
F-wave latency (F-Wave)	The time taken for the impulse to spread from the point of stimulation distally in the limb in a retrograde manner back to the anterior horn cell in the spinal cord and then back down to the recording electrodes; this latency is very dependent on the length of the limb
Insertional activity*	Refers to the initial potentials recorded on insertion of the needle into the muscle
Spontaneous activity*	Refers to abnormal muscle fibre activity such as fibrillation potentials, positive sharp waves and fasciculations seen in enervated muscle or the inflammatory myopathies
Recruitment*	Refers to how many motor units fire (recruit) with active muscle contraction

if the degree of compression is mild the NCS can be normal. Table H.2 lists the findings on NCS with increasing severity of median nerve compression in the carpal tunnel. It is important to note that the

> Normal NCS do not exclude a mild carpal tunnel syndrome and abnormal NCS that are in keeping with carpal tunnel syndrome may not explain the patient's symptoms.

NCS, even when positive, do NOT diagnose carpal tunnel syndrome; they simply localise the site of the problem to the region of the carpal tunnel in the wrist where carpal tunnel syndrome is the most likely cause. It is very important to correlate the clinical symptoms with the NCS findings. In patients with persistent symptoms following surgery, a comparison between the pre- and postoperative studies allows assessment of whether the median nerve compression in the carpal tunnel has been decompressed or not.

- NCS are very useful at confirming and localising the exact site of compression in ulnar nerve lesions [7, 8].
- NCS ± EMG is also usually diagnostic in patients with suspected peripheral neuropathy – a normal study virtually excludes this diagnosis (except with recent onset symptoms or with small fibre neuropathy, see Chapter 12, 'Back pain and

TABLE H.2   NCS findings in carpal tunnel syndrome with increasing severity of median nerve compression

Severity of carpal tunnel syndrome	Increasing severity of NCS findings*
Very mild or recent onset	Normal
Mild	Prolonged sensory latency, either palm to wrist or finger to wrist (with or without a reduction in the amplitude of the response) but only in comparison with the corresponding ulnar SNAP (> 0.3 ms difference)
Mild–moderate	Prolonged absolute sensory latency (palm to wrist)
Moderate	As above + prolonged median 2nd lumbrical to ulnar 4th interosseous latency (> 0.4 ms difference) [6]
Moderate–severe	• Prolonged median distal motor latency (DML) compared to corresponding ulnar DML (> 0.5 ms) ± absent median SNAP • Prolonged absolute median distal motor latency (> 4.7 ms)
Severe	• Absent median motor and sensory responses but retained lumbrical response • No response in the motor, sensory or lumbrical studies

*Note: This is similar to the severity rating scale proposed by Bland [4], except he does not refer to the absent responses or the median lumbrical studies. These latter studies are very useful and may help to confirm carpal tunnel syndrome in patients with coexistent peripheral neuropathy [5].

common leg problems with or without difficulty walking'). Occasionally NCS will detect subclinical neuropathy, particularly in diabetes [9].

- EMG is the test to order when looking for a disease of muscle such as polymyositis.
- NCS have a high sensitivity when a single nerve is damaged and in patients with a peripheral neuropathy. The exceptions to this are small fibre neuropathy, a common cause of burning feet syndrome where the NCS are normal and very early on in the course of AIDP where the initial NCS may be normal. Most protocols for electrophysiological examination of peripheral neuropathy require examination of motor and sensory nerves in at least two extremities [10].

> In patients with persistent neurological symptoms indicating a possible peripheral nerve lesion, particularly if there are objective neurological signs, the NCS will always be abnormal and a normal response would exclude that diagnosis.

- A condition where nerve conduction studies are often requested is impingement of the lateral cutaneous nerve of the thigh beneath the inguinal ligament, so-called meralgia paraesthetica (see Chapter 12, 'Back pain and common leg problems with or without difficulty walking'). It is important to warn the patient that the NCS are technically very difficult, the test is very painful with electric stimuli to the groin and the sensitivity and specificity are poor.
- NCS and EMG for cervical and lumbar radiculopathy, even in competent hands, have a variable sensitivity [11, 12] in patients with possible radiculopathy (29%) although results are a little better in patients with definite radiculopathy (72%) [11]. The most sensitive test is EMG [13].

- Repetitive stimulation studies are performed when myasthenia gravis or Lambert–Eaton Syndrome is suspected. [14]
- NCS for tarsal tunnel syndrome are technically very difficult and of uncertain sensitivity and specificity. [15]

What to do when the result is not what was anticipated

- A normal study essentially excludes the suspected diagnosis when there are objective abnormal signs of a peripheral neuropathy or peripheral nerve lesion unless it was of recent onset (1–2 weeks). If NCS are normal in a patient with clinically suspected peripheral neuropathy, somatosensory evoked potentials may be abnormal.
- In patients with intermittent symptoms a normal study does not exclude the diagnosis, particularly carpal tunnel syndrome. Approaches in this setting include wait-and-see with a repeat study in 3–6 months and if symptoms persist. If symptoms are severe and the patient is unable to tolerate them it is not unreasonable to recommend surgery in patients with classical carpal tunnel syndrome. However, as already alluded to, the results of surgery in the setting of normal NCS are less than optimal.
- In patients with atypical features of carpal tunnel syndrome and a normal NCS, the patient should be informed that there is no proof of the diagnosis, that some of the symptoms are not typical and may not resolve with surgery. The other alternative in this setting and probably the most useful is to seek a second opinion.

REFERENCES

1 American Association of Electrodiagnostic Medicine: American Academy of Neurology and American Academy of Physical Medicine and Rehabilitation. Practice parameter for electrodiagnostic studies in carpal tunnel syndrome: Summary statement, *Muscle Nerve* 25(6):918–922, 2002.
2 American Association of Electrodiagnostic Medicine: Guidelines in electrodiagnostic medicine. Practice parameter for electrodiagnostic studies in carpal tunnel syndrome, *Muscle Nerve Suppl* 8:S141–S167, 1999.
3 Schrijver HM, et al: Correlating nerve conduction studies and clinical outcome measures on carpal tunnel syndrome: Lessons from a randomized controlled trial, *J Clin Neurophysiol* 22(3):216–221, 2005.
4 Bland JD: A neurophysiological grading scale for carpal tunnel syndrome, *Muscle Nerve* 23(8):1280–1283, 2000.
5 Preston DC, Logigian EL: Lumbrical and interossei recording in carpal tunnel syndrome, *Muscle Nerve* 15(11):1253–1257, 1992.
6 Boonyapisit K, et al: Lumbrical and interossei recording in severe carpal tunnel syndrome, *Muscle Nerve* 25(1):102–105, 2002.
7 Kern RZ: The electrodiagnosis of ulnar nerve entrapment at the elbow, *Can J Neurol Sci* 30(4):314–319, 2003.
8 American Association of Electrodiagnostic Medicine: American Academy of Neurology, and American Academy of Physical Medicine and Rehabilitation. Practice parameter: Electrodiagnostic studies in ulnar neuropathy at the elbow, *Neurology* 52(4):688–690, 1999.
9 Liu MS, et al: [Clinical and neurophysiological features of 700 patients with diabetic peripheral neuropathy], *Zhonghua Nei Ke Za Zhi* 44(3):173–176, 2005.
10 American Association of Electrodiagnostic Medicine: Guidelines in electrodiagnostic medicine, *Muscle Nerve* 15:229–253, 1992.
11 Nardin RA, et al: Electromyography and magnetic resonance imaging in the evaluation of radiculopathy, *Muscle Nerve* 22(2):151–155, 1999.
12 Robinson LR: Electromyography, magnetic resonance imaging, and radiculopathy: It's time to focus on specificity, *Muscle Nerve* 22(2):149–150, 1999.
13 American Association of Electrodiagnostic Medicine and American Academy of Physical Medicine and Rehabilitation: Practice parameters for needle electromyographic evaluation of patients with suspected cervical radiculopathy: Summary Statement, *Muscle Nerve Supplement* 22(8):S211–S322, 1999.
14 American Association of Electrodiagnostic Medicine Quality Assurance Committee: Practice parameter for repetitive nerve stimulation and single fiber EMG evaluation of adults with suspected myasthenia gravis or Lambert–Eaton myasthenic syndrome: Summary statement, *Muscle Nerve* 24(9):1236–1238, 2001.
15 Patel AT, et al: Usefulness of electrodiagnostic techniques in the evaluation of suspected tarsal tunnel syndrome: An evidence-based review, *Muscle Nerve* 32(2):236–240, 2005.

Diagnostic Criteria for Multiple Sclerosis

(Chapter 14)

TABLE I.1   The 2005 revisions to the McDonald diagnostic criteria for multiple sclerosis [1]

Clinical presentation	Additional data needed for MS diagnosis
Two or more attacks;[a] objective clinical evidence of two or more lesions	No additional data required[b]
Two or more attacks; objective clinical evidence of one lesion	Dissemination in space, demonstrated by: • MRI[c] or • two or more MRI-detected lesions consistent with MS plus positive CSF[d] or • await further clinical attack implicating a different site
One attack; objective clinical evidence of two or more lesions	Dissemination in time, demonstrated by: • MRI[c] or • second clinical attack
One attack; objective clinical evidence of one lesion (monosymptomatic presentation; clinically isolated syndrome)	Dissemination in space, demonstrated by: • MRI[c] or • two or more MRI-detected lesions consistent with MS plus positive CSF[d] and dissemination in time, demonstrated by: • MRI[c] or • second clinical attack

Continued

TABLE I.1 The 2005 revisions to the McDonald diagnostic criteria for multiple sclerosis [1]–cont'd

Clinical presentation	Additional data needed for MS diagnosis
Insidious neurological progression suggestive of MS	One year of disease progression (retrospectively or prospectively determined) and two of the following: • positive brain MRI (nine T2 lesions or four or more to 2 L with positive VEP)[f] • positive spinal cord MRI (2 focal T2 lesions) • positive CSF[d]

CSF = cerebral spinal fluid; MRI = magnetic resonance imaging; MS = multiple sclerosis; VEP = visual evoked potential

[a]An attack is defined as an episode of neurological disturbance for which causative lesions are likely to be inflammatory and demyelinating in nature. There should be a subjective report (backed up by objective findings) or objective observation that the event lasts for at least 24 hours.

[b]No additional tests are required; however, if tests (MRI, CSF) are undertaken and are negative, extreme caution needs to be taken before making a diagnosis of MS. Alternative diagnoses must be considered. There must be no better explanation for the clinical picture and some objective evidence to support a diagnosis of MS.

[c]MRI demonstration of space dissemination must fulfill the criteria derived from Barkof et al and Tintore et al (see Box I.1).

[d]Positive CSF determined by oligoclonal bands detected by established methods (isoelectric focusing) different from any such bands in serum, or by an increased IgG index.

[e] MRI demonstration of time dissemination must fulfill the criteria in Box I.2.

[f]Abnormal VEP of the type seen in MS.

BOX I.1 The current magnetic resonance imaging (MRI) criteria to demonstrate brain abnormality and dissemination in space [2, 3]

Three of the following:
- at least one gadolinium-enhancing lesion or nine T2 hyperintense lesions if there this no gadolinium-enhancing lesion
- at least one infratentorial lesion (in the brainstem or cerebellum)
- at least one juxtacortical lesion (near the cortex)
- at least three periventricular lesions (adjacent to the lateral and 3rd ventricles)

BOX I.2 Magnetic resonance imaging (MRI) criteria to demonstrate dissemination of lesions in time

There are two ways to show dissemination in time using imaging:
- Detection of gadolinium enhancement at least 3 months after the onset of the initial clinical event, if not at the site corresponding to the initial event
- Detection of a new T2 lesion if it appears at any time compared with a reference scan done at least 30 days after the onset of the initial clinical event

REFERENCES
1   Polman CH, et al: Diagnostic criteria for multiple sclerosis: 2005 revisions to the "McDonald Criteria", *Ann Neurol* 58(6):840–846, 2005.
2   Barkhof F, et al: Comparison of MRI criteria at first presentation to predict conversion to clinically definite multiple sclerosis, *Brain* 120(Pt 11):2059–2069, 1997.
3   Tintore M, et al: Isolated demyelinating syndromes: Comparison of different MR imaging criteria to predict conversion to clinically definite multiple sclerosis, *AJNR Am J Neuroradiol* 21(4):702–706, 2000.

Glossary

Allodynia Hypersensitivity reaction to touch and gentle palpation (*allopathia* is sometimes used if the hypersensitivity is such as to lead to feelings of burning, electric shocks and excessive pins and needles)

Amaurosis fugax A fleeting loss of vision; if it occurs in one eye it is referred to as monocular amaurosis fugax (carotid territory); if it is bilateral it is vertebrobasilar territory (amaurosis is the Greek word for darkening, dark or obscure; fugax is related to fugitive/fleeing, fleeting or short-lived)

Amyotrophy Progressive wasting of muscle

Apraxia Total or partial loss of the ability to perform coordinated movements or manipulate objects in the absence of motor or sensory impairment

Aura The brief warning that may precede an actual seizure or headache; a peculiar sensation (visual, auditory, somatic or gustatory disturbance) forerunning the appearance of more definite symptoms [1]

Cerebral infarction Loss of brain tissue subsequent to the transient or permanent loss of circulation and/or oxygen delivery to that region of the brain

Chiari malformation Congenital malformation where the cerebellar tonsils protrude through the foramen magnum into the cervical spinal canal

Circumstantial evidence Information in the past, family and social history, that only increases the likelihood of a particular illness, it does not indicate the presence of that diagnosis

Clonus Upper motor neuron sign with repetitive contractions of muscles induced by a sudden movement

Déjà vu The experience of feeling sure that one has witnessed or experienced a new situation previously

Dermatome Area of the skin supplied by a specific spinal nerve root

Dysaesthesia Unpleasant sensation evoked by lightly stroking or touching the skin

Dysarthria Speech disorder in which the pronunciation is unclear although the meaning of what is said is normal

Dysphagia Difficulty swallowing

Dystonia Impairment of the ability to understand and use the symbols of language, both spoken and written

Epilepsy A condition characterised by recurrent seizures

Erb's point A site at the lateral root of the brachial plexus located 2–3 cm above the clavicle

Foramen magnum The opening in the occipital bone at the base of the skull, where the lower aspect of the brainstem becomes the upper aspect of the spinal cord

Herniation Brain tissue, cerebrospinal fluid and blood vessels are moved or pressed away from their usual position in the head, typically down through the tentorium

Ictus Strictly defined as a blow or sudden attack, it is another term used to describe a seizure

Intracerebral haemorrhage Haemorrhage inside the brain

Jamais vu A feeling of unfamiliarity, a sense of seeing the situation for the first time, despite rationally knowing that he or she has been in the situation before

Lacunar infarction Small area of cerebral infarction (diameter 0.2–1.5 cm) related to the occlusion of small arteries (30–300 *u*m)

Lewy body An eosinophilic intracytoplasmic neuronal inclusion

Ligamentum flavum Ligament that connects the lamina of adjacent vertebra, from the axis bone to the first segment of the sacrum

Likely pathology Established by eliciting the exact mode of onset and progression of symptoms

Lower motor neuron (LMN) Signs that indicate involvement of the peripheral nervous system

Meridians of longitude The descending motor pathway and the two ascending sensory pathways. Could also refer to the visual pathway from the eye to the occipital lobe and the vestibular pathway that arises in the inner ear and ends in the brainstem and cerebellum as these are long pathways with different abnormalities along those pathways that indicate the site of the problem

Myelopathy A disorder in which the tissue of the spinal cord is diseased or damaged; a disturbance or disease of the spinal cord

Myopathy Any of several diseases of muscle that are not caused by a disorder of the nerves

Myositis Inflammation of muscle

Myotome The muscles supplied by a particular spinal nerve root

Myotonia Tonic spasm of a muscle, typically seen in myotonic dystrophy where the patient has difficulty relaxing the muscle (e.g. after gripping an object the fingers are peeled slowly off the object)

Negative predictive value Concerned only with negative test results. For any diagnostic test, the positive predictive value will fall as the prevalence of the disease falls while the negative predictive value will rise

Paraesthesia Any subjective sensation, experienced as numbness, tingling or a 'pins-and-needles' feeling

Parallels of latitude The dermatomes, myotomes and reflexes in the limbs, the dermatomes on the trunk, the cranial nerves in the brainstem, the cerebellum and the cortical symptoms and signs in the cerebral hemispheres

Paraparesis Partial weakness affecting the lower limbs

Paraplegia Total weakness of the lower limbs

Pathognomonic A sign or symptom that is so characteristic of a disease that it makes the diagnosis

Periodic paralysis Intermittent episodes of muscle weakness, typically used to refer to the genetic muscle disorders hypokalaemic and hyperkalaemic periodic paralysis, also seen in hyperthyroidism

Phonophobia Increased sensitivity to noise

Photophobia Increased sensitivity to light

Photopsia Perceived flashes of light

Positive predictive value The chance that a positive test result will be correct. For any diagnostic test, the positive predictive value will fall as the prevalence of the disease falls, while the negative predictive value will rise. In practice, since most diseases have a low prevalence, even when the tests we use have apparently good sensitivity and specificity, the positive predictive value may be very low

Post-ictal Period of time immediately after the seizure

Primary prevention Measures taken to reduce the incidence of subsequent cerebral vascular disease before the first symptomatic event

Quadriparesis Partial weakness of all four limbs

Quadriplegia Total weakness of all four limbs, also referred to as tetraparesis

Radiculopathy Dysfunction of a nerve root that can cause weakness or sensory symptoms in a specific pattern corresponding to that nerve root. C, T, L and S are the abbreviations used to refer to the cervical, thoracic, lumbar and sacral regions, respectively. The number of the nerve root is placed after the letter, e.g. C6

Rhabdomyolysis Rapid disintegration of striated muscle tissue accompanied by the excretion of myoglobin in the urine

Secondary prevention Measures taken to reduce the incidence of subsequent cerebral vascular disease after the development of symptoms of cerebral vascular disease

Seizure Sudden change in behaviour due to an abnormal firing of nerve cells in the brain or symptoms of cerebral dysfunction resulting from paroxysmal discharges of neurons involving the cerebral cortex

Sensitivity Indication of how good a test is at correctly identifying people who have the disease

Specificity Indication of how good a test is at correctly excluding people who do not have the condition

Spondylolisthesis Forward dislocation of one vertebra over the one beneath

Spondylosis Degenerative arthritis, osteoarthritis of the spinal vertebrae in which osteophytes (abnormal bone outgrowths) cause a narrowing of the spinal canal and produce compression of the spinal cord and nerve roots

Subarachnoid haemorrhage (SAH) Bleeding within the head into the space between two membranes that surround the brain; the bleeding is beneath the arachnoid membrane and just above the pia mater (the arachnoid is the middle of three membranes around the brain while the pia mater is the innermost one)

Subdural haemorrhage Bleeding within the inner meningeal layer of the dura (the outer protective covering of the brain)

Subhyaloid haemorrhages Dark red, globular swellings around the optic disc that are thought to be caused by rapid venous engorgement secondary to the rapid increase in intracranial pressure that results from the initial subarachnoid haemorrhage

Tentorium Flap of the meninges separating the cerebral hemispheres from the brainstem and cerebellum in the posterior fossa

Tone Resistance to passive movement, increased with upper motor neuron problems and normal or decreased with lower motor neuron problems

Transient ischaemic attack (TIA) Sudden, focal neurological deficit that lasts for less than 24 hours, presumed to be of vascular origin, and confined to an area of the brain or eye

Upper motor neuron (UMN) Signs that indicate involvement of the central nervous system

Valsalva Forced expiration against a closed glottis, increasing intrathoracic pressure

Visual obscurations Inability to see in a particular part of the visual field for a period of time

Whiplash Injury to the neck (the cervical vertebrae) resulting from rapid acceleration or deceleration

REFERENCES

1 Dorland's medical dictionary, 31st edn Philadelphia. Elsevier; 2007.
2 Mosby's Dictionary of Medicine, Nursing & Health Professions, 2nd Australian and New Zealand Edition. Elsevier; 2009.

Index

Page references followed by 'f' denote figures; those followed by 't' denote tables.

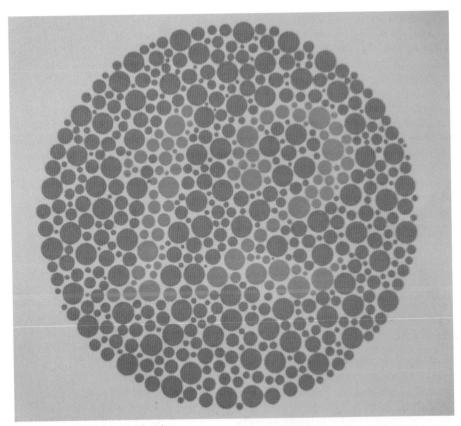

FIGURE 4.3 Ishihara sample chart

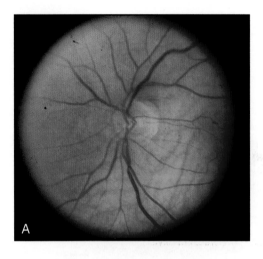

A

FIGURE 4.4
A Normal optic disc

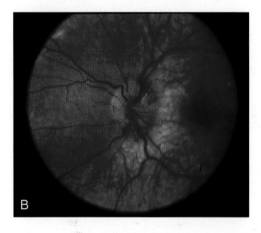

B

B Papilloedema
The visual acuity is normal unless the papilloedema is chronic, and the blind spot is enlarged. The pupillary responses are normal.

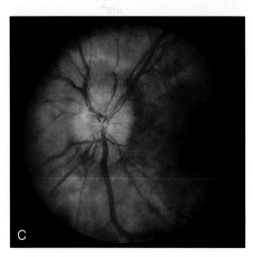

C

C Acute optic neuritis
The visual acuity is markedly impaired; colour vision is abnormal if the patient can read the chart (severe visual impairment will prevent the patient from seeing the numbers on the chart). The blind spot is enlarged. The direct pupillary response is slow and there is a Marcus–Gunn pupillary phenomenon (the pupil contracts promptly when the light is shone in the normal eye and when the light is shone in the abnormal eye the pupil initially dilates and then slowly contracts). Retrobulbar neuritis is the term applied to an inflammatory optic nerve lesion within the optic nerve but not affecting the optic nerve head, the part of the optic nerve that is visualised on examination of the fundus. In this situation, the visual acuity and colour vision are impaired, the visual field defect is usually a central scotoma although it may be a diffuse, lateral, superior or inferior defect. The fundus looks normal [3].

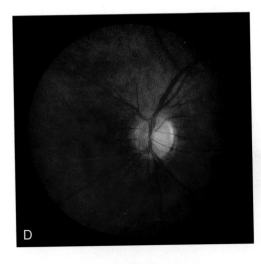

FIGURE 4.4 (cont'd)

D Long-standing optic neuritis with pallor of the optic disc

The visual acuity is reduced, colour vision is abnormal, and a Marcus–Gunn pupillary phenomenon is present (see 4C for an explanation of this abnormality).

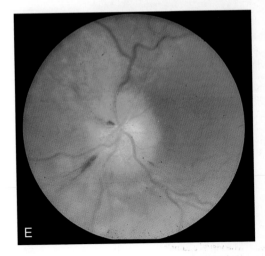

E Anterior ischaemic optic neuropathy (AION)

AION is the most common cause of acute optic neuropathy among older persons. It can be nonarteritic (nonarteritic anterior ischaemic optic neuropathy [NAION]) or arteritic, the latter being associated with giant cell arteritis. Visual loss usually occurs suddenly, or over a few days at most, and it is usually permanent. The optic disc is pale and swollen and there are flame haemorrhages.

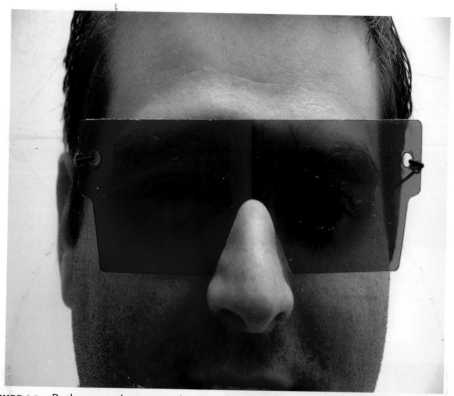

FIGURE 4.8   Red-green glasses used to test for diplopia

A light is shone into both eyes and the patient readily identifies the abnormal image by the colour of the image furthest from the midline. For example, in *figure 4.6* showing a right 3rd nerve palsy, when the patient is looking to the left the red image would be furthest to the left indicating weakness of the right medial rectus muscle. Whereas if the patient had a left fixed nerve palsy, the green image would be furthest from the midline.